Acute Encephalopathy and Encephalitis in Infancy and Its Related Disorders

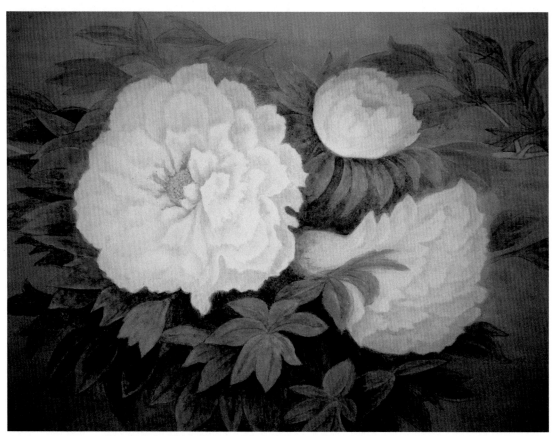

Frontispiece illustration provided courtesy of Mrs. Utako Yamanouchi.

Acute Encephalopathy and Encephalitis in Infancy and Its Related Disorders

HIDEO YAMANOUCHI, MD
President, International Symposium on Acute
Encephalopathy in Infancy and Its Related Disorders (ISAE2016)
Director, Saitama Medical University Hospital Comprehensive Epilepsy Center
Professor, Department of Pediatrics, Saitama Medical University, Saitama, Japan

SOLOMON L. MOSHÉ, MD
Charles Frost Chair In Neurosurgery and Neurology
Professor of Neurology, Neuroscience & Pediatrics
Vice-Chair, Dept. of Neurology
Director, Pediatric Neurology
Director, Clinical Neurophysiology
Einstein College of Medicine and Montefiore Medical Center
Bronx, NY, United States

AKIHISA OKUMURA, MD, PHD
Department of Pediatrics, Aichi Medical University
Nagakute, Japan

ELSEVIER

ELSEVIER

3251 Riverport Lane
St. Louis, Missouri 63043

Content Strategist: Kayla Wolfe
Content Development Manager: Taylor Ball
Content Development Specialist: Casey Potter
Publishing Services Manager: Deepthi Unni
Project Manager: Janish Ashwin Paul
Designer: Gopalakrishnan Venkatraman

Printed in United States of America

Last digit is the print number: 9   8   7   6   5   4   3   2   1

Working together
to grow libraries in
developing countries

www.elsevier.com • www.bookaid.org

List of Contributors

Mohamed Almuqbil, MD, FRCP (C)
Division of Genetics and Genomics
Boston Children's Hospital
Harvard Medical School
Boston, MA, USA
Division of Pediatric Neurology
King Saud bin Abdulaziz University for Health Sciences
Riyadh, Saudi Arabia
King Abdullah International Medical Research Center
King Abdullah Specialist Children's Hospital–Ministry of National Guard
Riyadh, Saudi Arabia

Hiroshi Arai, MD
Department of Pediatric Neurology
Bobath Memorial Hospital
Osaka, Japan

Hiroshi Baba, MD, PhD
Department of Neurosurgery and Epilepsy Center
Nishi-Isahaya Hospital
Isahaya, Nagasaki, Japan

Silvia Balosso, PhD
Department of Neuroscience
IRCCS-Istituto di Ricerche Farmacologiche Mario Negri
Milano, Italy

Ching-Shiang Chi, MD
Department of Pediatrics, Tungs' Taichung Metroharbor Hospital, Taichung, Taiwan
School of Medicine, Chung Shan Medical University, Taichung, Taiwan
Division of Nursing, Jen-Teh Junior College of Medicine, Nursing and Management, Miaoli, Taiwan

I-Jun Chou, MD
The CHEESE Study Group
Division of Pediatric Neurology
Chang Gung Children's Hospital and Chang Gung Memorial Hospital
Chang Gung University College of Medicine
Taoyuan, Taiwan
Chang Gung Children's Hospital Study Group for Children with Encephalitis/Encephalopathy-Related Status Epilepticus and Epilepsy (CHEESE)
Taoyuan, Taiwan

Russell C. Dale, MBChB, MSc, MRCPHCH, PhD
Professor of Paediatric Neurology
Children's Hospital at Westmead and University of Sydney
Sydney, NSW, Australia

Paola De Liso, MD, PhD
Neurology Unit
Bambino Gesù Paediatric Hospital
Rome, Italy

Aristea S. Galanopoulou, MD, PhD
Albert Einstein College of Medicine and Montefiore Medical Center,
Saul R. Korey Department of Neurology,
Dominick P. Purpura Department of Neuroscience,
Kennedy Center,
Bronx NY, United States

Judith Helen Cross, MBChB, PhD
Professor
The Prince of Wales's Chair of Childhood Epilepsy & Head of UCL-ICH Neurosciences Unit
ICH Developmental Neurosciences Prog
UCL GOS Institute of Child Health
London & Young Epilepsy
Lingfield, United Kingdom
Clinical Neurosciences
UCL-Institute of Child Health
London, United Kingdom

Satori Hirai, MD
Department of Pediatric Neurology
Morinomiya Hospital
Osaka, Japan

Shinichi Hirose, MD, PhD
Department of Pediatrics
School of Medicine
Fukuoka University
Fukuoka, Japan

Ryoko Honda, MD
Epilepsy Center and Department of Pediatrics
National Nagasaki Medical Center
Omura, Nagasaki, Japan

Asako Horino, MD
National Epilepsy Center
Shizuoka Institute of Epilepsy and Neurological
    Disorders, NHO
Shizuoka, Japan

Ai Hoshino, MD, PhD
Department of Developmental Medical Sciences
Graduate School of Medicine
The University of Tokyo
Tokyo, Japan

Takashi Ichiyama, MD
Vice Director
Department of Pediatrics
Tsudumigaura Medical Center for Children With
    Disabilities
Yamaguchi, Japan

George Imataka, MD, PhD, BA, PGDBA
Department of Pediatrics
Dokkyo Medical University
Tochigi, Japan

Atsushi Ishii, MD, PhD
Department of Pediatrics and Research Institute for
    the Molecular Pathomechanisms of Epilepsy
Fukuoka University
Fukuoka, Japan

Tomokazu Kimizu, MD
National Epilepsy Center
Shizuoka Institute of Epilepsy and Neurological
    Disorders, NHO
Shizuoka, Japan

Yukihiro Kitai, MD
Department of Pediatric Neurology
Morinomiya Hospital
Osaka, Japan

Takayoshi Koike, MD
National Epilepsy Center
Shizuoka Institute of Epilepsy and Neurological
    Disorders, NHO
Shizuoka, Japan

Hsiu-Fen Lee, MD, PhD
Department of Pediatrics, Taichung Veterans General
    Hospital, Taichung, Taiwan
School of Medicine, Chung Shan Medical University,
    Taichung, Taiwan
Division of Nursing, Jen-Teh Junior College of Medicine,
    Nursing and Management, Miaoli, Taiwan

Sooyoung Lee, MD, PhD
Department of Critical Care Medicine
Fukuoka Children's Hospital
Fukuoka, Japan
Department of Pediatrics
Graduate School of Medical Sciences
Kyushu University
Fukuoka, Japan
Emergency and Critical Care Center
Kyushu University Hospital
Fukuoka, Japan

Jainn-Jim Lin, MD
The CHEESE Study Group
Chang Gung Children's Hospital Study Group for
    Children with Encephalitis/Encephalopathy-
    Related Status Epilepticus and Epilepsy (CHEESE)
Taoyuan, Taiwan
Division of Pediatric Critical Care and Pediatric
    Neurocritical Care Center
Chang Gung Children's Hospital and Chang Gung
    Memorial Hospital
Chang Gung University College of Medicine
Taoyuan, Taiwan
Graduate Institute of Clinical Medical Sciences
College of Medicine, Chang Gung University,
    Taoyuan, Taiwan

Kuang-Lin Lin, MD
Division of Pediatric Neurology,
Chang Gung Children's Hospital and Chang Gung
    Memorial Hospital, Chang Gung University
    College of Medicine, Taoyuan, Taiwan
Chang Gung Children's Hospital Study Group for
    Children with Encephalitis/Encephalopathy-
    Related Status Epilepticus and Epilepsy (CHEESE),
    Taoyuan, Taiwan

Masashi Mizuguchi, MD, PhD
Department of Developmental Medical Sciences
Graduate School of Medicine
School of International Health
The University of Tokyo
Tokyo, Japan

Solomon L. Moshé, MD
Charles Frost Chair In Neurosurgery and Neurology
Professor of Neurology, Neuroscience & Pediatrics
Vice-Chair, Dept. of Neurology
Director, Pediatric Neurology
Director, Clinical Neurophysiology
Einstein College of Medicine and Montefiore Medical
    Center
Bronx, NY, United States

**Karthi Nallaswamy, MBBS, MD, DM
(Ped Crit Care)**
Assistant Professor
Critical Care Division
Department of Pediatrics & Advanced Pediatrics Centre
Post Graduate Institute of Medical Education and
    Research
Chandigarh, India

Takuji Nishida, MD, PhD
National Epilepsy Center
Shizuoka Institute of Epilepsy and Neurological
    Disorders, NHO
Shizuoka, Japan

Taikan Oboshi, MD
National Epilepsy Center
Shizuoka Institute of Epilepsy and Neurological
    Disorders, NHO
Shizuoka, Japan

Akihisa Okumura, MD
Department of Pediatrics
Aichi Medical University
Nagakute, Japan

Tomonori Ono, MD, PhD
Epilepsy Center and Department of Neurosurgery
National Nagasaki Medical Center
Omura, Nagasaki, Japan

Hirowo Omatsu, MD
National Epilepsy Center
Shizuoka Institute of Epilepsy and Neurological
    Disorders, NHO
Shizuoka, Japan

Hitoshi Osaka, MD, PhD
Department of Pediatrics
Jichi Medical School
Tochigi, Japan

Makiko Osawa, MD
Chairperson
Infantile Seizure Society (ISS), The Previous President
    of Japanese Society of Child Neurology (JSCN),
    The President of Japan Epilepsy Society (JES),
    Professor Emeritus
Tokyo Women's Medical University
Tokyo, Japan

Phillip L. Pearl, MD
Director of Epilepsy and Clinical Neurophysiology
Boston Children's Hospital
William G. Lennox Chair and Professor of Neurology
Harvard Medical School
Boston, MA, United States

Nicola Pietrafusa, MD
Rare and Complex Epilepsy Unit
Department of Neurosciences and Neurorehabilitation
"Bambino Gesù" Children's Hospital, IRCCSRome, Italy

Teresa Ravizza, PhD
Department of Neuroscience
IRCCS-Istituto di Ricerche Farmacologiche Mario Negri
Milano, Italy

**Arushi G. Saini, MD, DM (Pediatric
Neurology)**
Assistant Professor
Division of Pediatric Neurology and
    Neurodevelopment
Department of Pediatrics
Postgraduate Institute of Medical Education and
    Research
Chandigarh, India

Makiko Saitoh, MD, PhD
Department of Developmental Medical Sciences
Graduate School of Medicine
The University of Tokyo
Tokyo, Japan

Hiroshi Sakuma, MD, PhD
Project Leader
Department of Brain Development and Neural
    Regeneration
Tokyo Metropolitan Institute of Medical Science
Tokyo, Japan

Seda Salar, PhD
Albert Einstein College of Medicine,
Saul R. Korey Department of Neurology,
Kennedy Center,
Bronx NY, United States

Suvasini Sharma, MD, DM
Associate Professor
Neurology Division
Department of Pediatrics
Lady Harding Medical College and associated
    Kalawati Saran Children's Hospital
New Delhi, India

Masashi Shiomi, MD, PhD
Department of Pediatric, Aizenbashi Hospital
Osaka, Japan

Pratibha Singhi, MD, FIAP, FNAMS
Director, Pediatric Neurology, Department of
    Pediatrics, Medanta- the Medicity, Gurugram, NCR
Former Head and Chief Pediatric Neurology and
    Neurodevelopment
Department of Pediatrics
Advanced Pediatrics Centre
Post Graduate Institute of Medical Education and
    Research
Chandigarh, India

**Sunit Singhi, MBBS, MD, FIAP, FAMS, FISCCM,
FCCM**
Chairman, Department of Pediatrics, Medanta- the
    Medicity, Gurugram, NCR and
Professor Emeritus, Department Of Pediatrics, Post
    graduate Institute of Medical Education and
    Research, Chandigarh, India

Nicola Specchio, MD, PhD
Head of Rare and Complex Epilepsy Unit
Department of Neurosciences and Neurorehabilitation
"Bambino Gesù" Children's Hospital, IRCCSRome, Italy

Mary C. Spiciarich, MD
Assistant Professor of Neurology and Pediatrics
Saul R. Korey Department of Neurology
Division of Child Neurology
Montefiore Medical Center
Department of Pediatrics
Children's Hospital at Montefiore
Bronx, NY, United States

Yukitoshi Takahashi, MD, PhD
National Epilepsy Center
Shizuoka Institute of Epilepsy and Neurological
    Disorders, NHO
Shizuoka, Japan

Jun-ichi Takanashi, MD, PhD
Department of Pediatrics
Tokyo Women's Medical University
Tokyo, Japan
Yachiyo Medical Center
Yachiyo, Japan

Keisuke Toda, MD, PhD
Department of Neurosurgery
National Nagasaki-Kawatana Medical Center
Kawatana, Nagasaki, Japan

Hiroyuki Torisu, MD, PhD
Section of Pediatrics
Department of Medicine
Fukuoka Dental College
Fukuoka, Japan

Annamaria Vezzani, PhD
Lab Experimental Neurology
Unit of Pathophysiology of Neuron-Glia
    Communication, HeadDept Neuroscience
IRCCS-Mario Negri Institute for Pharmacological Research
Milano, Italy

Federico Vigevano, MD
Department of Neurosciences and Neurorehabilitation
"Bambino Gesù" Children's Hospital, IRCCS
Rome, Italy

Huei-Shyong Wang, MD
The CHEESE Study Group
Division of Pediatric Neurology
Chang Gung Children's Hospital and Chang Gung
    Memorial Hospital
Chang Gung University College of Medicine
Taoyuan, Taiwan
Chang Gung Children's Hospital Study Group for
    Children with Encephalitis/Encephalopathy-
    Related Status Epilepticus and Epilepsy (CHEESE)
Taoyuan, Taiwan

Tokito Yamaguchi, MD
National Epilepsy Center
Shizuoka Institute of Epilepsy and Neurological
    Disorders, NHO
Shizuoka, Japan

Hideo Yamanouchi, MD
President, International Symposium on Acute
    Encephalopathy in Infancy and Its Related
    Disorders (ISAE2016)
Director, Saitama Medical University Hospital
    Comprehensive Epilepsy Center
Professor, Department of Pediatrics, Saitama Medical
    University, Saitama, Japan

Tetsushi Yoshikawa, MD, PhD
Department of Pediatrics
Fujita Health University School of Medicine
Toyoake, Japan

Shinsaku Yoshitomi, MD
National Epilepsy Center
Shizuoka Institute of Epilepsy and Neurological
    Disorders, NHO
Shizuoka, Japan

Preface

It is our great honor to provide this book to all physicians and other medical personnel involved in infantile seizures and their related neurologic disorders. This book, entitled *Acute Encephalopathy and Encephalitis in Infancy and Its Related Disorders*, is comprised of chapters based on the excellent lectures from the International Symposium on Acute Encephalopathy in Infancy and Its Related Disorders (ISAE2016), held at the 18th annual meeting of the Infantile Seizure Society (ISS) in Tokyo on July 1–3, 2016. ISS is a professional organization, which was born in Japan in 1998, under the strong leadership by the late Prof. Yukio Fukuyama.

Pediatric healthcare programs supported by Japanese universal health insurance coverage have allowed Japanese pediatric neurologists to provide meticulous care without a rich-poor gap on all pediatric patients with intractable status epilepticus and other catastrophic epileptic conditions under careful observation. Quick and charge-free neuroradiological services, such as using leading-edge technology of magnetic resonance images, have offered sufficient and careful observations on these pediatric patients. Through abundant clinical information of pediatric critical neurologic disorders, we have established several novel encephalopathic categories such as acute necrotizing encephalopathy (ANE; Mizuguchi), acute encephalopathy with febrile convulsive status epilepticus (AEFCSE/AESD; Shiomi/Takanashi), and acute infantile encephalopathy predominantly affecting the frontal lobes (AIEF; Yamanouchi). In addition, the late Drs. Awaya and Fukuyama had reported the category of febrile infection–related epilepsy syndrome (FIRES) more than 10 years before the establishment.

In Japan, although we have been actively engaging in discussion and debates regarding these acute neurologic disorders, there has been little opportunity to share ideas with the international community. The motivation to organize this symposium ISAE2016 was stimulated by an apparent lack of discussion and collaboration worldwide. We felt that it was time to hold this inaugural event. As a result, ISAE2016 was a very successful event highlighting acute encephalopathy in infancy and childhood, consisting of 34 comprehensive reviews of recent scientific progress in these fields by excellent invited experts. All chapters in this book were written by these experts gathered in this symposium and exhibit comprehensive and very fruitful contents. We hope all readers of this book profoundly understand the recent updated knowledge of acute encephalopathy and encephalitis in infancy.

Lastly, we would like to express our sincere appreciation to the International League against Epilepsy (ILAE), Japan Medical Association (JMA), Asian and Oceanian Child Neurology Association (AOCNA), Japan Epilepsy Society (JES), and Japanese Society of Child Neurology (JSCN) for the strong endorsement to ISAE2016.

Hideo Yamanouchi, MD (corresponding author)
President, International Symposium on Acute Encephalopathy in Infancy and its Related Disorders (ISAE2016)
Professor, Department of Pediatrics,
Saitama Medical University
Saitama, Japan

Makiko Osawa, MD
Chairperson, Infantile Seizure Society (ISS)
The previous president of Japanese Society of Child neurology (JSCN)
The president of Japan Epilepsy Society (JES)
Professor emeritus, Tokyo Women's Medical University
Tokyo, Japan

Contents

CHAPTER 1

Overview and Definitions

HIDEO YAMANOUCHI, MD

DEFINITION

Acute encephalopathy in infancy and childhood is defined as a rapidly progressive dysfunction of the brain with noninflammatory edematous changes in infants and children. It is a neurologic syndrome causing rapid, accelerating, and protracted deterioration of consciousness, frequently following convulsive seizures triggered by febrile illness such as viral infections. The changes in the level of consciousness are often protracted. The guidelines of acute encephalopathy in infancy and childhood developed by the Japanese Society of Child Neurology propose that the impairment of consciousness in acute encephalopathy persists at least for 24 h with 11 points or less on the Glasgow coma scale (GCS) (Table 1.1). Even when the altered state of consciousness may be mild at the onset, with 12 points or more on the GCS, there is a possibility that the acute encephalopathy may progress into a more severe coma soon afterward. In contrast, transient impairments of consciousness, with complete recovery of consciousness within 24 h, are unlikely feature for acute encephalopathy in infancy and childhood.

CATEGORIES

The pathophysiologic mechanisms related with acute encephalopathy are discussed in this section. One of the most essentially pathologic features is noninflammatory acute brain edema. This pathologic feature causes increased intracranial pressure, leading to attenuation of cerebral perfusion pressure and finally to herniation syndromes and/or brainstem dysfunction associated with central nervous system (CNS)-related respiratory and circulatory failure. Two main types of mechanisms have been proposed for brain edema, i.e., cytotoxic edema and vasogenic edema. In cytotoxic edema, there is dysfunction of metabolism in the astrocytes and/or neurons, with increased influx into and/or decreased efflux from the intracellular spaces, causing water accumulation in astrocytes and/or neurons. On the other hand, dysfunction of

blood-brain barrier causes leakage of water and various macromolecules from the brain vessels into the extracellular spaces and vasogenic edema. Neuroradiological studies uniformly exhibit the widely distributed edematous changes of the brain. Diffusion-weighted magnetic resonance image (MRI) is a useful method to allow the distinction between cytotoxic edema and vasogenic edema (Chapter 8). The principal or predominant type of brain edema is based on the causative mechanisms relating to specific subtypes of acute encephalopathy.

Acute encephalopathy in infancy and childhood should be differentiated from other conditions that may cause a rapidly progressive and prolonged comatose state, such as febrile/nonfebrile convulsive status epilepticus, acute hypoxia and/or ischemia, traumatic brain injury, and cerebrovascular disorders (Table 1.2). CNS infections, such as acute encephalitis and meningitis, due to viral, rickettsial, or bacterial infections mimic acute encephalopathy in infancy and childhood on clinical presentation (see Chapters 22 and 23). One of the essential points for the differentiation from CNS infections is an absence of inflammatory processes in parenchymal CNS. Gram-negative sepsis due to gram-negative bacilli such as *Escherichia coli* and *Pseudomonas aeruginosa* or toxic shock syndrome due to *Staphylococcus aureus* cause conditions of coma as well as multiple organ failure and hypotension. Conditions with increased intracranial pressure such as brain tumors, brain abscess, and hydrocephalus are causative for severe impairment of consciousness and should be ruled out by neuroimaging studies. Heat stroke is a medical emergency with high mortality, involving CNS as well as other organs. Acute disseminated encephalomyelitis is caused by inflammatory demyelinating processes, showing multifocal CNS features with altered states of consciousness, which are commonly preceded by a viral or bacterial infection (Chapters 18–20). Anti-NMDA receptor encephalitis may present with a comatose state in a rapidly progressive manner following psychiatric manifestations, memory deficits, and autonomic instability (Chapter 21). This autoimmune encephalitis syndrome is confirmed by the detection of IgG antibodies to NR1 subunit of the NMDAR in serum or cerebrospinal fluid (CSF).

Acute encephalopathy in infancy and childhood is a heterogeneous syndrome and is categorized based on the plausible pathomechanism. Four types of categories were proposed (see Chapter 2 for details). The first category is a group of metabolic errors, including classic Reye syndrome as well as inherited metabolic disorders. The clinical picture may include slowly progressive or static features followed by the provocation of acute encephalopathic conditions including lethargy, behavioral changes, or gait disturbances provoked by infections or fasting states as acute encephalopathic crisis. These conditions are comprised of disorders in fatty acid β-oxidation, organic acid metabolism, amino acid metabolism glycolysis, and urea cycle (Table 1.3). Detailed laboratory studies are necessary when the patient has the following criteria: (1) acute crisis after fasting or infections; (2) peculiar facial appearance, skin lesions, strange odor of body or urine; (3) Kussmaul breathing or tachypnea; (4) mental retardation or growth failure; (5) cardiomyopathy and/or myopathy;

(6) hepatomegaly and/or splenomegaly; (7) multiple organ failure; (8) characteristic neuroimaging; and (9) family history of inborn error of metabolisms.

The second category is a group presenting with a cytokine storm. Hemorrhagic shock and encephalopathy syndrome,

TABLE 1.1
Glasgow Coma Scale

EYE OPENING (E)	
Spontaneous	4
To speech	3
To pain	2
None	1
VERBAL RESPONSE (V)	
Oriented	5
Confused conversation	4
Inappropriate words	3
Incomprehensible sounds	2
None	1
BEST MOTOR RESPONSE (M)	
Obeys	6
Localizes	5
Withdraws	4
Abnormal flexion	3
Abnormal extension	2
None	1
Total points	3–15

TABLE 1.2
Differential Diagnosis for Acute Encephalopathy in Infancy and Childhood

1. Epileptic conditions
   a. Febrile/nonfebrile convulsive status epilepticus
   b. Nonconvulsive status epilepticus
2. Acute hypoxia/ischemia
3. Traumatic brain injury
4. Cerebrovascular disorders
   a. Subdural, epidural, subarachnoid, and cerebral hemorrhage
   b. Shaken baby syndrome
   c. Arteriovenous malformation
   d. Sinus thrombosis
   e. Moyamoya disease
5. CNS infections
   a. Acute encephalitis
      i. Herpes simplex virus 1
      ii. Herpes simplex virus 2
      iii. Human herpes virus 6
      iv. Human herpes virus 7
      v. Varicella zoster virus
      vi. Ebstein-Barr virus
      vii. Cytomegalovirus
      viii. Measles virus
      ix. Rubella virus
      x. Mumps virus
      xi. Adenovirus 7
      xii. Enterovirus
      xiii. Japanese encephalitis virus
      xiv. West Nile virus
      xv. Lyme disease
      xvi. Rocky Mountain spotted fever
   b. Meningitis
      i. Bacterial meningitis
      ii. Tuberculosis meningitis
      iii. Fungal meningitis
   c. Brain abscess
   d. Subdural abscess
6. Systemic disorders
   a. Gram-negative sepsis
   b. Toxic shock syndrome
   c. Heat stroke
7. Immunologic CNS disorders
   a. Acute disseminated encephalomyelitis
   b. Postimmunization encephalopathy
   c. Anti-NMDA receptor encephalitis
8. Brain tumor

TABLE 1.2
Differential Diagnosis for Acute Encephalopathy in Infancy and Childhood—cont'd

9. Others
   a. Sudden infant death syndrome
   b. Hypertensive encephalopathy
   c. Myocarditis
   d. Arrhythmia
   e. Drug intoxication
      i. Immunosuppressive drugs
      ii. Anticonvulsants
      iii. Antidepressants
      iv. Antipsychotics

TABLE 1.3
Acute Encephalopathy Secondary to Inherited Metabolic Disorders

DISORDERS IN FATTY ACID TRANSPORT AND β-OXIDATION

Medium chain acyl-CoA dehydrogenase (MCAD) deficiency

Organic cation transporter 2 (OCTN2) deficiency

Mitochondrial trifunctional protein (TFP) deficiency

Carnitine palmitoyl transferase 1 (CPT1) deficiency

Carnitine palmitoyl transferase 2 (CPT2) deficiency

Carnitine-acylcarnitine translocase (CACT) deficiency

Systemic carnitine deficiency

DISORDERS IN ORGANIC ACID METABOLISM

Propionic acidemia

Methylmalonic acidemia

Isovaleric acidemia

Glutaric acidemia type 1

DISORDERS OF AMINO ACID METABOLISM

Maple syrup urine disease (MSUD)

Nonketotic hyperglycinemia

DISORDERS IN GLYCOLYSIS

Pyruvate dehydrogenase deficiency

Fructose-1,6-bisphosphatase deficiency

DISORDERS IN UREA CYCLE

Ornithine transcarbamoylase (OTC) deficiency

Carbamoyl phosphate synthetase 1 (CPS1) deficiency

Argininosuccinate synthetase (ASS) deficiency

Argininosuccinate lyase (ASL) deficiency

Arginase 1 (ARG1) deficiency

N-acetylglutamate synthase (NAGS) deficiency

Ornithine/citrulline antiporter (ORNT1) deficiency

as well as acute necrotizing encephalopathy (Chapter 13), are representative disorders in this category. The clinical features commonly show systemic inflammatory response syndrome with fulminant nature due to hypercytokinemia, causing vascular endothelial injury leading to severe damage of blood-brain barrier. The patients with this category may have systematic inflammatory response syndrome,[1] such as (1) core temperature of >38.5°C or <36°C, (2) tachycardia or bradycardia, (3) tachypnea or requiring mechanical ventilation, and (4) elevated or depressed leukocytes or 10% immature neutrophil.

The third category is a group of excitotoxic crisis. From the historical point of view, this subtype was initially termed as "acute encephalopathy with febrile convulsive status epilepticus" in Japanese literature; however, it was renamed as acute encephalopathy with biphasic seizures and late reduced diffusion[2] or acute infantile encephalopathy predominantly affecting the frontal lobes[3] according to the additional neuroradiological views of diffusion-weighted MRIs or cerebral blood flow images on single photon emission computed tomography. Hemiconvulsion-hemiplegia-epilepsy syndrome is included in this third category.

The last category is a group of obscure pathogeneses. Febrile infection–related epilepsy syndrome or acute encephalitis with refractory, repetitive partial seizures is suggested as one type of acute encephalopathy in infancy and childhood; however, their pathogenesis is as of now unknown (Section 6: Encephalopathy/ Encephalitis with Refractory Epileptic Status).

INITIAL STEPS LEADING TO THE FINAL DIAGNOSIS

The diagnostic strategy for acute encephalopathy in infancy and childhood is described in this section, including neuroimaging, electrophysiology, and specific markers helpful for the final diagnosis of each type. Here I briefly present the initial steps for the diagnosis focused on the initial laboratory tests. The subtype related with *inherited metabolic disorders* is suggested at the onset by the routine laboratory tests such as blood level of glucose, ammonia, lactate, and ketone bodies as well as plasma acid-base status. The final diagnosis is based on characteristic laboratory findings at the onset and/or static periods. Critical samples of blood, urine, and CSF at the provocation of acute encephalopathic conditions should be kept refrigerated for these specific tests for the final diagnosis. Hyperammonemia is one of the crucial conditions by inherited metabolic disorders causing acute encephalopathy in infancy and childhood. They are induced by metabolic disorders of urea cycle, organic acids, fatty acids, and mitochondria. Urea cycle disorders are one of the most crucial disorders and are differentiated from disorders of organic acids based on the normal blood levels of anion gap and glucose level. Maple syrup urine disease (MSUD) is one of representative amino acid metabolism abnormality causing acute encephalopathy. This disorder is caused by a defect in a branched-chain α-ketoacid dehydrogenase complex, which catalyzes the breakdown of three branched-chain ketoacids from the branched chain amino acids (leucine, isoleucine, and valine). This complex enzyme consists of four subunits, i.e., E1α, E1β, E2, and E3. Routine laboratory tests show hypoglycemia and metabolic acidosis with anion gap as well as increased levels of ketone bodies. Amino acid analysis shows marked elevations of leucine, isoleucine, valine, and alloisoleucine (pathognomonic amino acid for MSUD, not found in the normal conditions) and decreased levels of alanine. The severity of clinical status of CNS is correlated with blood level of leucine (leucine encephalopathy). Disorders of fatty acid β-oxidation mimic clinical and laboratory features in patients with Reye syndrome and/or Reye-like syndrome. Medium chain acyl-CoA dehydrogenase deficiency is one of the most common fatty acid oxidation disorders, which causes lethal encephalopathic crisis, but is completely preventive by carefully avoiding a fasting state. Routine laboratory tests show hypoketotic hypoglycemia without metabolic acidosis as well as abnormal liver functions, including elevations of liver enzymes, hyperammonia, and failure of coagulation functions such as prothrombin time and partial thromboplastin time. Additional laboratory tests may show decreased plasma levels of free carnitine and increased plasma levels of C8-C10 acylcarnitine as well as C6-C10 free fatty acids. Other disorders of fatty acid oxidation causing acute encephalopathic conditions are shown in Table 1.3.

The subtype related with *cytokine storm* is suspected by marked elevation of the serum and CSF concentrations of inflammatory cytokines such as tumor necrosis factor α and interleukin 6. Routine laboratory tests show marked elevations of ferritin, serum aminotransferase, pancreatic amylases, creatine kinase, creatinine, and uric acid nitrogen, as well as hematologic data presenting disseminated intravascular coagulation and hemophagocytic syndrome.

It is often difficult to make a quick diagnosis of the subtype of *excitotoxic crisis*, which may be similar to prolonged febrile seizure at the onset. There are no specific tests available so far as of this moment (Chapter 11). The delayed neuronal death or apoptosis after excess excitation of neurons during prolonged febrile convulsive episode is suspected, but why this will occur in some and not all infants and children with similar histories is unclear (Chapter 3). The diagnosis of subtype of excitotoxic crisis should be based on the clinical evidence such as a biphasic pattern of seizure and various degrees of altered states of consciousness as well as characteristic patterns of MRIs and cerebral flow images using single photon emission computed tomography (Chapter 8).

It should be pointed out that there are subtypes of acute encephalopathy in infancy and childhood, but their precise categorization remains undetermined. Dravet syndrome is an intractable epileptic disorder starting in infancy, when prolonged seizures are frequently provoked by febrile illness or triggered by hyperthermic states such as taking a hot bath tab. Clinical study has shown the high incidence of sudden death or provocation of acute encephalopathy mainly between the age of 1 and 4 years.[4,5] Acute encephalopathic condition may be provoked during the course of congenital adrenal hyperplasia (CAH). Diffuse or focal edematous changes are detected in the cerebrum on MRIs. Careful managements on CAH may be preventable for the encephalopathic conditions.[6]

In conclusion, acute encephalopathy in infancy and childhood is a rapidly progressive neurologic condition provoked by convulsive seizures and protracted comatose state. From the etiologic point of view, they are divided into subgroups of metabolic errors, cytokine storms, excitotoxic crisis, and others. It is important to be managed promptly and accurately to minimize the neurologic sequelae.

REFERENCES

1. Goldstein B, Giroir B, Randolph A. International pediatric sepsis consensus conference: definitions for sepsis and organ dysfunction in pediatrics. *Pediatr Crit Care Med.* 2005;6:2–8.
2. Takanashi J, Oba H, Barkovich AJ, et al. Diffusion MRI abnormalities after prolonged febrile seizures with encephalopathy. *Neurology.* 2006;66:1304–1309.
3. Yamanouchi H, Kawaguchi N, Mori M, et al. Acute infantile encephalopathy predominantly affecting the frontal lobes. *Pediatr Neurol.* 2006;34:93–100.
4. Okumura A, Uematsu M, Imataka G, et al. Acute encephalopathy in children with Dravet syndrome. *Epilepsia.* 2012;53:79–86.
5. Sakauchi M, Oguni H, Kato I, et al. Mortality in Dravet syndrome: search for risk factors in Japanese patients. *Epilepsia.* 2011;52(suppl 2):50–54.
6. Abe Y, Sakai T, Okumura A, et al. Manifestations and characteristics of congenital adrenal hyperplasia-associated encephalopathy. *Brain Dev.* 2016;38:638–647.

CHAPTER 2

Classification and Epidemiology of Acute Encephalopathy

MASASHI MIZUGUCHI, MD, PHD • AI HOSHINO, MD, PHD • MAKIKO SAITOH, MD, PHD

The word "encephalopathy" has various meanings. In the context of immune-mediated encephalitis/encephalopathy, this term denotes impairment of consciousness, either mild or severe.[1] Brain edema often represents the pathologic substrate of acute and severe impairment of consciousness.[2] Acute encephalopathy is usually defined as syndromes of acute central nervous system dysfunction due to diffuse or widespread, noninflammatory brain edema. The guideline for acute encephalopathy of childhood, published in July 2016 by the Japanese Society of Child Neurology, set the diagnostic criteria of acute encephalopathy, defining the severity of consciousness disturbance as "below or equal to 11 points on the Glasgow coma scale (GCS)" and its duration as "longer than 24 h."[3]

The incidence of acute encephalopathy is highest in infancy and early childhood. There usually is an antecedent infection, viral in most cases. The main symptoms are impaired consciousness, typically stupor or coma, often with signs of increased intracranial pressure. In many patients, there also are seizures, which are usually febrile and often prolonged (febrile status epilepticus).

Many studies in the last two decades (1995–2015) have elucidated the etiology and pathogenesis of acute encephalopathy. According to their findings, there are three pathogenetic mechanisms: metabolic error, cytokine storm, and excitotoxicity.[2] Many genetic and environmental factors leading to these abnormalities have been identified as the risk factors of acute encephalopathy (Fig. 2.1).[4–9]

CLASSIFICATION OF ACUTE ENCEPHALOPATHY

Acute encephalopathy is a heterogeneous group consisting of multiple syndromes. There are two ways of classification (Box 2.1). One is microbiologic classification based on the pathogenic viruses of the antecedent infection, such as influenza encephalopathy, human herpesvirus 6 (HHV-6) encephalopathy, and rotavirus encephalopathy. Another is syndromic classification based on the clinicopathologic features of encephalopathy, such as classic Reye syndrome, acute necrotizing encephalopathy (ANE), acute encephalopathy with biphasic seizures and late reduced diffusion (AESD), and mild encephalitis/encephalopathy with a reversible splenial lesion (MERS). The relationships between viruses and syndromes are nonspecific; any virus may cause any syndrome.[2] However, an epidemiologic study in Japan found a tendency that certain viruses are more likely to cause certain syndromes than other viruses. For example, influenza virus is the most common pathogen for ANE and MERS, and HHV-6 for AESD.[10]

Currently, ~10 syndromes of acute encephalopathy have been described and established. They are classified into four major groups according to their main pathomechanism: metabolic error, cytokine storm, excitotoxicity, and unknown mechanisms (Box 2.1).[2] The most typical syndromes of these groups are described below.

Classic Reye Syndrome

Established in 1963 as a clinicopathologic entity, Reye syndrome is an encephalopathy secondary to severe hepatic dysfunction, as well as a prototype of acute encephalopathy caused by metabolic error. The main diagnostic criteria include pathologic findings, such as microvesicular fatty metamorphosis of hepatocytes and abnormal morphology of mitochondria, and biochemical findings, such as hypoglycemia and hyperammonemia. In this syndrome, multiple genetic factors, such as mutation or polymorphism of mitochondrial enzymes, and environmental factors, such as infection, fasting, drugs, and toxins, are involved. Combination of these factors lead to a transient but significant deficiency in

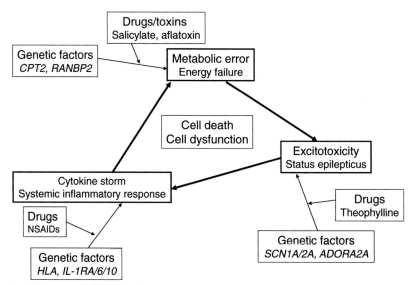

FIG. 2.1 Pathogenetic mechanism of acute encephalopathy. Acute encephalopathy is caused by three major events: metabolic error, cytokine storm, and excitotoxicity. For each of them, there are multiple risk factors: genetic factors such as gene mutations and polymorphisms, and environmental factors, such as drugs and toxins. The three events are mutually related and may form a vicious cycle in very severe cases.

BOX 2.1
Classification of Acute Encephalopathy

MICROBIOLOGIC CLASSIFICATION
- Influenza-associated encephalopathy
- HHV-6/7 encephalopathy
- Rotavirus encephalopathy
- Respiratory syncytial virus encephalopathy
- Herpes simplex virus encephalopathy
- Varicella-zoster virus encephalopathy
- Bacterial infection–associated encephalopathy (enterohemorrhagic *Escherichia coli*, *Salmonella*, *Bacillus cereus*, *Borrelia*, *Bordetella pertussis*, and others)
- Mycoplasma infection–associated encephalopathy
- Others

SYNDROMIC CLASSIFICATIONS
1. Acute encephalopathy due to metabolic error
   - Classic Reye syndrome
   - Encephalopathy secondary to inherited metabolic disorders
2. Acute encephalopathy caused by cytokine storm

- Encephalopathy with diffuse brain swelling (synonyms: Reyelike syndrome, sepsislike encephalopathy, and others)
- Hemorrhagic shock and encephalopathy syndrome
- Acute necrotizing encephalopathy (ANE)
3. Acute encephalopathy caused by excitotoxicity
   - Acute encephalopathy with biphasic seizures and late reduced diffusion (AESD) (subgroups: acute infantile encephalopathy predominantly affecting the frontal lobes, hemiconvulsion-hemiplegia-epilepsy syndrome)
4. Acute encephalopathy of obscure pathogenesis
   - Mild encephalitis/encephalopathy with a reversible splenial lesion (MERS)
   - Posterior reversible leukoencephalopathy syndrome
   - Febrile infection–related epilepsy syndrome (FIRES) (synonym: acute encephalitis with refractory, repetitive partial seizures)
   - Unclassified encephalopathy

the mitochondrial enzymatic activity of the liver and other organs, resulting in cellular energy failure and accumulation of toxic substances, which in turn cause encephalopathy and damage to systemic organs.[2]

Since the 1980s, the incidence of Reye syndrome has remarkably declined because of the decrease in the use of salicylates as an antipyretic and improvement in the differential diagnosis of inherited metabolic disorders. At present, Reye syndrome is nearly extinct; an epidemiologic study in Japan estimated its incidence as low as one case in entire Japan.[10]

Acute Necrotizing Encephalopathy

First described by Mizuguchi and collaborators in 1989–95 as a clinicopathologic entity,[11-13] ANE is a fulminant type of acute encephalopathy with severe

involvement of systemic organs, such as multiple organ failure and disseminated intravascular coagulation. ANE is seen worldwide but are most prevalent in East Asia. The most important finding for diagnosis is symmetric lesions in the bilateral thalamus (Fig. 2.2A and B). The main pathomechanism of ANE is an excessive systemic inflammatory response or cytokine storm. Systemic hypercytokinemia causes vascular endothelial injury and apoptosis of parenchymal cells in the brain and other target organs,[14] resulting in encephalopathy and damage to systemic organs.[2]

Acute Encephalopathy With Biphasic Seizures and Late Reduced Diffusion

AESD is the most prevalent syndrome of acute encephalopathy in Japan. In the 1990s, some Japanese

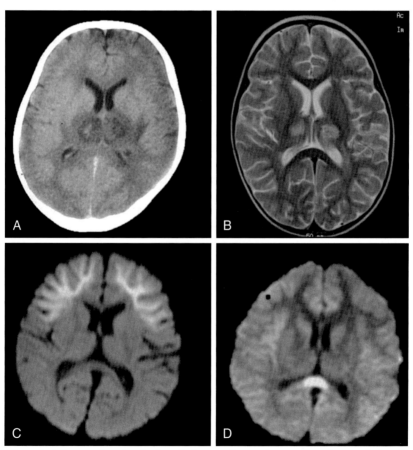

FIG. 2.2 Characteristic neuroimaging findings in three major syndromes of acute encephalopathy. **(A)** Computed tomography (CT) in acute necrotizing encephalopathy (ANE). **(B)** Magnetic resonance imaging (MRI) (T2-weighted image) in ANE. **(C)** MRI (diffusion-weighted image) in acute encephalopathy with biphasic seizures and late reduced diffusion. **(D)** MRI (diffusion-weighted image) in mild encephalitis/encephalopathy with a reversible splenial lesion.

pediatricians became aware of this type of encephalopathy. In 2000, Shiomi first described its clinical and radiologic features and proposed the term "acute encephalitis with febrile convulsive status epilepticus" (AEFCSE) in Japanese literature.[15] In 2006, Takanashi et al. first described this syndrome in an international, peer-reviewed journal, and named it as AESD.[16] Despite minor differences in their definition, AEFCSE and AESD are considered to be synonymous.[2]

Clinical picture of AESD is characterized by biphasic seizures consisting of early and late seizures. Early seizure is a febrile, generalized convulsion, prolonged in many cases (febrile status epilepticus) and followed by postictal alteration of consciousness for several hours to days. Patients then recover consciousness, but not to full alertness. Three to seven days later, there are late seizures, a cluster of brief partial seizures followed again by impairment of consciousness. When the second coma has gone, the patients show various signs of dysfunction of cerebral cortex, such as aphasia, agnosia, and loss of spontaneity. In convalescence, mild cases gradually regain cortical functions, but severe cases are left with intellectual and/or motor deficits.[2,15,16]

Radiologic features of AESD are not only characteristic but also essential for diagnosis. Immediately after the early seizure, head computed tomography (CT)/magnetic resonance imaging (MRI) findings are normal, except for mild swelling in the severest cases. Several days later, around the occurrence of late seizures, CT begins to show cerebral edema, whereas MRI demonstrates restricted diffusion of the cerebral subcortical white matter, so-called bright tree appearance (Fig. 2.2C).[15,16] The lesions have a low apparent diffusion coefficient (ADC), indicating cellular edema. Their distribution varies among patients but tends to be lobar, such as bilateral frontal and hemispheric, in typical cases.[2,17] Precentral and postcentral gyri are spared in the majority of patients.[15] The affected cortex remains to be edematous during the subacute period (for one to several weeks), then becomes atrophic during convalescence. The main pathomechanism of AESD is considered to be excitotoxicity. In the cerebral lesions, febrile status epilepticus causes an excessive release of glutamate, resulting in selective death of cortical neurons.[2]

Mild Encephalitis/Encephalopathy With a Reversible Splenial Lesion

In contrast to severe and often devastating syndromes such as ANE and AESD, the clinical course of MERS is mild, transient, and benign, consisting of mild impairment of consciousness, stupor or delirium, and brief seizures. The majority of patients show full recovery within a month. Diagnosis is based on the characteristic MRI findings: a lesion in the splenium of the

corpus callosum, ovoid or extended in shape, showing restricted diffusion with a low ADC (Fig. 2.2D).[18] This lesion is transient and disappears 3 days to 2 weeks later. Its pathologic substrate remains unclear; the possibility of intramyelinic edema has been postulated.

EPIDEMIOLOGY OF ACUTE ENCEPHALOPATHY

To date, cases of acute encephalopathy have been reported from many regions in the world: Asia, America, Europe, and Oceania. Based on their number, however, it is presumed that ANE, AESD, and influenza-associated encephalopathy are much more prevalent in East Asian countries, such as Japan, Korea, and Taiwan, than in the rest of the world.

In 2010, a research committee supported by the Japanese government conducted a nationwide survey on the epidemiology of acute encephalopathy. To date, it has been the only large-scale study in the world.[10] In this study, a questionnaire was sent to pediatric referral centers in Japan, to collect information of patients with acute encephalopathy during a 3-year period from April 2007 to June 2010. A total of 983 cases were reported. Taking the response rate (51.0%) into account, the annual incidence of acute encephalopathy in Japan (population: 130,000,000) was estimated to be 400–700 cases per year. The age at onset ranged from infancy to adulthood, but most commonly was under 5 years (mean $\pm$ SD, 4.0 ± 3.7 years; median, 3 years). There was no sex difference (male, 51%; female, 48%). Pathogens were most commonly influenza virus (27%), followed by HHV-6 (17%), rotavirus (4%), and respiratory syncytial virus (2%). Common syndromes were AESD (29%), MERS (16%), ANE (4%), and hemorrhagic shock and encephalopathy syndrome (2%). As many as 44% of the patients were not diagnosed with known syndromes. Outcome was full recovery in 56% of patients, mild to moderate neurologic sequelae in 22%, severe sequelae in 14%, and death in 6%.[10]

From an epidemiologic point of view, the syndromes were quite different from each other. First, regarding the age, the median age at onset was 1 year in AESD, 2 years in ANE, and 5 years in MERS. Onset at school age and adulthood was very rare in AESD, occasional in ANE, and common in MERS. Second, regarding antecedent infections, the most common virus was influenza virus in ANE and MERS but was HHV-6 in AESD. Third, the prognosis was very different. Fatality was high in ANE (28%), low in AESD (1%), and zero in MERS. Neurologic sequelae were common in ANE (56%) and AESD (60%), being often severe, but were rare in MERS (7%), being mild if any.[10]

REFERENCES

1. Krupp LB, Banwell B, Tenembaum S. International Pediatric MS Study Group. Consensus definitions proposed for pediatric multiple sclerosis and related disorders. *Neurology.* 2007;68:S7–S12.
2. Mizuguchi M, Yamanouchi H, Ichiyama T, Shiomi M. Acute encephalopathy associated with influenza and other viral infections. *Acta Neurol Scand.* 2007;115(4 Suppl):45–56.
3. Japanese Society of Child Neurology, ed. *Guideline for the Diagnosis and Treatment of Acute Encephalopathy in Children.* Tokyo: Shindan-To-Chiryo-Sha; 2016.
4. Shinohara M, Saitoh M, Takanashi JI, et al. Carnitine palmitoyl transferase II polymorphism is associated with multiple syndromes of acute encephalopathy with various infectious diseases. *Brain Dev.* 2011;33:512–517.
5. Saitoh M, Shinohara M, Hoshino H, et al. Mutations of the *SCN1A* gene in acute encephalopathy. *Epilepsia.* 2012;53:558–564.
6. Shinohara M, Saitoh M, Nishizawa D, et al. *ADORA2A* polymorphism predisposes children to encephalopathy with febrile status epilepticus. *Neurology.* 2013;80:1571–1576.
7. Saitoh M, Shinohara M, Ishii A, et al. Clinical and genetic features of acute encephalopathy in children taking theophylline. *Brain Dev.* 2015;37:463–470.
8. Saitoh M, Ishii A, Ihara Y, et al. Missense mutations in sodium channel *SCN1A* and *SCN2A* predispose children to encephalopathy with severe febrile seizures. *Epilepsy Res.* 2015;117:1–6.
9. Hoshino A, Saitoh M, Miyagawa T, et al. Specific HLA genotypes confer susceptibility to acute necrotizing encephalopathy. *Genes Immun.* 2016;17:367–369.
10. Hoshino A, Saitoh M, Oka A, et al. Epidemiology of acute encephalopathy in Japan, with emphasis on the association of viruses and syndromes. *Brain Dev.* 2012;34:337–343.
11. Mizuguchi M, Tomonaga M, Fukusato T, Asano M. Acute necrotizing encephalopathy with widespread edematous lesions of symmetrical distribution. *Acta Neuropathol.* 1989;78:108–111.
12. Mizuguchi M. Acute encephalopathy with necrosis of bilateral thalami. Clinical aspects. *Neuropathology.* 1993;13:327–331.
13. Mizuguchi M, Abe J, Mikkaichi K, et al. Acute necrotising encephalopathy of childhood: a new syndrome presenting with multifocal, symmetric brain lesions. *J Neurol Neurosurg Psychiatry.* 1995;58:555–561.
14. Nakai Y, Itoh M, Mizuguchi M, Becker LE, Itoh M, Takashima S. Apoptosis and microglial activation in influenza encephalopathy. *Acta Neuropathol.* 2003;105:233–239.
15. Shiomi M. A proposal of the clinical classification of influenza encephalopathy. *Jpn J Pediatr.* 2000;53:1739–1746. (in Japanese).
16. Takanashi J, Oba H, Barkovich AJ, et al. Diffusion MRI abnormalities after prolonged febrile seizures with encephalopathy. *Neurology.* 2006;66:1304–1309.
17. Yamanouchi H, Mizuguchi M. Acute infantile encephalopathy predominantly affecting the frontal lobes (AIEF): a novel clinical category and its tentative diagnostic criteria. *Epilepsy Res.* 2006;70:S263–S268.
18. Tada H, Takanashi J, Barkovich AJ, et al. Clinically mild encephalitis/encephalopathy with a reversible splenial lesion. *Neurology.* 2004;63:1854–1858.

CHAPTER 3

Translational Studies of Infantile Epileptic Encephalopathies

MARY C. SPICIARICH, MD • SOLOMON L. MOSHÉ, MD

INTRODUCTION

Translational studies of infantile epileptic encephalopathies have utilized animal models to better understand their pathophysiology. These models use an inciting event, typically a toxin, to induce an epilepsy phenotype. The expression of seizures in these models, and therefore the treatment of the subsequent epilepsy, differs depending on the developmental window during which the precipitating insult is introduced. In this review, we will discuss several of these models and how they have shaped our understanding of various infantile epilepsy syndromes.

SEIZURE CLASSIFICATION

In the prior International League Against Epilepsy classification of 1989, many infantile epileptic encephalopathies such as infantile spasms (IS) were classified as "generalized." We know now that there is often a focal onset to the epileptic spasms seen in IS and other syndromes, although they often quickly evolve to affect the bilateral hemispheres. As such, the 2016 classification places "epileptic spasms" in both the "focal" and "generalized" categories, reflecting this phenomenon. In addition, the new classification allows for multiple etiologies of a single epilepsy syndrome, for example, Tuberous Sclerosis, which has both genetic and structural etiologies. Recognition of the focal structural and metabolic etiologies of epileptic encephalopathies in infancy has allowed for the development of animal models to study these disorders.[1]

DESIGNING ANIMAL MODELS

Fig. 3.1 depicts the current schemata of the process of epileptogenesis and subsequent development of epilepsy as function of age, gender, and genetic predisposition. For epilepsy to develop, there is a theorized series of events that may occur and numerous variables that influence the outcome. Most often the proposed process relates to hippocampal-based epileptogenesis and epilepsy, because there is limited information to date for extrahippocampal epilepsies. In this approach, an initial event or etiology interacts with the genetics of a patient who is of particular age and sex, to produce the first seizure. Subsequently and again through interplay with genetics, age, and sex, the brain may undergo structural and/or functional changes, which lead to treatment-responsive epilepsy, refractory epilepsy, or no epilepsy at all (Fig. 3.1). The challenge lies in predicting which of these three outcomes will occur in a particular patient. In epileptic encephalopathies of infancy, animal models may help to elucidate this.[2]

The proposed mechanisms of epileptogenesis and the differences in neurotransmission we see in the developing brain provide the framework for developing animal models to study these disease processes. It is important to remember that these target mechanisms in the developing brain differ from those in the adult hippocampus, where cell loss and synaptic reorganization are thought to be the main targets.[2] In the developing brain, factors such as incomplete myelination, blood-brain barrier permeability, patterns of dendritic arborization, and "excitatory" effects of gamma-aminobutyric acid (GABA) are thought to be more influential (Table 3.1).

There are two peaks in the incidence of epilepsy based on age: one occurring early in life and the second in individuals over age 65 years.[3] In infants and children with structurally normal brains, there are numerous etiologies for the seizures including vascular, trauma, metabolic etiologies such as toxins and withdrawal, infectious, genetic predisposition, and perhaps also immune dysfunction. In infants and children with abnormal brains, immature brain epilepsy may develop secondary to developmental structural lesions or genetically determined diseases.[4]

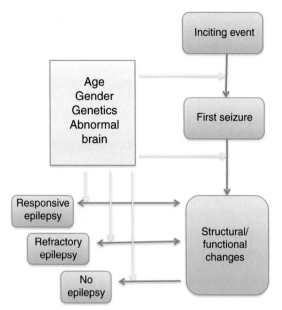

FIG. 3.1 **Epileptogenesis, the Development of Epi-lepsy, and Epilepsy-Related Outcomes as a Function of Etiology, Age, and Gender.** Although a seizure is often the symptom most readily identified, it may be the result of a previous inciting event, either remote or acute. Whether this inciting effect will generate a seizure depends on many factors including age, gender, genetic background, and the presence or absence of associated brain anomalies (subtle or overt). Recent studies suggest that inflammation may be a trigger. Whether a seizure is a single isolated event, heralds epilepsy, or leads to epilepsy depends on the same factors as discussed in this chapter. Indeed, under the same factors, on some occasions the seizure may induce additional structural or functional changes. The most prom-inent structural cell loss occurs in sensitive regions, such as the hippocampus, with increasing age as long as there is no genetic predisposition or associated brain anomaly. Finally, a combination of the same factors will determine whether the ensuing epilepsy is self-limited, responsive to antiseizure drugs, or refractory.

TABLE 3.1
Target Mechanisms of Epileptogenesis in the Adult Brain
Cell loss (e.g., hippocampal atrophy)
Axonal sprouting
Synaptic reorganization
Altered neuronal function (e.g., gene expression profiles, protein products)
Neurogenesis
Altered glial function and gliosis
Angiogenesis
Altered excitability and synchrony

Ideally, animal models would be created for all of these etiologies to conduct translational studies of epi-lepsy in the developing brain. However, many challenges exist in creating these models. For example, there are ani-mal models for ischemia and infectious and metabolic etiologies, but these animals do not necessarily develop epilepsy.[5-7] Additionally, many of these models have been created in adult animals,[6] and the findings are diffi-cult to extrapolate to infantile epilepsies because factors such as the immune response may vary with age.

Animal models must reflect the differing seizure susceptibility in various age groups. This is achieved by creating the model in animals of different ages and com-paring the phenotypes. The different neurologic mani-festations in these animals may be related to neuronal maturation and differ according to the developmental window during which the inciting event takes place. One example of this is in younger animals, where we see a greater tendency to develop multifocal seizures and sta-tus epilepticus as compared with older animals.[8,9]

To translate findings in rodent models to humans, it is important to be aware of the time course of devel-opmental milestones in these different species. In most studies, rats are considered neonatal at PN0-6; how-ever, comparisons of brain growth, cholesterol, GABA, and other objective parameters suggest that PN1-10 rats may be more similar to humans in the third trimester of gestation. This is further supported by the fact that rat pups begin to open their eyes only on PN13–15, a milestone that humans achieve on the day of birth. Rat pups can typically ambulate in the third week of life, whereas humans ambulate sometime shortly after the first year of life. These milestones serve as a marker of neuronal maturation and as such must be considered when studying models of developmental processes such as infantile epileptic encephalopathies.[10]

Although some translational studies have taken into account age differences in epilepsy phenotype and subsequent treatment, there have not been studies that account for gender differences. Translational studies to date have primarily been undertaken in male rats, leav-ing the question of gender difference in susceptibility and treatment unanswered.

MECHANISMS OF SEIZURES IN INFANCY

There are many factors that are believed to account for the occurrence and expression of seizures in the

TABLE 3.2
Proposed Mechanisms Involved in Epileptogenesis and Seizure Expression in the Immature Normal Brain

Injuries

Patterns of dendritic arborization and axon development

"Precocious" development of excitatory neurotransmission

Delayed development of inhibition

Depolarizing/"Excitatory" effects of GABA

Site specific maturation patterns of numerous channels such as HCN

Gap junctions

Incomplete myelination

Blood-brain barrier permeability

Late maturation of endogenous systems involved in seizure control such as SNr-based networks

Hormonal influences

Epigenetic factors

SNr, substantia nigra pars reticulata.

immature brain (Table 3.2). One common hypothesis for the mechanism of increased epileptogenicity in the immature brain is that there is a precocious development of excitatory neurotransmission and late development of inhibition in part due to a depolarizing excitatory effect of GABA. However, the available data[11–13] indicate that this theory may not be generalizable because different brain regions show specific patterns of equilibrium between excitation and inhibition, which are modified by discrete periods of development. The effects of sex and related hormonal alterations are an active area of investigation, and genetics also play a key role in seizure susceptibility.[14] Although many studies focus on neurons, the amount of myelination that has occurred and how well developed the blood-brain barrier is in a particular developmental stage also affect epileptogenicity. These factors increase the complexity of studies that need to be performed to understand the expression of seizures. One must keep these factors in mind when evaluating translational studies of this nature and therefore be mindful of the age of the animal, the brain region studied, gender, and other variables that may affect the findings and interpretation.

The presumed "excitatory" effect of the GABA A receptor (GABAAR) in the immature brain is not clear. In the mature brain, there is a higher proportion of K+/Cl− cotransporters, which export Cl− (KCC2), compared with Na+/K+/Cl− cotransporters, which import Cl− (NKCC1). As such, the extracellular Cl− concentration is tonically higher than the intracellular Cl− concentration. Therefore, under most physiologic conditions, activation of GABAAR induces hyperpolarization because of an intracellular influx of Cl− following the electrochemical gradient. Hyperpolarization is classically associated with decreased firing and thus with inhibition; therefore GABA is considered an inhibitory neurotransmitter in the mature brain.[15]

The activity of these transporters changes with maturation. In the immature brain, there is less KCC2[16] compared with NKCC1[17]; so the intracellular Cl− concentration is higher compared with that in mature cells. Thus, activation of GABAARs in immature neurons induces efflux of Cl− and triggers depolarizing potentials. The early depolarizing GABAAR signaling is essential for normal brain development, because it produces depolarization-induced activation of L-type voltage-sensitive calcium channels and NMDA receptors.[11] The precocious termination of the depolarizing GABA effect may have serious adverse effects in the way normal neurons develop and arborize to form synaptic connections.[18,19] It is worth noting that in the normal brain the GABAAR-mediated depolarizations are not necessarily excitatory, because they can still induce a weaker form of inhibition, shunting inhibition, when neuronal depolarization exceeds the reversal potential of GABAARs.[20]

The transition of GABA from a depolarizing to a hyperpolarizing neurotransmitter seems to occur at different developmental stages in different brain regions. This timing may also differ between genders. For example, in the GABAergic neurons of the substantia nigra pars reticulata (SNr), this occurs at 17 days of life in the male rat, whereas it occurs much earlier, at 10 days of life, in the female rat. In the hippocampus, this transition occurs even earlier in both genders with the female again maturing sooner than the male.[15,21,22]

The SNr plays a crucial role in the control of seizures and also in information processing, by way of a mechanism known as "dynamic gating." Normally, the SNr is tonically active and via GABAergic projections serves as an inhibitor of the excitatory pathways through the basal ganglia and prefrontal cortex. However, if GABA is decreased in the SNr, the cortex will be disinhibited and working memory improves. This phenomenon is age dependent, seen more prominently later in life.[23]

Accordingly, the ability of the SNr to control seizures changes with age and as a function of gender.

Our studies[24] have identified two regions in the SNr that mediate different effects. In adult male rats, following focal administration of GABAAergic agents, the anterior and posterior regions of the SNr mediate anticonvulsant and proconvulsant effects, respectively. These two distinct regions appear with time. In rats younger than 25 days, microinfusions of GABAAergic drugs produce proconvulsant effects irrespective of where the infusions are (anterior or posterior SNr). The two regions begin to produce opposite effects on seizures during adolescence, suggesting that this phenomenon is controlled by sex hormones. Indeed, in adult female rats there is only one effective region modulating seizures located in the anterior SNr and producing anticonvulsant effects, while similar infusions in the posterior SNr do not influence seizure control.[24] From the developmental point of view, studies in infant female rats have shown that microinfusions in the SNr initially have no effect on seizures and then the anticonvulsant region emerges. Interestingly, neonatal castration of male rats changes the ability of the SNr to control seizures, conferring features of the female SNr across the life span.[25]

ANIMAL MODELS

To understand the mechanisms involved in the expression and control of seizures, and their consequences as well as their responsivity to various therapeutic regimens, it is important to have realistic age-dependent animal models. In this section, we will review several key models that have advanced our knowledge of infantile epilepsies.

KINDLING

Kindling has been employed extensively as a chronic model of temporal lobe epilepsy with progression to bilateral clonic and occasionally tonic seizures.[8,26,27] The most common way of inducing kindling is using focal electrical brain stimulation, which results in the provocation of progressively more severe (intense) seizures. Additionally, this induces progressive change in response following repetitive stimulations as long as the stimuli are not delivered continuously.[9] The progression starts from the first effective stimulation with the appearance of a brief, low-frequency electrographic afterdischarge (AD) at the electrode tip, with little if any behavioral response. As the phenomenon becomes more complex, the responses evolve with the administration of the stimuli, eventually triggering long, high-frequency ADs associated with strong convulsive responses.[9] This progression occurs in all limbic and forebrain stimulation sites, but it is most dramatic from temporal lobe structures, such as the amygdala and adjacent cortices, including the piriform, perirhinal, insular, and entorhinal cortices.[28] It is the *progressive* increase in response severity in both the EEG and behavior that defines kindling. Ultimately, after many stimulations triggering kindled seizures, spontaneous seizures begin to appear without the application of the kindling stimulus. Kindling has been induced in many species, but it is most often produced in rodents.[29]

Kindling in developing rats has several unique features. As the brain of the infant rat rapidly grows, the kindling stimulations are delivered within a finite period of time, usually 48 h. The first protocol of amygdala kindling in infantile rats (PN15–18) was published by Moshé in 1981 using 1-h interstimulus intervals.[30] Subsequently, it was discovered that even shorter (15 min) interstimulus intervals were able to induce successful kindling, because of the lack of a refractory period.[9,31–34] With these paradigms, kindling can occur within 1 day, which is not the case in adult rats. Irrespective of the interstimulus intervals, kindling, once induced, is permanent and persists into adulthood in either the original kindling site or the contralateral site.[35]

There are some unique features of developmental kindling that have provided insights in understanding the biology of infantile seizures. These include age-related differences in the presence of a refractory period during which stimulations may not induce seizures, behavioral manifestations of kindled seizures and kindling rate (i.e., the number of stimulations required to develop bilateral seizures), the interaction between two foci kindled concurrently, and neuropathologic and metabolic sequelae. For example, the dorsal hippocampus kindles as fast as the amygdala and piriform cortex in 2-week-old rat pups, but in adults hippocampal kindling proceeds at a slower rate than in the other brain sites.[8,30] Because kindled seizures are semiologically different in infants than in adults, a modified seizure scoring scale has been created based on the seizures observed in PN15–18 rats undergoing amygdala kindling.[9] One difference from the adult scale is the appearance of alternating forelimb clonus in the same or consecutive seizure, which is indicative of bilateral seizures perhaps due to incomplete myelination of the corpus callosum.[8,30] Another significant feature of kindling in immature rats is the early appearance of severe kindled seizures consisting of wild running with jumping and vocalizations (stage 6 seizures) and sometimes tonus (stage 7 seizures).[9] These may occur early on, after only less than 30 stimulations, in adult rats whereas more than 100 stimulations may be required to induce these severe seizures in immature rats.[8]

PN15–17 rat pups are more prone to develop recurrent kindled seizures and status epilepticus than adult rats.[32] The absence of a postictal refractory period in infant rats has been proposed as a factor contributing to this increased propensity of the immature brain to develop status epilepticus or recurrent kindled seizures.[32] Interestingly, the duration of postictal refractoriness increases with age and is much longer in adulthood.[32] Also, in contrast to adult kindled rats, PN15–17 pups do not exhibit kindling antagonism.[8] Therefore, concurrent kindling of the amygdala and a second site, for example, the hippocampus, leads each site to develop accelerated kindling with rat pups exhibiting severe, and occasionally spontaneous, seizures.[8,9] These findings suggest that the immature brain is not yet capable of suppressing the development of multiple foci, explaining therefore the higher incidence of multifocal seizures in the immature brain.[8]

Imaging studies using deoxyglucose autoradiography have shown increased deoxyglucose uptake in rhinencephalic structures, but not in basal ganglia or neocortex in PN15–16 rats with stage 6 and 7 kindled seizures.[36] It has been proposed that the rapid propagation and increased severity of seizures at this age may reflect the immaturity of subcortical structures, such as the SNr, involved in seizure control.[8]

It is our experience that the development of kindling in Sprague-Dawley pups obtained from different sources may vary, suggesting that exogenous or genetic factors influence this process. The existence of strain differences in the development of kindling has been well documented in adult and infant Fast and Slow rats, a crossbreeding of Wistar and Long Evans rats.[28,37,38] This emphasizes the need to understand genetic influences in the expression of seizures.

STATUS EPILEPTICUS

Models of status epilepticus (SE) can be used to study the effects of severe, prolonged epileptic activity. The two most commonly used models involve the administration of either kainic acid[39] or lithium pilocarpine.[39,40] In adult rats, both agents induce brain injury,[41] which eventually leads to the appearance of spontaneous seizures.[42,43] In both models, status epilepticus can be induced in rat pups with lower doses of the convulsant agents as compared with adult rats.[42,43]

The studies using animal models of SE have two important findings. The first is that limbic injury including hippocampal injury (CA1 and CA3 hippocampal loss and synaptic reorganization in the dentate gyrus) is not often induced in rats less than PN21 with the intensity of neuronal loss increasing with the age of the animal at the time the convulsant was injected.[26,39,44] Although this is widely accepted and has been replicated, there have been studies that uncovered a degree of cell loss in some young animals, often in a different breed of rats, suggesting a genetic predisposition. For example, in Wistar rats, Sankar et al.[45] found early, milder structural injuries in immature rats, and Suchomelova et al.[46] found structural changes in the amygdala, hippocampus, and perirhinal cortex and enlargement of the lateral ventricles as well as reduced density of hilar neurons after status epilepticus in the PN10 rat of this breed. Kubova et al.[47] demonstrated neuronal loss in the mediodorsal nucleus of the thalamus in male Wistar albino PN12 rats. Lopez-Meraz et al.[48] also studied Wistar pups (of either sex) and found changes in the CA1 region of the hippocampus after SE. Wu et al.[49] observed changes in this same region in female Sprague-Dawley rats in addition to documenting spatial memory deficit in these animals. Nishimura et al.[50] induced status epilepticus in Sprague-Dawley rats at PN7–11 or PN30–34 and found structural changes such as change in arborization of dendrites in the younger group. Such changes in arborization were not seen in older animals because of the profound cell loss. Additionally, changes in the GABAAR subunit expression and function in hippocampal dentate granule neurons have been found in PN10 Sprague-Dawley pups that experienced SE via lithium pilocarpine. These rats, however, did not develop epilepsy in adulthood again, suggesting age-dependent differences in the effects of SE on brain structure and function.[51]

The second distinct feature of these models is that spontaneous recurrent seizures (SRS) occur only after a structural brain injury has been identified, for example, in the studies referenced above.[45–51] After SE is induced in adult and PN21 Sprague-Dawley rats, entorhinal and piriform cortices reveal MRI changes as early as 6 h later in those animals that went on to develop epilepsy. In addition, hippocampal signal change was seen 36–48 h later and worsened over time to sclerosis.[52]

Comorbidities after status epilepticus are also age dependent. Learning and behavior may be affected in young animals after experiencing status epilepticus. Deficits in spatial learning and increase in anxiety have been documented and replicated in animal studies.[53–55]

The age dependency of status induced injury and subsequent spontaneous seizures have led to studies aiming to identify biomarkers for the development of subsequent epilepsy. In a pioneer study, Roch et al.[56] performed MRIs in the 3-week-old (PN21) Sprague-Dawley rats at several time intervals between 2 h and 9 weeks after experiencing SE induced via the lithium-pilocarpine model. They found that at 2 h, blood-brain barrier breakdown was seen only in the thalamus, but this disappeared by 6 h. Furthermore, at 24 h after SE, changes were seen in the amygdala, piriform, and entorhinal cortices and neuronal loss was evident. At 48 h, hippocampal sclerosis was noted on imaging and pathology. Thereafter, three subgroups were identified based on imaging findings at 24 h after status epilepticus, two of which went on to develop epilepsy. The first of these groups had an MRI finding of hyperintense signal at the level of the piriform and entorhinal cortices, which began to disappear at 48–72 h after SE. In addition, these had a corresponding increase in T2 relaxation time. The second group displayed no signal change on MRI T2-weighted images, but was noted to have a moderate increase of the T2 relaxation time in the piriform cortex. The rats that had neither MRI abnormalities nor modification of the T2 relaxation time did not develop epilepsy.[56]

This study helped design the FEBSTAT study by Shinnar et al., which is a prospective study examining potential biomarkers that could be identified in testing obtained within 72 h after the onset of febrile status epilepticus (FSE) including EEG and brain MRI.[57] EEG revealed abnormalities in 45% of the children enrolled in the study. Focal slowing was the most common and appeared in 24% of children, followed by attenuation that was seen in 13%, typically over the temporal regions. In addition, epileptiform discharges were present in 6.5% of children.[58] However, MRI abnormalities were less frequent, with only 11.5% of children having certain or equivocal imaging abnormalities. Typically, this was increased T2 signal in the hippocampus or a developmental abnormality of the hippocampus. Overall, extrahippocampal imaging abnormalities were found in equal frequency in the case and control groups; however, extrahippocampal temporal abnormalities were more common in the FSE group. Hippocampal malrotation was the most common developmental abnormality, found in 7.5% of cases and 1% of controls.[59] After 1 year on repeat imaging, it was discovered that those patients with T2 hyperintensity on acute imaging were more likely to develop hippocampal sclerosis.[60] On cognitive testing at 1 month and 1 year post-FSE, patients with FSE did not appear to have significant cognitive impairment; however, children with MRI abnormalities were more likely to

have receptive language delay at 1 year.[61] These studies demonstrate the complexity of the possible etiologies of FSE. Fever and status epilepticus do not appear to be the key determinants; other factors such as genetic background, type of infection, prior injury, as discussed earlier maybe, gender, and, of course, the specific developmental window status epilepticus occurred.

LIPOPOLYSACCHARIDE-ASSOCIATED SEIZURES IN DEVELOPING RATS

Neuroinflammation is the nervous system's immune response to an external stimulus, which may or may not be infectious. This includes both innate and adaptive immune responses, which activate neutrophils and lymphocytes, respectively. Although both systems recruit neutrophils and macrophages to some degree and result in the production of proinflammatory cytokines, there are distinctions between the two immune responses. Innate immunity is nonspecific and engaged quickly, within hours. On the other hand, the adaptive response is more specialized and thus takes a longer period of time to develop.[62] This response may be protective or may result in pathology, including epileptogenesis. Studies have found that inflammation may decrease seizure threshold and also that seizures may cause neuroinflammation.[63]

Lipopolysaccharide (LPS) is a bacterial endotoxin that induces a broad, significant inflammatory reaction when injected intraperitoneally. It is recognized by Toll-like receptors (TLR), thereby activating a cascade that results in the production of cytokines, chemokines, and other proinflammatory molecules.[63] Furthermore, TLR sites in the CNS seem to increase after LPS injection, further mitigating inflammation.[64]

Febrile Seizures

A model of febrile seizures was created by Heida et al.[65] using LPS and kainic acid. This model produced febrile seizures at clinically relevant temperatures in 50% of PN14 rats. The seizure onset was ~60 min into the fever and the duration of the seizure was also ~60 min, constituting FSE. On postmortem H&E, there was no overt histopathologic change found in these animals.[65]

The long-term effects vary depending on the age at which the SE occurs. Most adult rats will develop SRS ~2 weeks after the SE. They also show significant learning and memory deficits when challenged with hippocampal-dependent tests. Cell loss is seen in the hippocampus, amygdala, thalamus, piriform, and entorhinal cortices. In prepubescent rats (PN19–30), SRSs are also observed although after a longer latent period of 3 weeks. The learning and memory deficits that they exhibit are less severe than those in the adult rat. Neuronal loss may occur in this group as well, but mainly in the hippocampus with the other regions relatively spared. In infant rats (PN11–17), SE rarely leads to SRS and when it does the seizures are nonconvulsive and the latency period is several months. Learning and memory deficits are even milder than those seen in prepubescent and adult rats. Studies examining neuronal loss in these animals have been inconsistent. Early postnatal rats (PN0–10) seem to tolerate SE well with the least amount of long-term sequelae. They do not experience SRS or neuronal cell loss and only rarely exhibit learning and memory deficits that are mild in nature.[66]

Effects of Lipopolysaccharide-Induced Inflammation on SE

Sankar et al. reported that when LPS was injected before the induction of status epilepticus in PN7 and PN14 rats, the hippocampal damage induced by lithium pilocarpine was exacerbated. There was no injury seen in animals that received LPS injections but did not have SE. They concluded that the effects of inflammation coupled with prolonged seizures in early life may impact the outcomes in neonatal seizures.[67] Another group induced febrile seizures by exposing the animals to hyperthermia with a heat lamp or hairdryer. They also demonstrated more severe seizures in those animals that had been injected with LPS as compared with those that had not, suggesting that inflammation coupled with hyperthermia exacerbates the seizure severity.[68] When Sankar's group controlled for body temperature, these findings were replicated, suggesting that perhaps the fever itself does not contribute to seizure severity. Furthermore, hippocampal injury was again demonstrated and further localized to the CA1 region.[69] When a kindling model was used in lieu of the lithium-pilocarpine model, enhanced epileptogenesis was also seen in the animals that undergo LPS injection before status epilepticus. This further supports the effects of inflammation on this process, because the kindling model does not cause the neurodegeneration seen in the lithium-pilocarpine model.[70] This may be secondary to increased baseline hippocampal excitability, rapid progression of rapid kindling, and/or the ability to retain kindling, which was seen in these animals.[71]

LIPOPOLYSACCHARIDE AND INFANTILE SPASMS

West syndrome is the classic epileptic encephalopathy of infancy and occurs secondary to a variety of etiologies including cortical and subcortical injury in early life. Galanopoulou and Scantlebury created a model of spasms by injecting LPS and doxorubicin focally in the cortex of rat pups at PN3 followed by an intraperitoneal injection of p-chlorophenylalanine at PN5. Flexion or extension spasms emerged at PN4 and lasted until PN11–12.[72] During the spasms, the ictal EEG findings consisted of multiple spikes at the onset of electrodecremental responses, which were at times followed by focally evolving discharges. The interictal EEG did not show hypsarrhythmia, but this a technical limitation, as it is not possible to place more than two intracranial electrodes on the very small skull of a PN6 rat and the mutifocality (a key feature of hypsarrhythmia) requires at least three electrodes. As the rats get older, spontaneous focal seizures emerged. The rats with spasms also demonstrated a cognitive decline, learning and memory deficits, and autistic-like behavior compared with controls.[72] Preliminary data were reported by Katsarou et al. at the annual American Epilepsy Society meeting in 2016, suggesting that there is a decreased number of GABAergic neurons in the cortex of these affected animals.

TREATMENT OF SEIZURES AND STATUS EPILEPTICUS IN THE DEVELOPING BRAIN

The models that have been created in the developing animal help us understand the pathophysiology of the seizures and also to explore potential treatment strategies. Hasson et al. induced status epilepticus for 1 h using either kainic acid or lithium pilocarpine in PN9, PN15, and PN21 rats.[73] These animals were then treated with varied doses of either diazepam (20–60 mg/kg) or pentobarbital (20–60 mg/kg). The results showed that at PN9 neither drug was effective in aborting the SE. In the older rats, however, both of the medications stopped the status epilepticus in a dose-dependent fashion with diazepam working significantly faster but at relatively higher doses. In the PN15 rats, diazepam at 20 mg/kg/dose aborted 63% of seizures, whereas at 60 mg/kg/dose 100% of seizures ceased. Similar dose-dependent results were found in the PN21 diazepam group and in the PN15 and PN21 animals treated with pentobarbital at these doses. Furthermore, if low-dose diazepam (20 mg/kg/dose) was initially ineffective, SE was always aborted with a subsequent low dose of pentobarbital (20 mg/kg/dose). This study suggested that high doses of diazepam or low doses of diazepam paired with pentobarbital may be needed to stop SE in developing rats, and furthermore these treatments may be less successful in the very young rats. As a result, the search for other treatments is ongoing, especially for the newborn.

As was discussed above, the relatively increased number of NKCC1 as compared with KCC2 cotransporters in the developing brain causes intracellular chloride concentration to be higher and GABA to be relatively "excitatory." Studies have implicated NKCC1 in the facilitation of seizures in the developing brain,[74] and this is a hypothesized reason why GABAergic agents work less well in aborting seizures in the developing brain. It also provides a rationale for the study of bumetanide, an NKCC1 blocker, in the treatment of these often-refractory seizures.[75] This compound was effective in treating seizures in these animals as well as enhancing the response to GABAergic agents such as phenobarbital.[76] However, one small open-label trial was conducted in neonates with seizures secondary to hypoxic ischemic encephalopathy and found bumetanide to be largely ineffective. Furthermore, several of the patients were left with hearing impairment, especially those who also received aminoglycosides.[77] Although there have been case reports suggesting safety and efficacy,[78] the discovery of hearing impairment as a potential adverse effect has limited the use of bumetanide in humans.

Topiramate has also been studied, and while it does not appear to abort status epilepticus in the developing rat, it does appear to prevent epileptogenesis when administered in PN15 and PN28 rats.[79]

Pretreatment with flupirtine in developing rats that have suffered ischemic injury has been shown to prevent hypoxic seizures[80]; however, this has not yet been studied as an administration after the onset of seizures, which is typically when antiseizure medication is given in humans.

The multiple hit model of ISs has introduced a novel paradigm to test the efficacy of putative treatments after the onset of the spasms and determine their effects not only on spasms but also on subsequent epileptogenesis, i.e. the development of additional seizures beyond the acute period following the initial insult. Galanopoulou et al. have created a standardized procedure that will allow drug trials in this condition.[81–84]

EFFECTS OF ANTISEIZURE DRUGS ON THE DEVELOPING BRAIN

Several studies have examined the effects of various antiseizure drugs (ASDs) on the developing brain in the rat. Most of the ASDs studied appear to induce apoptotic neurodegeneration when given to immature rats, for example, phenobarbital, phenytoin, diazepam, clonazepam, vigabatrin, and valproate.[85] It has been shown that these changes are age dependent, with the most prominent apoptosis occurring with exposure early in life around at PN7.[85] However, levetiracetam does not

produce such apoptotic changes[86] and zonisamide actually may have a neuroprotective effect in models of hypoxia ischemia.[87] Topiramate produced neurotoxicity at high doses (50 mg/kg), far above the accepted effective dose; therefore this may be a candidate for use in the developing brain.[88] These studies, however, were not performed at the time the animals were experiencing seizures, which is primarily when they would be used in humans. Indeed, Hasson et al. were not able to document any evidence of injury in the animals they treated with diazepam or pentobarbital after 1-h long SE.[73]

CONCLUSION

Epilepsy in the developing brain is caused by different etiologies and triggers, including structural and metabolic abnormalities, stroke, intracranial hemorrhage, infection, and others. These insults in isolation or in combination may cause the development of epileptic encephalopathies in the neonate and infant. It is difficult to create animal models to accurately simulate these conditions; several new models have been created using inflammation as a trigger. The currently available models have provided valuable information on the pathogenesis of seizures and epilepsy in young rats, treatments, and consequences. Future work will take advantage of these realistic models together with the development of new models and sophisticated drug testing akin to human clinical trials. The hope is that these studies will lead to subsequent investigations to treat or prevent epilepsy and its comorbidities in vulnerable children before it begins.

ACKNOWLEDGMENTS

Solomon L. Moshé is the Charles Frost Chair in Neurosurgery and Neurology and funded by grants from NIH NS43209 and 1U54NS100064, CURE Infantile Spasms Initiative, US Department of Defense (W81XWH-13-1-0180), the Heffer Family and the Segal Family Foundations and the Abbe Goldstein/Joshua Lurie and Laurie Marsh/Dan Levitz families.

DISCLOSURES

Mary C. Spiciarich, MD, has no disclosures. Solomon L. Moshé MD is serving as Associate Editor of Neurobiology of Disease and is on the editorial board of Brain and Development, Pediatric Neurology and Physiological Research. He receives from Elsevier an annual compensation for his work as Associate Editor in Neurobiology of Disease and royalties from two books he coedited. He received a consultant's fee from Eisai and UCB.

REFERENCES

1. Fisher RS, Acevedo C, Arzimanoglou A, et al. ILAE official report: a practical clinical definition of epilepsy. *Epilepsia.* 2014;55(4):475–482.

2. Haut SR, Velíšková J, Moshé SL. Susceptibility of immature and adult brains to seizure effects. *Lancet Neurol.* 2004;3(10):608–617.

3. Hauser WA, Kurland LT. The epidemiology of epilepsy in Rochester, Minnesota, 1935 through 1967. *Epilepsia.* 1975;16(1):1–66.

4. Scheffer IE, Berkovic S, Capovilla G, Connolly MB, French J, Guilhoto L, Hirsch E, Jain S, Mathern GW, Moshé SL, Nordli DR, Perucca E, Tomson T, Wiebe S, Zhang YH, Zuberi SM. ILAE classification of the epilepsies: Position paper of the ILAE Commission for Classification and Terminology, *Epilepsia.* 2017 Apr;58(4):512–521.

5. Jensen FE. An animal model of hypoxia-induced perinatal seizures. *Ital J Neurol Sci.* 1995;16(1–2):59–68.

6. Stewart KA, Wilcox KS, Fujinami RS, White HS. Development of post-infection epilepsy following theiler virus infection of C57BL/6 mice. *J Neuropathol Exp Neurol.* 2010;69(12):1210–1219.

7. Moshé SL, Albala BJ. Perinatal hypoxia and subsequent development of seizures. *Physiol Behav.* 1985;35(5):819–823.

8. Haas KZ, Sperber EF, Moshé SL. Kindling in developing animals: expression of severe seizures and enhanced development of bilateral foci. *Brain Res Dev Brain Res.* 1990;56(2):275–280.

9. Goddard GV, McIntyre DC, Leech CK. A permanent change in brain function resulting from daily electrical stimulation. *Exp Neurol.* 1969;25(3):295–330.

10. Katsarou AM, Moshe SL, Galanopoulou AS. Interneuronopathies and their role in early life epilepsies and neurodevelopmental disorders. *Epilepsia Open.* 2017;2(3):284–306.

11. Galanopoulou AS. GABA(A) receptors in normal development and seizures: friends or foes? *Curr Neuropharmacol.* 2008;6(1):1–20.

12. Insel TR, Miller LP, Gelhard RE. The ontogeny of excitatory amino acid receptors in rat forebrain–I. N-methyl-D-aspartate and quisqualate receptors. *Neuroscience.* 1990;35(1):31–43.

13. Galanopoulou AS, Moshé SL. In search of epilepsy biomarkers in the immature brain: goals, challenges and strategies. *Biomark Med.* October 2011;5(5):615–628.

14. Galanopoulou AS. Sex and epileptogenesis, introduction to the special issue. *Neurobiol Dis.* 2014;(72 Pt B):123–124.

15. Galanopoulou AS, Kyrozis A, Claudio OI, Stanton PK, Moshé SL. Sex-specific KCC2 expression and GABA(A) receptor function in rat substantia nigra. *Exp Neurol.* 2003;183(2):628–637.

16. Rivera C, Voipio J, Payne JA, et al. The K+/Cl– cotransporter KCC2 renders GABA hyperpolarizing during neuronal maturation. *Nature.* 1999;397(6716):251–255.

17. Plotkin MD, Snyder EY, Hebert SC, Delpire E. Expression of the Na-K-2Cl cotransporter is developmentally regulated in postnatal rat brains: a possible mechanism underlying GABA's excitatory role in immature brain. *J Neurobiol.* 1997;33(6):781–795.

18. Cancedda L, Fiumelli H, Chen K, Poo MM. Excitatory GABA action is essential for morphological maturation of cortical neurons in vivo. *J Neurosci.* 2007;27(19):5224–5235.

19. Wang DD, Kriegstein AR. Defining the role of GABA in cortical development. *J Physiol.* 2009;587(Pt 9):1873–1879.

20. Staley KJ, Mody I. Shunting of excitatory input to dentate gyrus granule cells by a depolarizing GABAA receptor-mediated postsynaptic conductance. *J Neurophysiol.* 1992;68(1):197–212.

21. Kyrozis A, Chudomel O, Moshé SL, Galanopoulou AS. Sex-dependent maturation of GABAA receptor-mediated synaptic events in rat substantia nigra reticulate. *Neurosci Lett.* 2006;398(1–2):1–5.

22. Galanopoulou AS, Dissociated gender-specific effects of recurrent seizures on GABA signaling in CA1 pyramidal neurons: role of GABA(A) receptors. *J Neurosci.* 2008;28(7):1557–1567.

23. O'Reilly RC. Biologically based computational models of high-level cognition. *Science.* 2006;314(5796):91–94.

24. Giorgi FS, Galanopoulou AS, Moshé SL. Sex dimorphism in seizure-controlling networks. *Neurobiol Dis.* 2014;72:144–152.

25. Velíšková J, Moshé SL. Sexual dimorphism and developmental regulation of substantia nigra function. *Ann Neurol.* 2001;50:596–601.

26. Haas KZ, Sperber EF, Opanashuk LA, Stanton PK, Moshé SL. Resistance of immature hippocampus to morphologic and physiologic alterations following status epilepticus or kindling. *Hippocampus.* 2001;11(6):615–625.

27. Haas KZ, Sperber EF, Moshé SL. Kindling in developing animals: interactions between ipsilateral foci. *Brain Res Dev Brain Res.* 1992;68(1):140–143.

28. McIntyre DC, Kelly ME, Dufresne C. FAST and SLOW amygdala kindling rat strains: comparison of amygdala, hippocampal, piriform and perirhinal cortex kindling. *Epilepsy Res.* 1999;35(3):197–209.

29. Ludvig N, Moshé SL. Deep prepiriform cortex lesion and development of amygdala kindling. *Epilepsia.* 1988;29(4):401–403.

30. Moshé SL. The effects of age on the kindling phenomenon. *Dev Psychobiol.* 1981;14(1):75–81.

31. Moshé SL, Sharpless NS, Kaplan J. Kindling in developing rats: variability of afterdischarge thresholds with age. *Brain Res.* 1981;211(1):190–195.

32. Moshé SL, Albala BJ. Maturational changes in postictal refractoriness and seizure susceptibility in developing rats. *Ann Neurol.* 1983;13(5):552–557.

33. Baram TZ, Hirsch E, Schultz L. Short-interval amygdala kindling in neonatal rats. *Brain Res Dev Brain Res.* 1993;73(1):79–83.

34. Sankar R, Auvin S, Kwon YS, Pineda E, Shin D, Mazarati A. Evaluation of development-specific targets for antiepileptogenic therapy using rapid kindling. *Epilepsia.* 2010; (51 suppl 3):39–42.

35. Moshé SL, Albala BJ. Kindling in developing rats: persistence of seizures into adulthood. *Brain Res.* 1982;256(1):67–71.

36. Ackermann RF, Moshé SL, Albala BJ. Restriction of enhanced [2-14C]deoxyglucose utilization to rhinencephalic structures in immature amygdala-kindled rats. *Exp Neurol.* 1989;104(1):73–81.

37. Velísková J, Claudio OI, Galanopoulou AS, et al. Seizures in the developing brain. *Epilepsia.* 2004;(45 suppl 8): 6–12.

38. Xu B, McIntyre DC, Fahnestock M, Racine RJ. Strain differences affect the induction of status epilepticus and seizure-induced morphological changes. *Eur J Neurosci.* 2004;20(2):403–418.

39. Albala BJ, Moshé SL, Okada R. Kainic-acid-induced seizures: a developmental study. *Brain Res.* 1984;315(1): 139–148.

40. Turski WA, Cavalheiro EA, Bortolotto ZA, Mello LM, Schwarz M, Turski L. Seizures produced by pilocarpine in mice: a behavioral, electroencephalographic and morphological analysis. *Brain Res.* 1984;321(2): 237–253.

41. Coppola A, Moshé SL. Animal models. *Handb Clin Neurol.* 2012;107:63–98.

42. André V, Marescaux C, Nehlig A, Fritschy JM. Alterations of hippocampal GABAergic system contribute to development of spontaneous recurrent seizures in the rat lithium-pilocarpine model of temporal lobe epilepsy. *Hippocampus.* 2001;11(4):452–468.

43. Lothman EW, Bertram EH. Epileptogenic effects of status epilepticus. *Epilepsia.* 1993;(34 suppl 1):S59–S70.

44. Sperber EF, Haas KZ, Stanton PK, Moshé SL. Resistance of the immature hippocampus to seizure-induced synaptic reorganization. *Brain Res Dev Brain Res.* 1991;60(1):88–93.

45. Sankar R, Shin DH, Liu H, Mazarati A, Pereira de Vasconcelos A, Wasterlain CG. Patterns of status epilepticus-induced neuronal injury during development and long-term consequences. *J Neurosci.* 1998;18(20):8382–8393.

46. Suchomelova L, Lopez-Meraz ML, Niquet J, Kubova H, Wasterlain CG. Hyperthermia aggravates status epilepticus-induced epileptogenesis and neuronal loss in immature rats. *Neuroscience.* 2015;305:209–224.

47. Kubova H, Druga R, Lukasiuk K, et al. Status epilepticus causes necrotic damage in the mediodorsal nucleus of the thalamus in immature rats. *J Neurosci.* 2001;21: 3593–3599.

48. Lopez-Meraz ML, Niquet J, Wasterlain CG. Distinct caspase pathways mediate necrosis and apoptosis in subpopulations of hippocampal neurons after status epilepticus. *Epilepsia.* 2010;(51 suppl 3):56–60.

49. Wu CL, Huang LT, Liou CW, et al. Lithium-pilocarpine-induced status epilepticus in immature rats result in long-term deficits in spatial learning and hippocampal cell loss. *Neurosci Lett.* 2001;312(2):113–117.

50. Nishimura M, Gu X, Swann JW. Seizures in early life suppress hippocampal dendrite growth while impairing spatial learning. *Neurobiol Dis.* 2011;44(2):205–214.

51. Zhang G, Raol YH, Hsu FC, Coulter DA, Brooks-Kayal AR. Effects of status epilepticus on hippocampal GABAA receptors are age-dependent. *Neuroscience.* 2004;125(2):299–303.

52. Roch C, Leroy C, Nehlig A, Namer IJ. Magnetic resonance imaging in the study of the lithium-pilocarpine model of temporal lobe epilepsy in adult rats. *Epilepsia.* 2002;43(4):325–335.

53. DaSilva AV, Regondi MC, Cavalheiro EA, Spreafico R. Disruption of cortical development as a consequence of repetitive pilocarpine-induced status epilepticus in rats. *Epilepsia.* 2005;(46 suppl 5):22–30.

54. Sayin U, Sutula TP, Stafstrom CE. Seizures in the developing brain cause adverse long-term effects on spatial learning and anxiety. *Epilepsia.* 2004;45(12):1539–1548.

55. Kleen JK, Wu EX, Holmes GL, Scott RC, Lenck-Santini PP. Enhanced oscillatory activity in the hippocampal-prefrontal network is related to short-term memory function after early-life seizures. *J Neurosci.* 2011;31(43): 15397–15406.

56. Roch C, Leroy C, Nehlig A, Namer IJ. Predictive value of cortical injury for the development of temporal lobe epilepsy in 21-day-old rats: an MRI approach using the lithium-pilocarpine model. *Epilepsia.* 2002;43(10):1129–1136.

57. Gomes WA, Shinnar S. Prospects for imaging-related biomarkers of human epileptogenesis: a critical review. *Biomark Med.* 2011;5(5):599–606.

58. Nordli DR Jr, Moshé SL, Shinnar S, et al. FEBSTAT Study Team, Acute EEG findings in children with febrile status epilepticus: results of the FEBSTAT study. *Neurology.* 2012;79(22):2180–2186.

59. Shinnar S, Bello JA, Chan S, et al. FEBSTAT Study Team, MRI abnormalities following febrile status epilepticus in children: the FEBSTAT study. *Neurology.* 2012;79(9):871–877.

60. Lewis DV, Shinnar S, Hesdorffer DC, et al. FEBSTAT Study Team, Hippocampal sclerosis after febrile status epilepticus: the FEBSTAT study. *Ann Neurol.* 2014;75(2):178–185.

61. Weiss EF, Masur D, Shinnar S, et al. FEBSTAT study team, cognitive functioning one month and one year following febrile status epilepticus. *Epilepsy Behav.* 2016;64(Pt A):283–288.

62. Chen GY, Nuñez G. Sterile inflammation: sensing and reacting to damage. *Nat Rev Immunol.* 2010;10(12):826–837.

63. Vezzani A, Granata T. Brain inflammation in epilepsy: experimental and clinical evidence. *Epilepsia.* 2005;46(11):1724–1743.

64. Rivest S, Lacroix S, Vallieres L, et al. How the blood talks to the brain parenchyma and the paraventricular nucleus of the hypothalamus during systemic inflammatory and infectious stimuli. *Proc Soc Exp Biol Med.* 2000;223:22–38.

65. Heida JG, Teskey GC, Pittman QJ. Febrile convulsions induced by the combination of lipopolysaccharide and low-dose kainic acid enhance seizure susceptibility, not epileptogenesis, in rats. *Epilepsia.* 2005;46(12):1898–1905.

66. Scantlebury MH, Heida JG, Hasson HJ, et al. Age-dependent consequences of status epilepticus: animal models. *Epilepsia.* 2007;(48 suppl 2):75–82.
67. Sankar R, Auvin S, Mazarati A, Shin D. Inflammation contributes to seizure-induced hippocampal injury in the neonatal rat brain. *Acta Neurol Scand Suppl.* 2007;186:16–20.
68. Eun BL, Abraham J, Mlsna L, Kim MJ, Koh S. Lipopolysaccharide potentiates hyperthermia-induced seizures. *Brain Behav.* 2015;5(8):e00348.
69. Auvin S, Shin D, Mazarati A, Nakagawa J, Miyamoto J, Sankar R. Inflammation exacerbates seizure-induced injury in the immature brain. *Epilepsia.* 2007;(48 suppl 5):27–34.
70. Auvin S, Mazarati A, Shin D, Sankar R. Inflammation enhances epileptogenesis in the developing rat brain. *Neurobiol Dis.* October 2010;40(1):303–310.
71. Auvin S, Shin D, Mazarati A, Sankar R. Inflammation induced by LPS enhances epileptogenesis in immature rat and may be partially reversed by IL1RA. *Epilepsia.* 2010;(51 suppl 3):34–38.
72. Scantlebury MH, Galanopoulou AS, Chudomelova L, Raffo E, Betancourth D, Moshé SL. A model of symptomatic infantile spasms syndrome. *Neurobiol Dis.* 2010;37(3):604–612.
73. Hasson H, Kim M, Moshé SL. Effective treatments of prolonged status epilepticus in developing rats. *Epilepsy Behav.* 2008;13(1):62–69.
74. Dzhala VI, Talos DM, Sdrulla DA, et al. NKCC1 transporter facilitates seizures in the developing brain. *Nat Med.* 2005;11(11):1205–1213.
75. Löscher W, Puskarjov M, Kaila K. Cation-chloride cotransporters NKCC1 and KCC2 as potential targets for novel antiepileptic and antiepileptogenic treatments. *Neuropharmacology.* 2013;69:62–74.
76. Dzhala VI, Brumback AC, Staley KJ. Bumetanide enhances phenobarbital efficacy in a neonatal seizure model. *Ann Neurol.* 2008;63(2):222–235.
77. Pressler RM, Boylan GB, Marlow N, et al. Bumetanide for the treatment of seizures in newborn babies with hypoxic ischaemic encephalopathy (NEMO): an open-label, dose finding, and feasibility phase 1/2 trial. *Lancet Neurol.* 2015;14(5):469–477.
78. Kahle KT, Barnett SM, Sassower KC, Staley KJ. Decreased seizure activity in a human neonate treated with bumetanide, an inhibitor of the Na(+)-K(+)-2Cl(-) cotransporter NKCC1. *J Child Neurol.* 2009;24(5):572–576.
79. Suchomelova L, Baldwin RA, Kubova H, Thompson KW, Sankar R, Wasterlain CG. Treatment of experimental status epilepticus in immature rats: dissociation between anticonvulsant and antiepileptogenic effects. *Pediatr Res.* 2006;59(2):237–243.
80. Sampath D, Shmueli D, White AM, Raol YH. Flupirtine effectively prevents development of acute neonatal seizures in an animal model of global hypoxia. *Neurosci Lett.* 2015;607:46–51.
81. Ono T, Moshé SL, Galanopoulou AS. Carisbamate acutely suppresses spasms in a rat model of symptomatic infantile spasms. *Epilepsia.* 2011;52(9):1678–1684.
82. Raffo E, Coppola A, Ono T, Briggs SW, Galanopoulou AS. A pulse rapamycin therapy for infantile spasms and associated cognitive decline. *Neurobiol Dis.* 2011;43(2):322–329.
83. Briggs SW, Mowrey W, Hall CB, Galanopoulou AS. CPP-115, a vigabatrin analogue, decreases spasms in the multiple-hit rat model of infantile spasms. *Epilepsia.* 2014;55(1):94–102.
84. Jequier Gygax M, Klein BD, White HS, Kim M, Galanopoulou AS. Efficacy and tolerability of the galanin analog NAX 5055 in the multiple-hit rat model of symptomatic infantile spasms. *Epilepsy Res.* 2014;108(1):98–108.
85. Bittigau P, Sifringer M, Genz K, et al. Antiepileptic drugs and apoptotic neurodegeneration in the developing brain. *Proc Natl Acad Sci USA.* 2002;99:15089–15094.
86. Manthey D, Asimiadou S, Stefovska V, et al. Sulthiame but not levetiracetam exerts neurotoxic effect in the developing rat brain. *Exp Neurol.* 2005;193:497–503.
87. Topçu Y, Bayram E, Ozbal S, et al. Zonisamide attenuates hyperoxia-induced apoptosis in the developing rat brain. *Neurol Sci.* 2014;35(11):1769–1775.
88. Glier C, Dzietko M, Bittigau P, Jarosz B, Korobowicz E, Ikonomidou C. Therapeutic doses of topiramate are not toxic to the developing brain. *Exp Neurol.* 2004;185:403–409.

CHAPTER 4

Ictogenic and Epileptogenic Mechanisms of Neuroinflammation: Insights From Animal Models

SILVIA BALOSSO, PHD • TERESA RAVIZZA, PHD • ANNAMARIA VEZZANI, PHD

INTRODUCTION

Neuroinflammation still lacks a consensus definition; therefore it is important to define beforehand what do we mean when describing this phenomenon.[1] We specifically refer to molecules with inflammatory properties, the biosynthesis and release of which chiefly involve brain-resident cells, including activated microglia and astrocytes, neurons, and endothelial cells of the blood-brain barrier (BBB), as well as blood-borne macrophages.[2] The broader definition of inflammation includes phenomena associated with the activation of both innate and adaptive immunity cells (i.e., lymphocytes) in response to noxious stimuli, leading to the production of inflammatory cytokines and related effector molecules. It represents a key homeostatic mechanism of defense against infections or sterile (noninfectious) tissue injuries, which is instrumental for initiating programs for tissue repair. Neuroinflammation is more specifically related to activation of innate immunity and local mechanisms of inflammation in injured brain tissue.

It is well established that the inflammatory response requires a rapid resolution to avoid tissue damage and dysfunction. Resolution of inflammation is an active process that involves the generation of proresolving antiinflammatory proteins and lipids.[3] There is experimental evidence, validated in surgical brain specimens from pharmacoresistant epilepsy patients, that the mechanisms of resolution are inefficient in epilepsy, therefore potentially contributing to the detrimental effects of a persistent inflammatory response to epileptogenic injuries or to recurrent seizures.[4] In particular, IL-1 receptor antagonist (IL-1Ra) that controls IL-1β signaling, CD59 that modulates complement activation, or the transcriptional factor ATF3 that controls TLR4 expression is induced only moderately compared with their respective proinflammatory partners.[5-9]

Key determinants of a pathogenic role of (neuro) inflammation are the cells targeted by the inflammatory molecules because they express the relevant receptors. In this context, there is evidence for the upregulation of receptors for cytokines, chemokines, danger signals, prostaglandins, and complement factors in neuronal cells, glia, and cell components of the BBB in epileptogenic brain areas from animal models and in human epilepsies (e.g., temporal lobe epilepsy, focal cortical dysplasia type 2b, tuberous sclerosis, glioneuronal tumors, Rasmussen's encephalitis). These findings, together with evidence for induction of endogenous cognate ligands and receptor-related cell signaling pathways,[9-15] underscore the existence of both autocrine and paracrine effects of inflammatory molecules released in epileptogenic brain tissue, thus fostering additional investigations on the consequences of the activation of these pathways for neuronal network excitability and cell survival.

INFLAMMATORY PATHWAYS INVOLVED IN ICTOGENESIS AND EPILEPTOGENESIS

To unveil the potential role of inflammatory signals in epilepsy, two main approaches have been commonly taken: (1) Intrinsic seizure susceptibility to chemoconvulsants, or the development of epilepsy following status epilepticus, was tested in mice with genetic deletion or amplification of specific inflammatory pathways. (2) Molecules or drugs mimicking or blocking inflammatory signal activation were either intracerebrally or systemically injected to animals before provoking acute seizures or during recurrent spontaneous seizures in chronic epilepsy, or after exposing the animal to epileptogenic insults. The main outcome measures were the onset, frequency, and duration of seizures. When testing epileptogenesis, neurologic comorbidities were

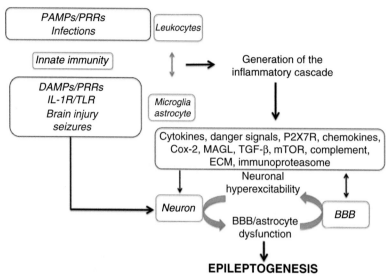

FIG. 4.1 **Schematic Representation of the Evidence-Based Cascade of Inflammatory Events Contributing to Epileptogenesis.** Activation of innate immunity cells can occur following infections or sterile injuries. PAMPs (pathogen-associated molecular patterns) expressed by microbes are recognized by PPRs (pattern-recognition receptors) expressed by leukocytes (or microglia) to initiate the inflammatory tissue response apt to remove the pathogen. Similarly, PRRs are activated in microglia and astrocytes by DAMPs (damage-associated molecular pattern) released by injured tissue, in the absence of infection, to ignite homeostatic mechanisms of repair. The inflammatory response to infection or injury may become detrimental, thus provoking tissue damage and dysfunction, if it is not timely and efficiently resolved by endogenous antiinflammatory peptides and lipids. In epilepsy, these resolution mechanisms are inefficient, therefore promoting persistent brain inflammation. Several inflammatory mediators have been reported to play a significant role in seizure generation and epileptogenesis in experimental models. The activation of ictogenic/epileptogenic inflammatory pathways has been validated in human brain tissue resected at surgery from pharmacoresistant forms of epilepsy such as temporal lobe epilepsy, focal cortical dysplasia, tuberous sclerosis, Rasmussen's encephalitis, and following epileptogenic events such as stroke and neurotrauma. The interactions between glia, neurons and the blood brain barrier (BBB), and peripheral immune cells, mediated by aberrant inflammatory responses, contribute to determine pathologic molecular, structural, and functional changes in the brain. This creates a vicious cycle that promotes neuronal network hyperexcitability that underlies seizure generation and disease progression.

often assessed, in particular, cognitive deficits and anxiety, as well as neuroprotection by evaluating neuronal cell loss.[14]

IL-1R/TLR signaling. The activation of the interleukin (IL)-1 receptor/Toll-like receptor (TLR) signaling in glial cells is the upstream generator of the neuroinflammatory cascade. TLRs are part of the family of pattern recognition receptors (PRRs) that recognize molecular patterns expressed by pathogens (PAMPs) during infections or damage-associated molecular patterns (DAMPs) motifs expressed by danger signals, which are molecules that are released by injured cells in the absence of infections, thereby eliciting *sterile* inflammation. Activation of PRRs by DAMPs (or PAMPs) results in the transcriptional activation

of NFkB-sensitive inflammatory genes, leading to the generation and rapid amplification of the inflammatory cascade (Fig. 4.1).

IL-1R type 1 (IL-1R1) and PRRs (in particular, TLR3 and TLR4) are induced in brain cells following various experimental epileptogenic insults, such as status epilepticus, stroke, neurotrauma, CNS infection, as well as during recurring seizures. Their endogenous ligands include IL-1β, ATP, High Mobility Group Box 1 (HMGB1), Heat Shock Proteins (HSP), S100β, formyl peptides, mitochondrial DNA that are released from injured neurons, or activated microglia and astrocytes. The production of breakdown products of the extracellular matrix (ECM), such as hyaluronates, also activates PRRs.[16,17] There is evidence for upregulation of key signaling molecules of the IL-1R1-TLR4 axis in epileptogenic areas surgically resected from patients with structural/lesional pharmacoresistant epilepsies,[18–20] therefore prompting further investigations for understanding the pathophysiologic consequences of such activation.

Pharmacologic and genetic studies carried out in experimental models have demonstrated that the IL-1R1 and TLR4 pathways, respectively activated by IL-1β and HMGB1, have a permissive role in seizure generation and epileptogenesis (i.e., the development and extension of brain tissue capable of generating spontaneous seizures[21]) (Fig. 4.1).

In particular, the data showed that the activation of the IL-1R1/TLR4 pathway exacerbates seizures by increasing their frequency and accelerating their onset time; accordingly, inhibitors of this signaling (e.g., IL-1Ra; caspase-1 inhibitors; TLR4 antagonists) mediated significant antiseizure effects also against seizures unresponsive to classic antiepileptic drugs.[18,20,22–25] Recent evidence has shown that IL-1R1/TLR4 signaling plays a role in status epilepticus–induced cell loss, epileptogenesis, and the progression of the disease after the onset of spontaneous seizures.[16,18,26–30] In the context of PRRs, genetic ablation of TLR3,[30] TLR4,[18,20] or IL-1R1[23,31] drastically reduced evoked or spontaneous recurrent seizures in animal models and dramatically improved the disease outcomes in models of status epilepticus–induced epileptogenesis.

A key driver of neuroinflammation is the *P2X7 receptor*, an ATP-gated ionotropic purinergic receptor, predominantly expressed in microglia but also in presynaptic nerve terminals where it regulates glutamate release. Activation of P2X7 receptors in microglia is pivotal for the assembly of the inflammasome, a macromolecular complex comprising caspase-1, which is instrumental for the biosynthesis of the biologically active and mature IL-1β and the release of HMGB1. Previous studies found increased expression of the P2X7 receptor in experimental and human epilepsy, and their antagonism significantly reduced status epilepticus and spontaneous seizures in animal models.[32–35]

Other inflammatory signals. Increasing evidence points to the pathologic involvement of several inflammatory mediators in epilepsy. We briefly report the salient features of some inflammatory pathways by focusing on those that were found to be upregulated also in brain specimens from human pharmacoresistant epilepsies (Fig. 4.1).

Arachidonic acid–related pathways. Reduction of cell loss, improved survival, and rescue of neurologic comorbidities were beneficial effects observed in animals when neuronal cyclooxygenase-2 (*COX-2)*

activation or prostaglandin E2 (PGE2) receptors (EP1 and EP2) were antagonized during epileptogenesis evoked by status epilepticus.[36,37] In addition to PGE2, several prostaglandins have been implicated in acute seizures; however, their involvement in epileptogenesis is mostly unknown,[12,28] and so far conflicting results have been reported related to prophylactic administration of different COX-2 inhibitors after status epilepticus in rodents.[38–40] *Monoacylglycerol lipase,* the key enzyme in the hydrolysis of the endocannabinoid 2-arachidonoylglycerol (2-AG), represents the major source of arachidonic acid and eicosanoids in the CNS and is an emerging potential target for drug development in epilepsy.[41]

Additional targets. (1) TNF-α activating p55 (type 1) receptors promote ictogenesis and favor kindling epileptogenesis[42–45]; (2) *the immunoproteasome,* a proteasome isoform, is induced during inflammation with different immune-related functions as compared with the standard proteasome. In particular, the β5i subunit is induced in neurons and glia in human and experimental epilepsy brain tissue and is involved in ictogenesis.[46–48] (3) The *mTOR pathway* has been extensively studied for its involvement in seizures and possibly in epileptogenesis, as shown in rat models of temporal lobe epilepsy[49,50] and malformations of cortical development such as tuberous sclerosis and focal cortical dysplasia.[51] (4) *Various chemokines* (CCL2 [MCP-1], CCL3 [MIP-1α], CCL4 [MIP-1β], and CCL5 [RANTES]) and their receptors have also been studied for their effects related not only to leukocyte recruitment but also to neuromodulation. In particular, CCR5 receptors activated by MIP-1α and RANTES contribute to neuroinflammation, cell loss, acute seizures, and BBB damage in experimental models. Similarly, CCR2 activated by CCL2 contributes to spontaneous seizures in mice, and to their exacerbation by lipopolysaccharide (LPS), a TLR4 agonist that mimics bacterial infections.[52]

Transforming growth factor (TGF)-β signaling and BBB dysfunction. BBB permeability strictly regulates the reciprocal blood-to-brain exchange of molecules and immune cells, and its integrity is instrumental for protecting the brain from the entry of xenobiotics or potentially dangerous molecules. BBB dysfunction occurs in epilepsy as in other neurologic disorders, such as stroke and trauma. Consequently, blood-borne molecules and immune cells enter the brain and may induce an inflammatory response leading to neuropathology.[53,54] In particular, serum albumin enters the brain parenchyma because of BBB dysfunction and is sensed by astrocytes via activation of TGF-β receptors. Astrocytes exposed to albumin or IgG become reactive and proliferate, releasing TGF-β1 and several proinflammatory cytokines that are induced by transcriptional activation programs. The ultimate result is the alteration of neural physiology and network connectivity (reactive synaptogenesis),[55] which promotes seizure occurrence (Fig. 4.1).

MECHANISTIC INSIGHTS

Reactive gliosis is commonly observed during epileptogenesis and is associated with chronic spontaneous seizures in animal models and in human epileptogenic *foci*.[56] These cells display an inflammatory phenotype together with functional changes including, but not limited to, reduced K^+, water and glutamate buffering capacity (*for comprehensive review see* Ref. 57), a plethora of phenomena, which concur to generate neuronal hyperexcitability, and seizures. Recently, brain exposure to albumin was shown to induce the degradation of perineuronal nets, a protective ECM structure that provide synaptic stability and restrict reorganization of inhibitory interneurons, via activation of TGF-β signaling.[58] Consistent with this evidence, blockade of TGF signaling interfered with epileptogenesis and reduced chronic seizures.[59]

The *inflammasome*-dependent cellular release of HMGB1 and IL-1β is induced by intracellular ionic changes that are produced during glioneuronal network activation (i.e., K^+ and Cl^- efflux, Na^+ influx). This evidence implies that a state of enhanced neuronal activity may promote the production of inflammatory molecules.[60] PRRs and IL-1R1 activation in neurons can rapidly increase neuronal excitability via posttranslational modification of receptor-gated or voltage-dependent ion channels, mostly mediated by activation of protein kinase C and tyrosine kinase (Src) family of protein kinases.[16,61] The net result is an increased Ca^{2+} influx into neurons, which mediates excitotoxicity. TNF-α is another cytokine that affect neuronal responses to glutamate by inducing membrane expression of AMPA receptors lacking the GLUR2 subunit, thus promoting a receptor configuration more permissive for Ca^{2+} influx.[62] In the context of neuromodulatory effects of cytokines and chemokines, there is evidence that both IL-1β and fractalkine/CX3CL1 modulate GABA-A receptor currents in human temporal lobe epilepsy by protein kinase–mediated mechanisms.[10,63] In particular, IL-1β decreased the GABA-evoked current amplitude in specimens from patients with TLE but not in control tissues. This evidence suggests that this cytokine contributes to seizure generation in human TLE also by reducing GABA-mediated neurotransmission.[10]

Epigenetic effects mediated by DAMPs, such as HMGB1, should also be considered. HMGB1 is a constitutive protein physiologically bound to nuclei in every cell type, where it regulates gene transcription. On various cellular stressor events, including epileptogenic insults or seizures, it can rapidly translocate to the cytoplasm from where it can be extracellularly released. Recent evidence showed that after HMGB1 cytoplasmatic translocation in macrophages and fibroblasts, their cell phenotype was significantly altered (Marco Bianchi, *personal communication*). If the same effects are induced in brain cells, then HMGB1 translocation during epileptogenesis may lead to epigenetic changes in neurons and glia with a possible impact on long-term disease outcomes.[64] Notably, extracellular HMGB1 can be oxidized to its disulfide isoform in the presence of oxidative stress, and both phenomena occur during epileptogenesis. Disulfide HMGB1 is proinflammatory and ictogenic and promotes cell loss by activating TLR4.[65] Therefore HMGB1 can be considered as a nodal molecule linking neuroinflammation to oxidative stress during epileptogenesis.[66]

CONSEQUENCES OF NEUROINFLAMMATION ON IMMATURE BRAIN EXCITABILITY

Febrile-like seizures induced in immature rodents (PN7–14) by heat or systemic LPS or Poly I:C (a TLR3 agonist mimicking viral infections) trigger a systemic inflammatory response associated with neuroinflammation in forebrain, which includes the release of cytokines from microglia and astrocytes[67,68] and HMGB1 from neurons.[69] The data proved that seizures, but not the increment in brain temperature, provoked neuroinflammation. The temperature threshold for evoking febrile-like seizures in mice lacking IL-1R1 was significantly increased, while treatment with intracerebroventricular IL-1β before inducing hyperthermia lowered seizure threshold.[70] Noteworthy, there was a strict association between persistent neuroinflammation in the hippocampus and development of epilepsy in rats exposed to febrile seizures of which only 30% developed the disease.[68] These data provide proof-of-concept evidence that neuroinflammation determines the threshold for the occurrence of experimental febrile seizures and may contribute to the ensuing epilepsy. Febrile seizures in children often occur in the context of an ongoing systemic infection. To mimic this condition and the associated fever, immature rodents were exposed to systemic LPS or Poly I:C. This inflammatory challenge decreased seizure threshold to various chemoconvulsants[67,71] and facilitated electrical kindling;[72] notably, the increased susceptibility to seizures was maintained until animal's adulthood,[73] thus denoting a long-lasting modification of brain excitability similar to a priming-like effect.[74] In accordance, preexposure of immature rodents to LPS increased the severity of epilepsy when the animal was exposed to status epilepticus in adulthood.[73]

Prevention of the neuroinflammatory response using minocycline, an inhibitor of microglia activation, or intraventricular administration of IL-1Ra or TNF-α inactivating antibody precluded both the acute and long-term reduction in seizure threshold, as well as the neurologic comorbidities (anxiety-like behavior, learning and memory deficits) that developed in animal's adulthood.[67,71] Considering that brain inflammation has been implicated in several neuropsychiatric disorders, it is conceivable that inflammatory processes that are triggered in the brain by an immune or epileptogenic insult may, concurrently with seizures, lead to the development of neurobehavioral abnormalities.[14]

Interestingly, the transient inflammatory challenge imposed to immature rodent brain induced long-term changes in glutamate receptor subtypes expression and the K^+/Cl^- cotransporter in the rat hippocampus and cortex,[75,76] two phenomena that may contribute to pathologic changes in brain function.

CONCLUSIONS

Mechanistic studies and pharmacologic interventions on neuroinflammation pathways activated in experimental models of epilepsy have increased our understanding of this complex response to brain injury and helped to identify anticonvulsive and/or antiepileptogenic properties of target-specific antiinflammatory drugs. Notably, some of these drugs are already in medical use for other clinical indications such as in autoinflammatory or autoimmune diseases. These drugs may therefore be considered for preventing or treating pharmacoresistant seizures. Treating therapy-resistant patients with specific antiinflammatory drugs already approved for other indications has shown signs of clinical efficacy (Table 4.1). This may foster further clinical translation of laboratory findings because these treatments target inflammatory mechanisms involved in experimental seizure in animal models.[29,77] Importantly, adverse events of antiinflammatory drugs, in particular, susceptibility to infections, have to be closely monitored, and combination of antiinflammatory treatments may be considered as one therapeutic option because of the reverberant inflammatory cascade. It is also worth considering that there are therapeutic interventions in pharmacoresistant epilepsies, such as the use of steroids, the ketogenic diet, the vagal nerve stimulation, and the cannabinoids, that display antiinflammatory mechanisms of action, which may mediate some of their therapeutic effects.

Patient selection for clinical studies of antiinflammatory drugs should be considered based on evidence of neuroinflammation, such as temporal lobe epilepsy, cortical dysplasia, and tuberous sclerosis. Recently, PET imaging of neuroinflammation has been developed using the translocator protein 18 kDa ligands to detect microglia activation in epileptogenic areas of patients.[78,79]

TABLE 4.1
Molecular Pathways Activated in Epilepsy With a Pathogenic Role in Seizure Mechanisms: Clinical Translation

Pathway	Clinical Study	References
IL-1β system/inflammasome	**VX09-765-401**: focal epilepsy	80
• IL-1β/IL-1R1	(*Caspase-1 inhibitor*)	
• Caspase-1	**Kineret**: FIRES	81
• P2X7	**Kineret**: intractable epilepsy	82
• HMGB1/TLR4	(*IL-1R1 antagonist*)	
TNF-α	**Adalimumab**: RE (*inactivating Ab*)	83
Arachidonic acid pathways		
• COX-2/PGE2		
• EP1/EP2		
• MAGL/2-AG/cannabinoids	**Cannabidiol**	84

Continued

TABLE 4.1
Molecular Pathways Activated in Epilepsy With a Pathogenic Role in Seizure Mechanisms:
Clinical Translation—cont'd

Pathway	Clinical Study	References
Immunoproteasome • β5 inducible		
Chemokines • CCL2 (MIP-1)/CCR2 • CCL5 (RANTES), CCL3,CCL4/CCR5		
TGF-β • TGF-β R1/2 • Albumin		
mTOR • mTORC1 • mTORC2	**Rapamycin, Sirolimus, Everolimus:** TS (*inhibitors*)	85
Adhesion molecules	**Natalizumab:** RE, MS (anti-α2 integrin Ab)	86,87
Microglia	**Minocycline:** astrocytoma (*cell activation inhibitor*) Nowak 2012	88

Pathways have been characterized by immunohistochemistry, RTqPCR, and western blot in epileptogenic brain areas in experimental and human epilepsy. Pharmacologic studies in animal models or the use of transgenic mice showed the pathway's involvement in seizure mechanisms (for reviews see Refs. 12, 14, 15, 46–48, 51, 54, 89, 90).
FIRES, febrile infection-related epilepsy syndrome; *MS*, multiple sclerosis; *RE*, Rasmussen's encephalitis.

The design of preventing or disease-modifying antiinflammatory interventions in epilepsy requires deep insights into the dynamic changes of neuroinflammation during epileptogenesis to determine the best target and therapeutic window for intervention. We also need to unequivocally distinguish homeostatic from pathologic inflammatory signaling triggered by the various epileptogenic insults to block the latter without interfering with the repair mechanisms. In this frame, boosting resolution mechanisms of inflammation may be a safer strategy than inhibiting the process itself.

The progress in elucidating the mechanisms underlying the pathogenic effects of neuroinflammation in epilepsy is critical for developing safe and effective drugs with potential disease-modifying, and not purely symptomatic, therapeutic effects.

ACKNOWLEDGMENTS

We are grateful to Citizen United for Research in Epilepsy (CURE), RING14 International, and European Union's Seventh Framework Programme (FP7/2007–13) under grant agreement n602102 (EPITARGET), for supporting our research on the role of inflammation in epilepsy.

REFERENCES

1. Filiou MD, Arefin AS, Moscato P, Graeber MB. 'Neuroinflammation' differs categorically from inflammation: transcriptomes of Alzheimer's disease, Parkinson's disease, schizophrenia and inflammatory diseases compared. *Neurogenetics.* 2014;15(3):201–212.
2. Varvel NH, Neher JJ, Bosch A, et al. Infiltrating monocytes promote brain inflammation and exacerbate neuronal damage after status epilepticus. *Proc Natl Acad Sci USA.* 2016;113(38):E5665–E5674.
3. Serhan CN, Chiang N, Van Dyke TE. Resolving inflammation: dual anti-inflammatory and pro-resolution lipid mediators. *Nat Rev Immunol.* 2008;8(5):349–361.
4. Vezzani A, French J, Bartfai T, Baram TZ. The role of inflammation in epilepsy. *Nat Rev Neurol.* 2011;7(1):31–40.
5. De Simoni MG, Perego C, Ravizza T, et al. Inflammatory cytokines and related genes are induced in the rat hippocampus by limbic status epilepticus. *Eur J Neurosci.* 2000;12(7):2623–2633.
6. Eriksson C, Van Dam AM, Lucassen PJ, Bol JG, Winblad B, Schultzberg M. Immunohistochemical localization of interleukin-1beta, interleukin-1 receptor antagonist and interleukin-1beta converting enzyme/caspase-1 in the rat brain after peripheral administration of kainic acid. *Neuroscience.* 1999;93(3):915–930.
7. Eriksson C, Tehranian R, Iverfeldt K, Winblad B, Schultzberg M. Increased expression of mRNA encoding interleukin-1beta and caspase-1, and the secreted isoform of

interleukin-1 receptor antagonist in the rat brain following systemic kainic acid administration. *J Neurosci Res.* 2000;60(2):266–279.

8. Pernhorst K, Herms S, Hoffmann P, et al. TLR4, ATF-3 and IL8 inflammation mediator expression correlates with seizure frequency in human epileptic brain tissue. *Seizure.* 2013;22(8):675–678.

9. Aronica E, Boer K, van Vliet EA, et al. Complement activation in experimental and human temporal lobe epilepsy. *Neurobiol Dis.* 2007;26(3):497–511.

10. Roseti C, van Vliet EA, Cifelli P, et al. GABA currents are decreased by IL-1beta in epileptogenic tissue of patients with temporal lobe epilepsy: implications for ictogenesis. *Neurobiol Dis.* 2015;82:311–320.

11. Tan CC, Zhang JG, Tan MS, et al. NLRP1 inflammasome is activated in patients with medial temporal lobe epilepsy and contributes to neuronal pyroptosis in amygdala kindling-induced rat model. *J Neuroinflammation.* 2015;12(1):18.

12. Rojas A, Jiang J, Ganesh T, et al. Cyclooxygenase-2 in epilepsy. *Epilepsia.* 2014;55(1):17–25.

13. Meng XF, Tan L, Tan MS, et al. Inhibition of the NLRP3 inflammasome provides neuroprotection in rats following amygdala kindling-induced status epilepticus. *J Neuroinflammation.* 2014;11:212.

14. Vezzani A, Aronica E, Mazarati A, Pittman QJ. Epilepsy and brain inflammation. *Exp Neurol.* 2013;244: 11–21.

15. Vezzani A, Friedman A, Dingledine RJ. The role of inflammation in epileptogenesis. *Neuropharmacology.* 2013;69: 16–24.

16. Vezzani A, Maroso M, Balosso S, Sanchez MA, Bartfai T. IL-1 receptor/Toll-like receptor signaling in infection, inflammation, stress and neurodegeneration couples hyperexcitability and seizures. *Brain Behav Immun.* 2011;25(7):1281–1289.

17. Bianchi ME. DAMPs, PAMPs and alarmins: all we need to know about danger. *J Leukoc Biol.* 2007;81(1):1–5.

18. Iori V, Maroso M, Rizzi M, et al. Receptor for Advanced Glycation Endproducts is upregulated in temporal lobe epilepsy and contributes to experimental seizures. *Neurobiol Dis.* 2013;58:102–114.

19. Zurolo E, Iyer A, Maroso M, et al. Activation of TLR, RAGE and HMGB1 signaling in malformations of cortical development. *Brain.* 2011;134(4):1015–1032.

20. Maroso M, Balosso S, Ravizza T, et al. Toll-like receptor 4 and high-mobility group box-1 are involved in ictogenesis and can be targeted to reduce seizures. *Nat Med.* 2010;16(4):413–419.

21. Pitkanen A, Engel J Jr. Past and present definitions of epileptogenesis and its biomarkers. *Neurotherapeutics.* 2014;11(2):231–241.

22. Vezzani A, Conti M, De Luigi A, et al. Interleukin-1beta immunoreactivity and microglia are enhanced in the rat hippocampus by focal kainate application: functional evidence for enhancement of electrographic seizures. *J Neurosci.* 1999;19(12):5054–5065.

23. Vezzani A, Moneta D, Conti M, et al. Powerful anticonvulsant action of IL-1 receptor antagonist on intracerebral injection and astrocytic overexpression in mice. *Proc Natl Acad Sci USA.* 2000;97(21):11534–11539.

24. Ravizza T, Lucas SM, Balosso S, et al. Inactivation of caspase-1 in rodent brain: a novel anticonvulsive strategy. *Epilepsia.* 2006;47(7):1160–1168.

25. Maroso M, Balosso S, Ravizza T, et al. Interleukin-1beta biosynthesis inhibition reduces acute seizures and drug resistant chronic epileptic activity in mice. *Neurotherapeutics.* 2011;8(2):304–315.

26. Noé FM, Polascheck N, Frigerio F, et al. Pharmacological blockade of IL-1beta/IL-1 receptor type 1 axis during epileptogenesis provides neuroprotection in two rat models of temporal lobe epilepsy. *Neurobiol Dis.* 2013;59:183–193.

27. Kwon YS, Pineda E, Auvin S, Shin D, Mazarati A, Sankar R. Neuroprotective and antiepileptogenic effects of combination of anti-inflammatory drugs in the immature brain. *J Neuroinflammation.* 2013;10:30.

28. Iori V, Iyer A, Ravizza T, et al. Blockade of the IL-1R1/TLR4 pathway mediates disease-modification therapeutic effects in a model of acquired epilepsy. *Neurobiol Dis.* 2017;99:12–23.

29. Vezzani A. Anti-inflammatory drugs in epilepsy: does it impact epileptogenesis? *Expert Opin Drug Saf.* 2015;14(4):583–592.

30. Gross A, Benninger F, Madar R, et al. Toll-like receptor 3 deficiency decreases epileptogenesis in a pilocarpine model of SE-induced epilepsy in mice. *Epilepsia.* 2017;58(4):586–596.

31. Vezzani A, Balosso S, Maroso M, Zardoni D, Noé F, Ravizza T. ICE/caspase 1 inhibitors and IL-1beta receptor antagonists as potential therapeutics in epilepsy. *Curr Opin Investig Drugs.* 2010;11(1):43–50.

32. Henshall DC, Diaz-Hernandez M, Miras-Portugal MT, Engel T. P2X receptors as targets for the treatment of status epilepticus. *Front Cell Neurosci.* 2013;7:237.

33. Jimenez-Pacheco A, Mesuret G, Sanz-Rodriguez A, et al. Increased neocortical expression of the P2X7 receptor after status epilepticus and anticonvulsant effect of P2X7 receptor antagonist A-438079. *Epilepsia.* 2013;54(9): 1551–1561.

34. Jimenez-Pacheco A, Diaz-Hernandez M, Arribas-Blazquez M, et al. Transient P2X7 receptor antagonism produces lasting reductions in spontaneous seizures and gliosis in experimental temporal lobe epilepsy. *J Neurosci.* 2016;36(22):5920–5932.

35. Wei YJ, Guo W, Sun FJ, et al. Increased expression and cellular localization of P2X7R in cortical lesions of patients with focal cortical dysplasia. *J Neuropathol Exp Neurol.* 2016;75(1):61–68.

36. Rojas A, Ganesh T, Lelutiu N, Gueorguieva P, Dingledine R. Inhibition of the prostaglandin EP2 receptor is neuroprotective and accelerates functional recovery in a rat model of organophosphorus induced status epilepticus. *Neuropharmacology.* 2015;93:15–27.

37. Rojas A, Bueorguieva P, Lelutiu N, Quan Y, Shaw R, Dingledine R. The prostaglandin EP1 receptor potentiates kainate receptor activation via a protein kinase C pathway and exacerbates status epilepticus. *Neurobiol Dis.* 2014;70:74–89.

38. Jung KH, Chu K, Lee ST, et al. Cyclooxygenase-2 inhibitor, celecoxib, inhibits the altered hippocampal neurogenesis with attenuation of spontaneous recurrent seizures following pilocarpine-induced status epilepticus. *Neurobiol Dis.* 2006;23(2):237–246.

39. Holtman L, van Vliet EA, van Schaik R, Queiroz CM, Aronica E, Gorter JA. Effects of SC58236, a selective COX-2 inhibitor, on epileptogenesis and spontaneous seizures in a rat model for temporal lobe epilepsy. *Epilepsy Res.* 2009;84(1):56–66.

40. Polascheck N, Bankstahl M, Loscher W. The COX-2 inhibitor parecoxib is neuroprotective but not antiepileptogenic in the pilocarpine model of temporal lobe epilepsy. *Exp Neurol.* 2010;224(1):219–233.

41. von Rüden EL, Bogdanovic RM, Wotjak CT, Potschka H. Inhibition of monoacylglycerol lipase mediates a cannabinoid-1 receptor dependent delay of kindling progression in mice. *Neurobiol Dis.* 2015;77:238–245.

42. Balosso S, Ravizza T, Perego C, et al. Tumor necrosis factor-alpha inhibits seizures in mice via p75 receptors. *Ann Neurol.* 2005;57(6):804–812.

43. Balosso S, Ravizza T, Pierucci M, et al. Molecular and functional interactions between TNF-alpha receptors and the glutamatergic system in the mouse hippocampus: implications for seizure susceptibility. *Neuroscience.* 2009;161(1):293–300.

44. Balosso S, Ravizza T, Aronica E, Vezzani A. The dual role of TNF-alpha and its receptors in seizures. *Exp Neurol.* 2013;247C:267–271.

45. Weinberg MS, Blake BL, McCown TJ. Opposing actions of hippocampus TNFalpha receptors on limbic seizure susceptibility. *Exp Neurol.* 2013;247:429–437.

46. Mishto M, Ligorio C, Bellavista E, et al. Immunoproteasome expression is induced in mesial temporal lobe epilepsy. *Biochem Biophys Res Commun.* 2011;408(1):65–70.

47. Mishto M, Raza M, De Biase D, et al. The immunoproteasome β5i subunit is key contributor to ictogenesis in a rat model of chronic epilepsy. *Brain Behav Immun.* 2015;49: 188–196.

48. van Scheppingen J, Broekaart D, Scholl T, et al. Dysregulation of the (immuno)proteasome pathway in malformations of cortical development. *J Neuroinflammation.* 2016;13(1):202.

49. Galanopoulou AS, Gorter JA, Cepeda C. Finding a better drug for epilepsy: the mTOR pathway as an antiepileptogenic target. *Epilepsia.* 2012;53(7):1119–1130.

50. van Vliet EA, Forte G, Holtman L, et al. Inhibition of mammalian target of rapamycin reduces epileptogenesis and blood-brain barrier leakage but not microglia activation. *Epilepsia.* 2012;53(7):1254–1263.

51. Crino PB. The mTOR signalling cascade: paving new roads to cure neurological disease. *Nat Rev Neurol.* 2016;12(7): 379–392.

52. Cerri C, Genovesi S, Allegra M, et al. The Chemokine CCL2 mediates the seizure-enhancing effects of systemic inflammation. *J Neurosci.* 2016;36(13):3777–3788.

53. Friedman A, Kaufer D, Heinemann U. Blood-brain barrier breakdown-inducing astrocytic transformation: novel targets for the prevention of epilepsy. *Epilepsy Res.* 2009;85 (2–3):142–149.

54. Heinemann U, Kaufer D, Friedman A. Blood-brain barrier dysfunction, TGFbeta signaling, and astrocyte dysfunction in epilepsy. *Glia.* 2012;60(8):1251–1257.

55. Weissberg I, Wood L, Kamintsky L, et al. Albumin induces excitatory synaptogenesis through astrocytic TGF-beta/ALK5 signaling in a model of acquired epilepsy following blood-brain barrier dysfunction. *Neurobiol Dis.* 2015;78:115–125.

56. Aronica E, Ravizza T, Zurolo E, Vezzani A. Astrocyte immune response in epilepsy. *Glia.* 2012;60(8):1258–1268.

57. Devinsky O, Vezzani A, Najjar S, De Lanerolle NC, Rogawski MA. Glia and epilepsy: excitability and inflammation. *Trends Neurosci.* 2013;36(3):174–184.

58. Kim SY, Porter BE, Friedman A, Kaufer D. A potential role for glia-derived extracellular matrix remodeling in postinjury epilepsy. *J Neurosci Res.* 2016;94(9):794–803.

59. Kim SY, Buckwalter M, Soreq H, Vezzani A, Kaufer D. Blood-brain barrier dysfunction-induced inflammatory signaling in brain pathology and epileptogenesis. *Epilepsia.* 2012;(53 suppl 6):37–44.

60. Xanthos DN, Sandkuhler J. Neurogenic neuroinflammation: inflammatory CNS reactions in response to neuronal activity. *Nat Rev Neurosci.* 2014;15(1):43–53.

61. Vezzani A, Viviani B. Neuromodulatory properties of inflammatory cytokines and their impact on neuronal excitability. *Neuropharmacology.* 2015;96(Pt A):70–82.

62. Stellwagen D, Beattie EC, Seo JY, Malenka RC. Differential regulation of AMPA receptor and GABA receptor trafficking by tumor necrosis factor-alpha. *J Neurosci.* 2005;25(12):3219–3228.

63. Roseti C, Fucile S, Lauro C, et al. Fractalkine/CX3CL1 modulates GABAA currents in human temporal lobe epilepsy. *Epilepsia.* 2013;54(10):1834–1844.

64. Kobow K, Blumcke I. Epigenetic mechanisms in epilepsy. *Prog Brain Res.* 2014;213:279–316.

65. Balosso S, Liu J, Bianchi ME, Vezzani A. Disulfide-containing High Mobility Group Box-1 promotes N-methyl-d-aspartate receptor function and excitotoxicity by activating Toll-like receptor 4-dependent signaling in hippocampal neurons. *Antioxid Redox Signal.* 2014;21(12):1726–1740.

66. Pauletti A, Terrone G, Shekh-Ahmad T, et al. Targeting oxidative stress improves disease outcomes in a rat model of acquired epilepsy. *Brain.* 2017;140(7):1885–1899.

67. Galic MA, Riazi K, Pittman QJ. Cytokines and brain excitability. *Front Neuroendocrinol.* 2012;33(1):116–125.

68. Dubé CM, Ravizza T, Hamamura M, et al. Epileptogenesis provoked by prolonged experimental febrile seizures: mechanisms and biomarkers. *J Neurosci.* 2010;30(22): 7484–7494.

69. Choy M, Dubé CM, Patterson K, et al. A novel, noninvasive, predictive epilepsy biomarker with clinical potential. *J Neurosci*. 2014;34(26):8672–8684.

70. Dubé C, Vezzani A, Behrens M, Bartfai T, Baram TZ. Interleukin-1beta contributes to the generation of experimental febrile seizures. *Ann Neurol*. 2005;57(1):152–155.

71. Riazi K, Galic MA, Pittman QJ. Contributions of peripheral inflammation to seizure susceptibility: cytokines and brain excitability. *Epilepsy Res*. 2010;89(1):34–42.

72. Dupuis N, Mazarati A, Desnous B, et al. Pro-ictogenic effects of viral-like inflammation in both mature and immature brains. *J Neuroinflammation*. 2016;13(1):307.

73. Auvin S, Mazarati A, Shin D. Inflammation enhances epileptogenesis in immature rat brain. *Neurobiol Dis*. 2010;40(1):303–310.

74. Bilbo SD, Schwarz JM. The immune system and developmental programming of brain and behavior. *Front Neuroendocrinol*. 2012;33(3):267–286.

75. Reid AY, Riazi K, Campbell Teskey G, Pittman QJ. Increased excitability and molecular changes in adult rats after a febrile seizure. *Epilepsia*. 2013;54(4):e45–e48.

76. Riazi K, Galic MA, Kentner AC, Reid AY, Sharkey KA, Pittman QJ. Microglia-dependent alteration of glutamatergic synaptic transmission and plasticity in the hippocampus during peripheral inflammation. *J Neurosci*. 2015;35(12):4942–4952.

77. Vezzani A, Lang B, Aronica E. Immunity and inflammation in epilepsy. *Cold Spring Harb Perspect Med*. 2015;6(2).

78. Gershen LD, Zanotti-Fregonara P, Dustin IH, et al. Neuroinflammation in temporal lobe epilepsy measured using positron emission tomographic imaging of translocator protein. *JAMA Neurol*. 2015;72(8):882–888.

79. Butler T, Li Y, Tsui W, et al. Transient and chronic seizure-induced inflammation in human focal epilepsy. *Epilepsia*. 2016;57(9):e191–e194.

80. Bialer M, Johannessen SI, Levy RH, Perucca E, Tomson T, White HS. Progress report on new antiepileptic drugs: a summary of the Eleventh Eilat Conference (EILAT XI). *Epilepsy Res*. 2013;103(1):2–30.

81. Kenney-Jung DL, Vezzani A, Kahoud RJ, et al. Febrile infection-related epilepsy syndrome treated with anakinra. *Ann Neurol*. 2016;80:939–945.

82. Jyonouchi H, Geng L. Intractable epilepsy (IE) and responses to anakinra, a human recombinant IL-1 receptor antagonist (IL-1Ra): case reports. *J Clin Cell Immunol*. 2016;7(5):456–460.

83. Lagarde S, Villeneuve N, Trébuchon A, et al. Anti-tumor necrosis factor alpha therapy (adalimumab) in Rasmussen's encephalitis. An open pilot study. *Epilepsia*. 2016;57:956–966.

84. Devinsky O, Marsh E, Friedman D, et al. Cannabidiol in patients with treatment-resistant epilepsy: an open-label interventional trial. *Lancet Neurol*. 2016;15(3):270–278.

85. Sasongko TH, Ismail NF, Zabidi-Hussin Z. Rapamycin and rapalogs for tuberous sclerosis complex. *Cochrane Database Syst Rev*. 2016;13(7):CD011272.

86. Bittner S, Simon OJ, Gobel K, Bien CG, Meuth SG, Wiendel H. Rasmussen encephalitis treated with natalizumab. *Neurol*. 2013;81:395–397.

87. Sotgiu S, Murrighile MR, Constantin G. Treatment of refractory epilepsy with natalizumab in a patient with multiple sclerosis. Case report. *BMC Neurol*. 2010;10:84.

88. Nowak M, Strzelczyk A, Reif PS, et al. Minocycline as potent anticonvulsivant in a patient with astrocytoma and drug resistant epilepsy. *Seizure*. 2012;21:227–228.

89. Pernice HF, Schieweck R, Kiebler MA, Popper B. mTOR and MAPK: from localized translation control to epilepsy. *BMC Neurosci*. 2016;17(1):73.

90. Bozzi Y, Caleo M. Epilepsy, seizures, and inflammation: role of the C-C motif ligand 2 chemokine. *DNA Cell Biol*. 2016;35(6):257–260.

CHAPTER 5

Neuroinflammation in the Pathogenesis of Early Life Epileptic Encephalopathies

SEDA SALAR, PHD • ARISTEA S. GALANOPOULOU, MD, PHD

Epileptic encephalopathies (EEs) were first introduced in the epilepsy classification of the International League Against Epilepsy (ILAE) in 2001.[1] They comprise a group of disorders where epileptiform activity is thought to be the main factor that precipitates progressive cognitive dysfunction and behavioral impairments.[1-4] The adverse impact of epileptic activities on cognition and behavior is expected to outweigh the impact of the underlying structural or pathologic abnormalities (e.g., malformations). EEs are more common in the early years of life,[3,5,6] when they may have severe, progressive, and drug-resistant course. Suppression of seizures or epileptiform activities in patients may improve cognitive impairments underlining the importance of early intervention. The availability of animal models for EEs is critical in accelerating progress in better understanding and treating these conditions, given the challenges of testing new therapies in pediatric populations.[7-9]

TYPES AND ETIOLOGIES OF EARLY LIFE EPILEPTIC ENCEPHALOPATHIES

EEs are heterogeneous group of disorders with variable pathologies and etiologies.[5,7-13] Genetic defects (e.g., in voltage-gated sodium channel genes 1A or 1B, SCN1A or SCN1B; copy number variations), structural cortical (e.g., focal cortical dysplasia, polymicrogyria) or subcortical (e.g., basal ganglia) abnormalities, and possible alterations in synaptic connections (e.g., pathologic changes in up and down states during slow-wave activity) have been suggested to underlie EE pathology. Increasing interest has been gathered around the putative contribution of neuroinflammatory pathways, based on both clinical evidence and convergence of the signaling pathways implicated in EEs around neuroinflammatory cascades (for summary, Table 5.1).

In this chapter, we review the role of neuroinflammation in the pathology and treatment of EEs.

ROLE OF INFLAMMATION IN EPILEPTIC ENCEPHALOPATHIES

Neuroinflammation is a chain of brain responses triggered by classic intruders of homeostasis such as infections, autoimmunity, and toxins or increased neurogenic (neuroinflammatory) signaling due to insults such as epileptic seizures.[14] Several studies have indicated the role of inflammation in seizure and/or epilepsy etiology (e.g., increased seizure susceptibility),[15,16] their consequences (e.g., seizure-induced injury),[17,18] and their long-term prognosis (e.g., epilepsy, drug resistance in epilepsy, and comorbidities)[15,19-21] or in targeting inflammatory pathways (e.g., Toll-like receptor 4 [TLR4] and high-mobility group box 1 [HMGB1]) to treat seizures and/or epilepsies.[5,22-28] Clinical information from patients and experimental evidence from animal models for EEs provide valuable insights about both pathologic and protective mechanisms of inflammation.[4,7-9,11,14]

The benefit for EE patients from the use of adrenocorticotropic hormone (ACTH) and steroids reinforces the role of inflammation in EE pathology.[22-24,29] Likewise, few antiseizure drugs may interfere with inflammatory pathways.[30] Vigabatrin, a gamma aminobutyric acid (GABA) aminotransferase inhibitor, reduces proconvulsive interleukin-1β (IL-1β), IL-6, and antigen-presenting cells in an allergic encephalitis model,[31] whereas carbamazepine decreases IL-1β and tumor necrosis α (TNFα) in adult male rats.[32] As a beneficial add-on and also a single therapy for some EE patients,[33-35] ketogenic diet is indicated to have antiinflammatory properties (i.e., mitigation of the fever response, decrease in proinflammatory IL-1β, and

TABLE 5.1
Neuroinflammatory Pathway Involvement in Epileptic Encephalopathies (EEs): Clinical and Experimental Evidence

EEs	Inflammatory Pathway Involvement
Infantile spasms/West syndrome	**Clinical evidence** • Decreased IgA, IgG, and IgM in serum (10% of the WS patients in the study, PHB with nitrazepam, clonazepam, or VPA)[69] • Normal/low IgA and increased IgG and IgM, in serum (including LGS and MIS patients,during ACTH free period vs. controls)[71] • Normal IgA, increased IgG and IgM, lower κ/λ of IgG and IgM in serum (including LGS patients, VPA with/out nitrazepam)[70] • Decrease in CD3+, CD4+, and CD4+/CD8+ in serum (pre-ACTH vs. healthy controls, including LGS and MIP patients)[71] • Decrease in CD3+ CD25+, CD19+, CD19+ CD95+ in serum (pre-ACTH vs. healthy controls)[73] • Low IL-1β in CSF (low ELISA sensitivity, pretreatment vs. controls)[76] • Normal IL-1β, IL-6, and TNFα, reduced IL-1Ra in CSF (pre-ACTH)[77] • Normal IL-6 in CSF (pretreatment)[78] • Increased IL-1Ra and decreased IL-1β in serum (post-ACTH and antiseizure treatments)[79] • Increased IL-1Ra, IL-5, IL-6, IL-15, eotaxin, bFGF, IP10 in serum (pre-ACTH), reduced IL-1β, IL-12, MIP-1β in serum (post-ACTH)[73] • No change in IFNα in CSF[80] • Increased IL-2, TNFα, IFNα in serum (post-ACTH and antiseizure drugs)[81] • Expression changes in TNFα, NF-kB cell adhesion molecules,[82] IL-1β,[83] inflammatory genes[84] in tubers in TSC (from RS) • VGKC antibodies[67] • IS triggered by ketotifen or oxatomide administration[89,91] • TNFAIP6, SQSTM1 CD46, and IL-27RA mutations[105] • STS3GAL3 mutations[106] **Animal models** • Suppression of spasms, cognitive amelioration, and reduction in pS6 expression with Rapamycin (mTORC1 inhibitor) in multiple-hit model[42] • Overactivation of NF-kB pathway and iinhibition of spasms by celastrol in multiple-hit model[100] • LPS-only induction of spasms in multiple-hit model[101] • Suppression of spasms by IgG in NMDA-induced spasms model[103] • Cognitive deficits and allergic eosinophilic airway inflammation St3gal3−/− mice (but no spasms reported in this model)[108,109]
Dravet syndrome	**Clinical evidence** • Increased CD70[135] **Animal models** • Suppression of seizures by clemizole in Scn1Lab zebrafish mutants[136] • Effect of ketogenic diet on metabolic amelioration in Scn1Lab zebrafish mutants[137] • After antiseizure treatment reduced hyperthermia-induced seizure threshold in KO and KI models[142–145]
Lennox-Gastaut syndrome	**Clinical evidence** • Decreased IgG (1 patient)[69] • Normal IgA, increased IgG and IgM, lower κ/λ of IgG and IgM (including WS patients, VPA with/out nitrazepam)[70] • Increased HLA-7[116] • Increased HLA-DR5[117]
LKS/LKSV and EE with CSWS	**Clinical evidence** • Autoantibodies against central, and peripheral myelin[129] • Autoantibodies against cerebellum, auditory cortex layer V, and brainstem[131]

TNFα levels) in lipopolysaccharide (LPS)-treated adult male rats.[36]

Moreover, related to the cognitive abnormalities in EE patients, some neuroinflammatory pathways may intercede with cognitive dysfunction. IL-1β and TNF inhibit long-term potentiation in the hippocampus,[37–39] and cerebral administration of HMGB1 abolishes novel object recognition in mice.[40] The mechanistic target of rapamycin, also known as mammalian target of rapamycin (mTOR) signaling pathway, plays roles in cognition, while inhibition of the mTOR pathway improves cognitive dysfunction.[41–49] Cyclooxygenase 2 (COX-2) inhibition impairs memory formation.[50] On the other hand, there are also reports indicating amelioration in cognitive deficits after COX-2 inhibition or deletion.[51,52] COX-2 is released from neurons following N-methyl-D-aspartate (NMDA) receptor–dependent synaptic activity and seizures and, as in peripheral tissues, its release can be blocked by glucocorticoids.[53]

The timing and context within which interventions targeting such pathways take place may, however, be important in determining the final outcome. For example, mTOR pathway inhibition may have opposite cognitive effects in a model of infantile spasms (IS) compared with naïve animals, as mentioned later on for the multiple-hit model of IS.[42] Prostaglandin E$_2$ receptor (EP2) activation may promote survival in neurons[54]; however, EP2 inhibition may be neuroprotective but only if done at specific time points after the status epilepticus induction.[53,55]

Neuroinflammatory pathway activation is also seen in patients with autism. Inflammation in cerebral cortex, white matter, and cerebellum[56]; increased blood levels of HMGB1 and S100 calcium binding protein A9 (S100A9), two cell membrane *Receptor for Advanced Glycation End* products (RAGE) ligands[57,58]; increased reactivity of TLR2 and 4 expressing monocytes[59]; and activation of mTOR pathway[60] are all reported in patients with autism.

As a common mechanism of EEs, here, we discuss the role of neuroinflammation specifically in IS seen in West syndrome (WS), Lennox-Gastaut syndrome (LGS), Landau-Kleffner syndrome (LKS), and continuous spike-waves in sleep (CSWS) and Dravet syndrome (DS).

Infantile Spasms/West Syndrome

WS was first described by Dr. West in 1894 to seek help for his son's condition.[61] It manifests with epileptic spasms and developmental arrest. Ictal EEG pattern shows generalized electrodecremental response, whereas interictally a disorderly high-amplitude background with multifocal spikes and sharp waves is present. Hypsarrhythmia is not always present, because two of the three features (IS, hypsarrhythmia, mental retardation) are sufficient for the diagnosis of WS. A majority of the patients (~60%) have structural or metabolic etiologies while 10% carry genetic alterations and the rest of the patients have unknown causes.[8,13,24,62] Corticosteroids are one of the effective treatment strategies in patients with WS. In fact, the use of ACTH was suggested for treatment of IS and hypsarrhythmia in infants long ago,[22] and it is now considered as the first-line treatment of IS.[23,24,63,64] However, the determination of the etiology may divert the treatment choices and give information about the prognosis of the disease. As in IS due to tuberous sclerosis complex (TSC), for example, vigabatrin is used as a first-line treatment, and it is known that patients with the structural/metabolic alterations such as TS have the poorest outcome.[26]

The fact that numerous etiologies lead to a similar phenotype or syndromic features in patients points toward a common mechanism or network involved in the pathogenesis of IS. From the therapeutic perspective, the identification of a common pathway would allow for the design of treatments that can benefit patients with IS across various etiologies or pathologies. In light of the recent evidence, neuroinflammation could be a good candidate. Activation of neuroinflammatory pathways are seen in some IS etiologies such as infectious diseases (e.g., bacterial meningitis or encephalitis),[65] TSC (mTOR),[10] cortical dysplasias or malformations (may be due to overactivation of downstream mTOR targets),[66] autoantibodies (e.g., antibodies against voltage-gated potassium channel complex [VGKC]),[67] and hypoxic ischemic encephalopathy.[68]

Clinical data from WS patients show decreased immunoglobulin A (IgA), IgG, and IgM levels (although contradictory evidence such as normal or low IgA levels and increased IgG and IgM levels are also reported), indicating an abnormality in immune response in these patients.[69–72] Along with Ig changes, CD3+ and CD4+ cells as well as CD4+/CD8+ ratio may decrease, while CD8+ cells increase during the ACTH-free period in a study containing mostly WS patients but also patients with LGS and multifocal independent spike syndrome (MIS).[71] A more recent study comparing both T and B cells only in WS patients during both pre-ACTH and post-ACTH period and against controls finds reduction in CD3+ CD25+, CD19+, and CD19+ CD95+ cells in pre-ACTH period compared with healthy controls.[73] When compared with post-ACTH group, pre-ACTH group have higher CD4+ and CD4+ cells and CD4+/CD8+ ratio. Interleukin 2 receptor α+ (CD25+) regulatory T cells, which are important for self-tolerance and control of susceptibility to viral or other infectious agents, are also diminished in patients before ACTH treatment compared with healthy controls.[73] On the other hand, spontaneous remission of spasms has been reported after viral infections[74]; however, four drug-resistant EE patients presenting with epileptic spasms gained temporary seizure freedom following an acute febrile illness as reported in a case report.[75] These changes indicate that both humoral and cellular immunity may be affected during the course of WS. In addition, inflammatory insults may potentially have pathogenic or protective effects, depending on the context or inflammatory processes activated.

Clinically, cytokine system also seems to be affected although the data from reports are conflicting possibly because of variable underlying pathology. In a study by Baram et al. (1992), IL-1 levels were too low to be detected in the cerebrospinal fluid (CSF) in patients with IS and hypsarrhythmia before treatment or in controls.[76] However, the sensitivity of the ELISA assay used in this early study was not high enough to detect differences from controls or IL-1β levels within the range detected at subsequent studies. In a subsequent study, IL-1β levels along with IL-6 and TNFα levels were unchanged while IL-1 receptor antagonist (IL-1Ra) was reduced in the CSF of patients before ACTH treatment was started.[77] Tekgul et al. reported that IL-6 levels in CSF were not significantly elevated in IS patients before treatment when compared with CSF from two groups of patients with either bacterial meningitis or post-traumatic seizures, both of which had very high levels of this cytokine.[78] Following ACTH and antiseizure drug treatment, Yamanaka et al. reported increased serum IL-1Ra and decreased IL-1β in 13 patients who responded to treatment.[79] Shiihara et al. found higher serum levels of IL-1Ra in the ACTH pretreatment group compared with controls and reduced levels of IL-1β after ACTH treatment although no changes in IL-1Ra were reported.[73] The discrepancy in IL-1Ra changes caused by treatment found in these two studies was suggested to be due to the time point when the samples were collected: in the first study the blood samples were taken a week after ACTH treatment, whereas in the latter they were obtained within a month.[73,79] Furthermore, it is also possible that the IL-1Ra reduction in the Yamanaka study might be due to the fact that these patients responded to treatment, while in the Shiihara study (no change in IL-1Ra after the treatment) it is not clear whether patients had responded to

treatment or not. Shiihara et al. also noted increased IL-5, IL-6, IL-15, eotaxin, basic fibroblast growth factor (bFGF), and interferon gamma (IFNγ)-induced protein 10 (IP-10) levels in plasma in untreated patients against controls and reduced IL-12 and macrophage inflammatory protein 1β (MIP-1β) in plasma of the ACTH-treated patients compared with pretreatment values. Although long before no change was seen in CSF IFNα levels in patients with IS,[80] elevated serum IL-2, TNFα, and IFNα are measured in the serum of patients treated with ACTH followed by antiseizure drugs when compared with that of controls.[81] In addition to these alterations, data from tuber or brain tumor resection from TSC patients show expression changes in TNFα, nuclear factor kappa-light-chain-enhancer of activated B cells (NF-kB), and cell adhesion molecules[82]; involvement of complement system and IL-1β signaling[83]; and expression of inflammatory genes.[84] Autoimmunity may also play a role in the etiology in WS. A case report revealed antibodies against VGKC proteins in a female patient with IS and developmental delay, while treatment of the patient with steroids led to partial amelioration.[67] In addition to these clinical findings, a ketogenic diet, an effective therapy for some IS patients,[34,35] is shown to have anti-inflammatory properties in LPS-treated rats[36] as well as to inhibit mTOR pathway in kainate-induced epilepsy model.[85] Perturbations in cytokine signaling have also been implicated in processes important in cognition (i.e., synaptic plasticity, long-term potentiation in the hippocampus),[37–39] supporting a possible involvement in cognitive dysfunction associated with WS.

Interestingly, the histaminergic system, which is not only closely related with immune reactions but also plays roles in sleep-wake cycle, memory, appetite control, and stress responses,[86–88] is also reported to be linked to WS pathology.[89–91] Yasuhara et al. described two boys in whom spasms are triggered 8 and 10 days after the administration of ketotifen, a centrally acting histamine H1 receptor (H1R) antagonist.[89] Likewise, a girl started having spasms 8 days after she received oxatomide (also an H1R antagonist) therapy for atopic dermatitis.[91] One of the male patients and the female patient were both responsive to ACTH.[89–91]

Along with the clinical data, a number of acute and chronic animal models for IS also contribute to the understanding of the role of inflammation in the underlying etiology.[8] A chronic model of IS in which inflammation is one of the inducing pathologies is the multiple-hit rat model.[92] IS in this model are triggered by injections of doxorubicin (DOX) into the right lateral ventricle and LPS into the right parietal cortex of

Sprague-Dawley rats on postnatal day 3 (PN3).[92] Doxorubicin is a chemotherapeutic cytotoxic agent, whereas LPS injures white matter and induces inflammatory responses when injected intracerebrally.[93,94] Behavioral spasms in this model are apparent beginning from PN4 and lasting until PN13. The intraperitoneal injection of p-chlorophenylalanine (PCPA; a serotonin depleter)[95] on PN5 was added because of reports of altered serotonin metabolism in WS patients[96] but is not needed for IS to occur. This model features ictal electrodecremental responses with the spasms, interictal epileptiform EEG bilaterally, seizure evolution, and behavioral and cognitive abnormalities reminiscent of the human clinical condition.

The multiple-hit model has also provided a screening platform to test the efficacy of new therapies. ACTH is not effective in this model and vigabatrin only partially and transiently reduces spasms for a day but at doses that eventually are lethal. Therefore, this model is considered as a model of drug-resistant IS. CPP-115, a vigabatrin analogue with higher affinity for GABA aminotransferase that exhibits lower risk for retinal toxicity in animal studies, decreases spasms with better and longer efficacy and improved tolerability in the multiple-hit model.[97] CPP-115 is currently an orphan drug with indication for IS in the United States and has been recently used for the treatment of an infant with IS.[98] It shows improved efficacy and tolerability at much lower doses than vigabatrin, confirming, in this case report, the animal data in the multiple-hit model. Carisbamate showed acute suppression of spasms in the multiple-hit model,[99] evident within the first hour of administration, which is interesting because ACTH and vigabatrin take a few days to show a therapeutic effect. Interestingly, in this nongenetic model of IS, rapamycin, an mTOR complex 1 (mTORC1) inhibitor, suppresses spasms and normalizes the cortical expression of phosphorylated S6 ribosomal protein (pS6), a marker of mTOR pathway overactivation.[42,48] Rapamycin also improved cognitive deficits in this model; however, mTORC1 inhibition with rapamycin in control animals deteriorated cognition, indicating that the stable functioning of this pathway is vital for maintaining normal cognitive performance. These findings also provide an example of how targets identified in IS with genetic etiology can be used for the treatment of IS due to acquired etiologies. Overactivation of NF-kB pathway has recently been shown in this model, and celastrol, an inhibitor of NF-kB activation, reduces spasms.[100] A direct evidence that cortical inflammation in immature rats may suffice to induce IS was provided by Ono et al. who demonstrated that intracerebral LPS

application on PN3 also triggers spasms in Sprague-Dawley rats.[101] LPS, an activator of TLR4, is known to stimulate IL-1β, TNFα, and COX-2 expression.[21,102] In addition to the multiple-hit model, in a pilot study using the NMDA-induced status epilepticus model,[103] seizures (not specifically limited to spasms) and hippocampal neurotoxicity were suppressed by IgG from postpartum rats.[104]

Although genetic etiologies are less common in IS compared with metabolic and structural alterations, an increasing number of genetic variants have been linked with IS.[8,10,13,105] Out of the reported rare de novo mutations identified by whole exome sequencing in IS patients by Michaud et al., six are directly related with immune system. Single nucleotide variations in TNFα-induced protein 6 (TNFAIP6), sequestosome 1 (SQSTM1), myosin 9B (MYO9B), proline-rich coiled coil protein 2B (PRRC2B), a frameshift deletion in IL-27 receptor α (IL-27RA), and CD46 are each associated with the phenotype in unidentified IS cases, and except CD46 mutation all are indicated to be deleterious by online bioinformatics tools.[105] In a consanguineous family, homozygous β-galactoside-α-2,3-sialyltransferase-III (ST3GAL3) mutations are found in three children with IS.[106] The explicit link of this mutation to IS pathology is not known. However, this enzyme is in charge of terminal sialylation of brain gangliosides[107] and St3gal3 null mice show cognitive deficits.[108] Interestingly, increased allergic eosinophilic airway inflammation in both St3gal3 null mice and mice carrying only one allele of St3gal3 is also reported.[109]

Both the clinical evidence and findings from animal studies evidently point out the inflammatory pathway involvement in the etiology of IS. More research is needed to clarify the precise connection between neuroinflammatory alterations and IS.

Lennox-Gastaut Syndrome

LGS presents with various seizure types, EEG with diffuse slow spikes and waves (1–2.5 Hz), and cognitive dysfunction.[110,111] As in the etiology of WS, LGS may result from variable pathologies and no clear etiology has been defined for LGS.[112] Cortical malformations, anoxic episodes, hemorrhage, and encephalitis play a role in the etiology.[112] LGS may also evolve from WS.[113] The similar phenotypical changes and the efficacy of ACTH and corticosteroids[114,115] in some LGS patients also bring up a common mechanism.

Clinically, increased frequency of human leukocyte antigen serotype 7 (HLA-7) is indicated in LGS patients and also their families, giving a hint of the involvement of inflammatory system.[116] In addition, more recently a human leukocyte antigen-antigen D related 5 (HLA-DR5) is found to be elevated in LGS patients.[117] This major histocompatibility complex (MHC) class II cell surface receptor together with its peptide ligand is a binding point for T cell receptors and mainly plays a role in transplant rejections. Immunoglobulins are also affected because they are in the pathology of WS. Serum levels of IgG and IgM were found to be increased in LGS patients, while IgG and M kappa to lambda light chain (κ/λ) ratio are reduced and κ/λ ratio of IgA and IgA levels remain unaltered.[70] In line with these findings, LGS and also some WS patients benefit from intravenous immunoglobulin therapy (IVIG).[118,119]

Although official animal models for this syndrome do not exist, the AY-9944 model exhibits atypical absences that are seen in LGS patients. AY-9944 is a cholesterol biosynthesis inhibitor and when applied subcutaneously to Long Evans hooded rat pups, atypical absence seizures manifesting with 4–6 Hz spike waves in EEG develop.[120,121] In rodents, these are considered as slow spike waves because the rodent equivalent of the typical absences is 7–8 Hz spike wave discharges seen in animal models of absence epilepsy.[122] These rats also show cognitive dysfunction, which could not be overcome by inhibiting spike waves using ethosuximide.[123] On the contrary, although not having an effect on spike waves, CGP35348, a GABAB receptor inhibitor, improves cognitive outcome.[124] These results give insights about involvement and interaction of different pathways in the development of key features of LGS.

Landau-Kleffner Syndrome/Continuous Spike Waves in Sleep

LKS[147] and CSWS[148] manifest language or cognitive and behavioral regression, respectively, in response to the appearance of epileptic discharges in the EEG of the patients.[4–6,11] ACTH and/or corticosteroids are considered as a treatment option[125] and may improve both EEG and language or neurodevelopmental deficits.

No animal model for these types of EE has been developed.[9] Although mutations in glutamate ionotropic receptor NMDA type subunit 2A (GRIN2A) are suggested to be involved in the pathology,[126] autoimmune pathology is also considered for LKS.[72] Autoantibodies against both central and peripheral myelin are detected in three LKS patients during the time when speech exacerbation is observed where steroid treatment normalizes this autoimmune reaction in the same patients.[127] Antibodies against brain endothelial cells are present in serum of patients with LKS variant (LKSV) disease, LKS involving abnormalities in social skills (autism-like

phenotype).[128] Autoantibodies against cerebellum, auditory cortex layer V, and brainstem are also observed in serum from patients with LKS/LKSV and CSWS.[129]

Dravet Syndrome

DS or severe myoclonic epilepsy of infancy was first reported in 1978.[130] Patients present with prolonged clonic or hemiclonic febrile seizures that progress into myoclonus, atypical absences, and focal or generalized seizures. The majority of the patients carry genetic mutations, mostly in SCN1A gene occurring de novo or recurrently. Mutations in other genes such as SCN1B, GABA receptor A gamma 2 (GABRG2), and protocadherin 19 (PCDH19) are also involved in DS pathology. Seizures in DS were thought to be triggered by vaccination; therefore DS was named as vaccine encephalopathy. However, recent studies showed that the majority of patients whose seizures are triggered after vaccination carry SCN1A mutations.[131] Vaccines might decrease the age of the first seizure onset but has no interference to the disease course.[132]

A recent study shows increased CD70 in lymphocytes from DS patients, a marker for lymphocyte proliferation and activation. In the same study, authors also find, although not statistically significant, a slight increase in peroxisome proliferator activated receptor gamma (PPAR-γ) and proinflammatory cytokines. Both results indicate an immune involvement.[133]

A number of animal models for DS give insights about the pathology and treatment of this syndrome.[8] One of these models is a zebrafish model carrying mutations in voltage-gated sodium channel 1 (Scn-1Lab) gene. This gene shows 77% identity to human SCN1A gene, and mutations lead to spontaneous, convulsive, and drug-resistant seizures in zebrafish.[134] Interestingly, clemizole, a U.S. Food and Drug administration (FDA)-approved H1R antagonist and hepatitis C virus nonstructural protein 4B (NS4B) RNA binding inhibitor, suppresses seizures in this model. However, the fact that a couple of other H1R antagonists used in the same study showed no seizure suppression and the IS-provoking effect of certain H1R antagonists, as we have discussed in the WS/IS section, suggests a different mechanism of action for clemizole that is yet to be discovered. In addition to these findings, also in the zebrafish Scn1Lab model, a modified ketogenic diet ameliorates the decreased glycolytic rate and oxygen consumption rate seen in these mutants.[135] In addition, considering the role of inflammation in fever and fever-induced seizures,[136–139] modification of hyperthermia-induced seizure thresholds and also mitigation of cognitive and behavioral outcome by different drugs in various knock-out and knock-in DS models indirectly provide evidence to the involvement of inflammatory systems.[8,140–143]

Both the clinical data and limited data from animal models give clues about immune system involvement in the pathology of DS. However, these alterations were found in patients already diagnosed with DS and, therefore, may represent secondary manifestations of seizures. More research is needed to shine light into the role of inflammation in DS pathology.

CONCLUSIONS AND FUTURE PERSPECTIVES

Neuroinflammation is a common mechanism shared in EEs and along with systemic inflammation contributes to the pathology.[144] Elucidating the roles of this common mechanism may lead to discover new diagnostic markers and therapeutic targets. This is of great importance because early intervention may improve cognitive dysfunction and developmental outcome[145,146] and prevent possible evolution of a new symptom or comorbidity (i.e., increased autism risk after IS).[113]

There is a complex interplay within neuroinflammatory mechanisms. Although inflammation is a robust response of a body against intruders such as infections or insults such as epileptic seizures, its secondary effects can be either compensatory or pathologic. We discussed in the previous sections not only the evidence that inflammatory processes may precipitate and worsen epileptic seizures and their comorbidities, but also clinical evidence that spasms may remit or transiently stop after certain febrile illnesses. Such effects may depend on the context of the disease, the timing, type, and magnitude of inflammatory response, and further research is needed to elucidate these factors and design rationale treatments for the these epileptic disorders. The availability of animal models of early life epileptic encephalopathies may help increase our understanding of their pathophysiology and their possible treatments.

LIST OF ABBREVIATIONS

ACTH   Adrenocorticotropic hormone
bFGF   Basic fibroblast growth factor
CSF   Cerebrospinal fluid
COX-2   Cyclooxygenase 2
CSWS   Continuous spike-wave in sleep
DOX   Doxorubicin
DS   Dravet syndrome
GABA   Gamma aminobutyric acid
GABRG2   GABA receptor A gamma 2
GRIN2A   Glutamate ionotropic receptor NMDA type subunit 2A
EE   Epileptic encephalopathies
EP2   Prostaglandin E2 receptor
FDA   U.S. Food and Drug Administration
H1R   Histamine H1 receptor
HLA-7   Human leukocyte antigen serotype 7
HLA-DR5   Human leukocyte antigen-antigen D related 5
HMGB1   High-mobility group box 1
IFNα   Interferon alpha
IFNγ   Interferon gamma
Ig   Immunoglobulin
IL   Interleukin
IL-1β   Interleukin 1beta
IL-1Ra   IL-1 receptor antagonist
IL-27RA   IL-27 receptor α
ILAE   International League against Epilepsy
IS   Infantile spasms
IP-10   IFNγ-induced protein 10
IVIG   Intravenous immunoglobulin therapy
LGS   Lennox-Gastaut syndrome
LKS   Landau-Kleffner syndrome
LKSV   Landau-Kleffner syndrome variant
LPS   Lipopolysaccharide
MHC   Major histocompatibility complex
MIP-1β   Macrophage inflammatory protein 1β
MIS   Multifocal independent spike syndrome
mTOR   Mammalian target of rapamycin
MTORC1   mTOR complex 1
MYO9B   Myosin 9B
NF-kB   Nuclear factor kappa-light-chain-enhancer of activated B cells
NMDA   N-methyl-D-aspartate
NS4B   Nonstructural protein 4B
PCDH19   Protocadherin 19
PCPA   p-Chlorophenylalanine
PN   Postnatal day
pS6   Phosphorylated S6 ribosomal protein
PPAR-γ   Peroxisome proliferator activated receptor gamma
PRRC2B   Proline-rich coiled coil protein 2B
RAGE   Receptor for advanced glycation end products
RS   Resection surgery
S100A9   S100 calcium binding protein A9
SCN1A   Voltage-gated sodium channel gene 1α, human
SCN1B   Voltage-gated sodium channel gene 1β, human
Scn1Lab   Voltage-gated sodium channel gene 1, zebrafish
SQSTM1   Sequestosome 1
ST3GAL3   β-Galactoside-α-2,3-sialyltransferase-III
TLR4   Toll-like receptor 4

TNFAIP6 TNFα-induced protein 6
TNFα Tumor necrosis alpha
TSC Tuberous sclerosis complex
VGKC Voltage-gated potassium channel complex
VPA Valproic acid
WS West syndrome
κ/λ ratio Kappa to lambda light chain ratio

ACKNOWLEDGMENTS

ASG has been supported by research grants from NINDS-NS91170, NINDS-1U54NS100064, Department of Defense (W81XWH-13-1-0180), and the Infantile Spasms Initiative from CURE (Citizens United for Research in Epilepsy) and also acknowledges research funding from the Heffer Family and the Segal Family Foundations and the Abbe Goldstein/Joshua Lurie and Laurie Marsh/Dan Levitz families.

REFERENCES

1. Engel Jr J. International League Against E. A proposed diagnostic scheme for people with epileptic seizures and with epilepsy: report of the ILAE Task Force on Classification and Terminology. *Epilepsia*. 2001;42(6):796–803.
2. Engel Jr J. Report of the ILAE classification core group. *Epilepsia*. 2006;47(9):1558–1568.
3. Berg AT, Berkovic SF, Brodie MJ, et al. Revised terminology and concepts for organization of seizures and epilepsies: report of the ILAE Commission on Classification and Terminology, 2005-2009. *Epilepsia*. 2010;51(4):676–685.
4. Covanis A. Epileptic encephalopathies (including severe epilepsy syndromes). *Epilepsia*. 2012;(53 suppl 4):114–126.
5. Galanopoulou AS, Bojko A, Lado F, Moshé SL. The spectrum of neuropsychiatric abnormalities associated with electrical status epilepticus in sleep. *Brain Dev*. 2000;22(5):279–295.
6. Guerrini R, Pellock JM. Age-related epileptic encephalopathies. *Handb Clin Neurol*. 2012;107:179–193.
7. Galanopoulou AS. Basic mechanisms of catastrophic epilepsy – overview from animal models. *Brain Dev*. 2013;35(8):748–756.
8. Galanopoulou AS, Moshe SL. Pathogenesis and new candidate treatments for infantile spasms and early life epileptic encephalopathies: a view from preclinical studies. *Neurobiol Dis*. 2015;79:135–149.
9. Shao LR, Stafstrom CE. Pediatric epileptic encephalopathies: pathophysiology and animal models. *Semin Pediatr Neurol*. 2016;23(2):98–107.
10. Epi KC, Epilepsy Phenome/Genome P, Allen AS, et al. De novo mutations in epileptic encephalopathies. *Nature*. 2013;501(7466):217–221.
11. Lado FA, Rubboli G, Capovilla G, Avanzini G, Moshe SL. Pathophysiology of epileptic encephalopathies. *Epilepsia*. 2013;(54 suppl 8):6–13.
12. Stafstrom CE, Kossoff EM. Epileptic encephalopathy in infants and children. *Epilepsy Curr*. 2016;16(4):273–279.
13. Paciorkowski AR, Thio LL, Dobyns WB. Genetic and biologic classification of infantile spasms. *Pediatr Neurol*. 2011;45(6):355–367.
14. Xanthos DN, Sandkuhler J. Neurogenic neuroinflammation: inflammatory CNS reactions in response to neuronal activity. *Nat Rev Neurosci*. 2014;15(1):43–53.
15. Galic MA, Riazi K, Heida JG, et al. Postnatal inflammation increases seizure susceptibility in adult rats. *J Neurosci*. 2008;28(27):6904–6913.
16. Galic MA, Riazi K, Henderson AK, Tsutsui S, Pittman QJ. Viral-like brain inflammation during development causes increased seizure susceptibility in adult rats. *Neurobiol Dis*. 2009;36(2):343–351.
17. Auvin S, Shin D, Mazarati A, Nakagawa J, Miyamoto J, Sankar R. Inflammation exacerbates seizure-induced injury in the immature brain. *Epilepsia*. 2007;(48 suppl 5):27–34.
18. Sankar R, Auvin S, Mazarati A, Shin D. Inflammation contributes to seizure-induced hippocampal injury in the neonatal rat brain. *Acta Neurol Scand*. 2007;115(suppl 4):16–20.
19. Riazi K, Galic MA, Kuzmiski JB, Ho W, Sharkey KA, Pittman QJ. Microglial activation and TNFalpha production mediate altered CNS excitability following peripheral inflammation. *Proc Natl Acad Sci USA*. 2008;105(44):17151–17156.
20. Marchi N, Betto G, Fazio V, et al. Blood-brain barrier damage and brain penetration of antiepileptic drugs: role of serum proteins and brain edema. *Epilepsia*. 2009;50(4):664–677.
21. Vezzani A, French J, Bartfai T, Baram TZ. The role of inflammation in epilepsy. *Nat Rev Neurol*. 2011;7(1):31–40.
22. Sorel L, Dusaucy-Bauloye A. [Findings in 21 cases of Gibbs' hypsarrhythmia; spectacular effectiveness of ACTH]. *Acta Neurol Psychiatr Belg*. 1958;58(2):130–141.
23. Baram TZ, Mitchell WG, Tournay A, Snead OC, Hanson RA, Horton EJ. High-dose corticotropin (ACTH) versus prednisone for infantile spasms: a prospective, randomized, blinded study. *Pediatrics*. 1996;97(3):375–379.
24. Pellock JM, Hrachovy R, Shinnar S, et al. Infantile spasms: a U.S. consensus report. *Epilepsia*. 2010;51(10):2175–2189.
25. Nabbout R. Autoimmune and inflammatory epilepsies. *Epilepsia*. 2012;(53 suppl 4):58–62.
26. Pardo CA, Nabbout R, Galanopoulou AS. Mechanisms of epileptogenesis in pediatric epileptic syndromes: rasmussen encephalitis, infantile spasms, and febrile infection-related epilepsy syndrome (FIRES). *Neurotherapeutics*. 2014;11(2):297–310.

27. Klein R, Livingston S. The effect of adrenocorticotropic hormone in epilepsy. *J Pediatr.* 1950;37(5):733–742.

28. Maroso M, Balosso S, Ravizza T, et al. Toll-like receptor 4 and high-mobility group box-1 are involved in ictogenesis and can be targeted to reduce seizures. *Nat Med.* 2010;16(4):413–419.

29. Snead 3rd OC, Benton JW, Myers GJ. ACTH and prednisone in childhood seizure disorders. *Neurology.* 1983;33(8):966–970.

30. Mlodzikowska-Albrecht J, Steinborn B, Zarowski M. Cytokines, epilepsy and epileptic drugs–is there a mutual influence? *Pharmacol Rep.* 2007;59(2):129–138.

31. Bhat R, Axtell R, Mitra A, et al. Inhibitory role for GABA in autoimmune inflammation. *Proc Natl Acad Sci USA.* 2010;107(6):2580–2585.

32. Gomez CD, Buijs RM, Sitges M. The anti-seizure drugs vinpocetine and carbamazepine, but not valproic acid, reduce inflammatory IL-1beta and TNF-alpha expression in rat hippocampus. *J Neurochem.* 2014;130(6):770–779.

33. Nordli Jr DR, Kuroda MM, Carroll J, et al. Experience with the ketogenic diet in infants. *Pediatrics.* 2001;108(1):129–133.

34. Kossoff EH, Pyzik PL, McGrogan JR, Vining EPG, Freeman JM. Efficacy of the ketogenic diet for infantile spasms. *Pediatrics.* 2002;109(5):780–783.

35. Hong AM, Turner Z, Hamdy RF, Kossoff EH. Infantile spasms treated with the ketogenic diet: prospective single-center experience in 104 consecutive infants. *Epilepsia.* 2010;51(8):1403–1407.

36. Dupuis N, Curatolo N, Benoist JF, Auvin S. Ketogenic diet exhibits anti-inflammatory properties. *Epilepsia.* 2015;56(7):e95–e98.

37. Bellinger FP, Madamba S, Siggins GR. Interleukin 1β inhibits synaptic strength and long-term potentiation in the rat CA1 hippocampus. *Brain Res.* 1993;628(1–2):227–234.

38. Cunningham AJ, Murray CA, O'Neill LAJ, Lynch MA, O'Connor JJ. Interleukin-1β (IL-1β) and tumour necrosis factor (TNF) inhibit long-term potentiation in the rat dentate gyrus in vitro. *Neurosci Lett.* 1996;203(1):17–20.

39. Schneider H, Pitossi F, Balschun D, Wagner A, del Rey A, Besedovsky HO. A neuromodulatory role of interleukin-1beta in the hippocampus. *Proc Natl Acad Sci USA.* 1998;95(13):7778–7783.

40. Mazarati A, Maroso M, Iori V, Vezzani A, Carli M. High-mobility group box-1 impairs memory in mice through both toll-like receptor 4 and receptor for advanced glycation end products. *Exp Neurol.* 2011;232(2):143–148.

41. Ehninger D, Han S, Shilyansky C, et al. Reversal of learning deficits in a Tsc2+/– mouse model of tuberous sclerosis. *Nat Med.* 2008;14(8):843–848.

42. Raffo E, Coppola A, Ono T, Briggs SW, Galanopoulou AS. A pulse rapamycin therapy for infantile spasms and associated cognitive decline. *Neurobiol Dis.* 2011;43(2):322–329.

43. Stoica L, Zhu PJ, Huang W, Zhou H, Kozma SC, Costa-Mattioli M. Selective pharmacogenetic inhibition of mammalian target of Rapamycin complex I (mTORC1) blocks long-term synaptic plasticity and memory storage. *Proc Natl Acad Sci USA.* 2011;108(9):3791–3796.

44. Way SW, Rozas NS, Wu HC, et al. The differential effects of prenatal and/or postnatal rapamycin on neurodevelopmental defects and cognition in a neuroglial mouse model of tuberous sclerosis complex. *Hum Mol Genet.* 2012;21(14):3226–3236.

45. Wong M. A critical review of mTOR inhibitors and epilepsy: from basic science to clinical trials. *Expert Rev Neurother.* 2013;13(6):657–669.

46. Crino PB. The mTOR signalling cascade: paving new roads to cure neurological disease. *Nat Rev Neurol.* 2016;12(7):379–392.

47. Jeong A, Wong M. mTOR inhibitors in children: current indications and future directions in neurology. *Curr Neurol Neurosci Rep.* 2016;16(12):102.

48. Galanopoulou AS, Gorter JA, Cepeda C. Finding a better drug for epilepsy: the mTOR pathway as an antiepileptogenic target. *Epilepsia.* 2012;53(7):1119–1130.

49. Hoeffer CA, Klann E. mTOR signaling: at the crossroads of plasticity, memory and disease. *Trends Neurosci.* 2010;33(2):67–75.

50. Teather LA, Packard MG, Bazan NG. Post-training cyclooxygenase-2 (COX-2) inhibition impairs memory consolidation. *Learn Mem.* 2002;9(1):41–47.

51. Gobbo OL, O'Mara SM. Post-treatment, but not pre-treatment, with the selective cyclooxygenase-2 inhibitor celecoxib markedly enhances functional recovery from kainic acid-induced neurodegeneration. *Neuroscience.* 2004;125(2):317–327.

52. Levin JR, Serrano G, Dingledine R. Reduction in delayed mortality and subtle improvement in retrograde memory performance in pilocarpine-treated mice with conditional neuronal deletion of cyclooxygenase-2 gene. *Epilepsia.* 2012;53(8):1411–1420.

53. Yamagata K, Andreasson KI, Kaufmann WE, Barnes CA, Worley PF. Expression of a mitogen-inducible cyclooxygenase in brain neurons: regulation by synaptic activity and glucocorticoids. *Neuron.* 1993;11(2):371–386.

54. Jiang J, Dingledine R. Prostaglandin receptor EP2 in the crosshairs of anti-inflammation, anti-cancer, and neuroprotection. *Trends Pharmacol Sci.* 2013;34(7):413–423.

55. Jiang J, Yang MS, Quan Y, Gueorguieva P, Ganesh T, Dingledine R. Therapeutic window for cyclooxygenase-2 related anti-inflammatory therapy after status epilepticus. *Neurobiol Dis.* 2015;76:126–136.

56. Vargas DL, Nascimbene C, Krishnan C, Zimmerman AW, Pardo CA. Neuroglial activation and neuroinflammation in the brain of patients with autism. *Ann Neurol.* 2005;57(1):67–81.

57. Boso M, Emanuele E, Minoretti P, et al. Alterations of circulating endogenous secretory RAGE and S100A9 levels indicating dysfunction of the AGE-RAGE axis in autism. *Neurosci Lett.* 2006;410(3):169–173.

58. Emanuele E, Boso M, Brondino N, et al. Increased serum levels of high mobility group box 1 protein in patients with autistic disorder. *Prog Neuropsychopharmacol Biol Psychiatry.* 2010;34(4):681–683.

59. Enstrom AM, Onore CE, Van de Water JA, Ashwood P. Differential monocyte responses to TLR ligands in children with autism spectrum disorders. *Brain Behav Immun.* 2010;24(1):64–71.

60. Sato A. mTOR, a potential target to treat autism spectrum disorder. *CNS Neurol Disord – Drug Targets.* 2016;15(5):533–543.

61. Cone Jr TE. On a peculiar form of infantile convulsions (hypsarrhythmia) as described in his own infant son by Dr. W.J. West in 1841. *Pediatrics.* 1970;46(4):603.

62. Hrachovy RA, Frost JD. Infantile epileptic encephalopathy with hypsarrhythmia (infantile spasms/West syndrome). *J Clin Neurophysiol.* 2003;20(6):408–425.

63. Go CY, Mackay MT, Weiss SK, et al. Evidence-based guideline update: medical treatment of infantile spasms. Report of the Guideline Development Subcommittee of the American Academy of Neurology and the Practice Committee of the Child Neurology Society. *Neurology.* 2012;78(24):1974–1980.

64. Shumiloff NA, Lam WM, Manasco KB. Adrenocorticotropic hormone for the treatment of West Syndrome in children. *Ann Pharmacother.* 2013;47(5):744–754.

65. Riikonen R. Infantile spasms: infectious disorders. *Neuropediatrics.* 1993;24(5):274–280.

66. Becker AJ, Urbach H, Scheffler B, et al. Focal cortical dysplasia of Taylor's balloon cell type: mutational analysis of the TSC1 gene indicates a pathogenic relationship to tuberous sclerosis. *Ann Neurol.* 2002;52(1):29–37.

67. Suleiman J, Brenner T, Gill D, et al. Immune-mediated steroid-responsive epileptic spasms and epileptic encephalopathy associated with VGKC-complex antibodies. *Dev Med Child Neurol.* 2011;53(11):1058–1060.

68. Kato T, Okumura A, Hayakawa F, et al. Prolonged EEG depression in term and near-term infants with hypoxic ischemic encephalopathy and later development of West syndrome. *Epilepsia.* 2010;51(12):2392–2396.

69. Montelli TC, Mota NG, Peracoli MT, Torres EA, Rezkallah-Iwasso MT. Immunological disturbance in West and Lennox-Gastaut syndromes. *Arq Neuropsiquiatr.* 1984;42(2):132–139.

70. Haraldsson Á, van Engelen BGM, Renier WO, Bakkeren JAJM, Weemaes CMR. Light chain ratios and concentrations of serum immunoglobulins in children with epilepsy. *Epilepsy Res.* 1992;13(3):255–260.

71. Montelli TC, Soares AM, Peracoli MT. Immunologic aspects of West syndrome and evidence of plasma inhibitory effects on T cell function. *Arq Neuropsiquiatr.* 2003;61(3B):731–737.

72. Carvalho KS, Walleigh DJ, Legido A. Generalized Epilepsies: Immunologic and inflammatory mechanisms. *Semin Pediatr Neurol.* 2014;21(3):214–220.

73. Shiihara T, Miyashita M, Yoshizumi M, Watanabe M, Yamada Y, Kato M. Peripheral lymphocyte subset and serum cytokine profiles of patients with West syndrome. *Brain Dev.* 2010;32(9):695–702.

74. Hattori H. Spontaneous remission of spasms in West syndrome – implications of viral infection. *Brain Dev.* 2001;23(7):705–707.

75. Pintaudi M, Eisermann MM, Ville D, Plouin P, Dulac O, Kaminska A. Can fever treat epileptic encephalopathies? *Epilepsy Res.* 2007;77(1):44–61.

76. Baram TZ, Mitchell WG, Snead 3rd OC, Horton EJ, Saito M. Brain-adrenal axis hormones are altered in the CSF of infants with massive infantile spasms. *Neurology.* 1992;42(6):1171–1175.

77. Haginoya K, Noguchi R, Zhao Y, et al. Reduced levels of interleukin-1 receptor antagonist in the cerebrospinal fluid in patients with West syndrome. *Epilepsy Res.* 2009;85(2–3):314–317.

78. Tekgul H, Polat M, Tosun A, Serdaroglu G, Kutukculer N, Gokben S. Cerebrospinal fluid interleukin-6 levels in patients with West syndrome. *Brain Dev.* 2006;28(1):19–23.

79. Yamanaka G, Kawashima H, Oana S, et al. Increased level of serum interleukin-1 receptor antagonist subsequent to resolution of clinical symptoms in patients with West syndrome. *J Neurol Sci.* 2010;298(1–2):106–109.

80. Dussaix E, Lebon P, Ponsot G, Huault G, Tardieu M. Intrathecal synthesis of different alpha-interferons in patients with various neurological diseases. *Acta Neurol Scand.* 1985;71(6):504–509.

81. Liu Z-S, Wang Q-W, Wang F-L, Yang L-Z. Serum cytokine levels are altered in patients with West syndrome. *Brain Development.* 2001;23(7):548–551.

82. Maldonado M, Baybis M, Newman D, et al. Expression of ICAM-1, TNF-α, NFκB, and MAP kinase in tubers of the tuberous sclerosis complex. *Neurobiol Dis.* 2003;14(2):279–290.

83. Boer K, Jansen F, Nellist M, et al. Inflammatory processes in cortical tubers and subependymal giant cell tumors of tuberous sclerosis complex. *Epilepsy Res.* 2008;78(1):7–21.

84. Boer K, Crino PB, Gorter JA, et al. Gene expression analysis of tuberous sclerosis complex cortical tubers reveals increased expression of adhesion and inflammatory factors. *Brain Pathol.* 2010;20(4):704–719.

85. McDaniel SS, Rensing NR, Thio LL, Yamada KA, Wong M. The ketogenic diet inhibits the mammalian target of rapamycin (mTOR) pathway. *Epilepsia.* 2011;52(3):e7–e11.

86. Jutel M, Watanabe T, Klunker S, et al. Histamine regulates T-cell and antibody responses by differential expression of H1 and H2 receptors. *Nature.* 2001;413(6854):420–425.

87. Brown RE, Stevens DR, Haas HL. The physiology of brain histamine. *Prog Neurobiol.* 2001;63(6):637–672.

88. Haas HL, Sergeeva OA, Selbach O. Histamine in the nervous system. *Physiol Rev.* 2008;88(3):1183–1241.

89. Yasuhara A, Ochi A, Harada Y, Kobayashi Y. Infantile spasms associated with a histamine H1 antagonist. *Neuropediatrics.* 1998;29(6):320–321.

90. Yokoyama H. The role of central histaminergic neuron system as an anticonvulsive mechanism in developing brain. *Brain Dev-jpn.* 2001;23(7):542–547.

91. Yamashita Y, Isagai T, Seki Y, Ohya T, Nagamitsu S, Matsuishi T. West syndrome associated with administration of a histamine H1 antagonist, oxatomide. *Kurume Med J.* 2004;51(3–4):273–275.

92. Scantlebury MH, Galanopoulou AS, Chudomelova L, Raffo E, Betancourth D, Moshe SL. A model of symptomatic infantile spasms syndrome. *Neurobiol Dis.* 2010;37(3):604–612.

93. Siegal T, Melamed E, Sandbank U, Catane R. Early and delayed neurotoxicity of mitoxantrone and doxorubicin following subarachnoid injection. *J Neurooncol.* 1988;6(2):135–140.

94. Pang Y, Cai Z, Rhodes PG. Disturbance of oligodendrocyte development, hypomyelination and white matter injury in the neonatal rat brain after intracerebral injection of lipopolysaccharide. *Brain Res Dev Brain Res.* 2003;140(2):205–214.

95. Rattray M, Baldessari S, Gobbi M, Mennini T, Samanin R, Bendotti C. p-Chlorphenylalanine changes serotonin transporter mRNA levels and expression of the gene product. *J Neurochem.* 1996;67(2):463–472.

96. Silverstein F, Johnston MV. Cerebrospinal fluid monoamine metabolites in patients with infantile spasms. *Neurology.* 1984;34(1):102–105.

97. Briggs SW, Mowrey W, Hall CB, Galanopoulou AS. CPP-115, a vigabatrin analogue, decreases spasms in the multiple-hit rat model of infantile spasms. *Epilepsia.* 2014;55(1):94–102.

98. Doumlele K, Conway E, Hedlund J, Tolete P, Devinsky O. A case report on the efficacy of vigabatrin analogue (1S, 3S)-3-amino-4-difluoromethylenyl-1-cyclopentanoic acid (CPP-115) in a patient with infantile spasms. *Epilepsy Behav Case Rep.* 2016;6:67–69.

99. Ono T, Moshe SL, Galanopoulou AS. Carisbamate acutely suppresses spasms in a rat model of symptomatic infantile spasms. *Epilepsia.* 2011;52(9):1678–1684.

100. Shandra O, Wang Y, Mowrey W, Moshe SL, Galanopoulou AS. Effects of celastrol and edavarone in the multiple-hit rat model of infantile spasms. #2.048. In: *AES 69th Annual Meeting December 4–8, 2015, Philadelphia, PA, USA; 2015.* Available at: https://www.aesnet.org/meetings_events/annual_meeting_abstracts/view/2327525.

101. Ono T, Briggs SW, Chudomelova L, Raffo E, Moshe SL, Galanopoulou AS. Intracortical injection of lipopolysaccharide induces epileptic spasms in neonatal rats: another animal model of symptomatic infantile spasms. #3.058. In: *AES 65th Annual Meeting December 2–6, 2011, Baltimore, MD, USA. Epilepsy Currents; 2012; 12(s1):1–418.*

102. Vezzani A, Granata T. Brain inflammation in epilepsy: experimental and clinical evidence. *Epilepsia.* 2005;46(11):1724–1739.

103. Mareš P, Velíšek L. (NMDA)-induced seizures in developing rats. *Dev Brain Res.* 1992;65(2):185–189.

104. Zou LP, Zhang WH, Wang HM, Zen M, Chen K, Mix E. Maternal IgG suppresses NMDA-induced spasms in infant rats and inhibits NMDA-mediated neurotoxicity in hippocampal neurons. *J Neuroimmunol.* 2006;181(1–2):106–111.

105. Michaud JL, Lachance M, Hamdan FF, et al. The genetic landscape of infantile spasms. *Hum Mol Genet.* 2014;23(18):4846–4858.

106. Edvardson S, Baumann AM, Muhlenhoff M, et al. West syndrome caused by ST3Gal-III deficiency. *Epilepsia.* 2013;54(2):e24–e27.

107. Sturgill ER, Aoki K, Lopez PH, et al. Biosynthesis of the major brain gangliosides GD1a and GT1b. *Glycobiology.* 2012;22(10):1289–1301.

108. Yoo SW, Motari MG, Susuki K, et al. Sialylation regulates brain structure and function. *FASEB J.* 2015;29(7): 3040–3053.

109. Kiwamoto T, Brummet ME, Wu F, et al. Mice deficient in the St3gal3 gene product alpha2,3 sialyltransferase (ST3Gal-III) exhibit enhanced allergic eosinophilic airway inflammation. *J Allergy Clin Immunol.* 2014;133(1): e241–243. 240–247.

110. Lennox WG, Davis JP. Clinical correlates of the fast and the slow spike-wave electroencephalogram. *Pediatrics.* 1950;5(4):626–644.

111. Gastaut H, Roger J, Soularyol R, et al. Childhood epileptic encephalopathy with diffuse slow spike-waves (otherwise known as "petit mal variant") or Lennox syndrome. *Epilepsia.* 1966;7(2):139–179.

112. Blume WT. Pathogenesis of Lennox-Gastaut syndrome: considerations and hypotheses. *Epileptic Disord.* 2001;3(4): 183–196.

113. Saemundsen E, Ludvigsson P, Rafnsson V. Risk of autism spectrum disorders after infantile spasms: a population-based study nested in a cohort with seizures in the first year of life. *Epilepsia.* 2008;49(11):1865–1870.

114. Yamatogi Y, Ohtsuka Y, Ishida T, et al. Treatment of the Lennox syndrome with ACTH: a clinical and electroencephalographic study. *Brain Dev.* 1979;1(4):267–276.

115. Roger J, Dravet C, Bureau M. The Lennox-Gastaut syndrome. *Cleve Clin J Med.* 1989;(56 suppl Pt 2):S172–S180.

116. Smeraldi E, Smeraldi RS, Cazzullo CL, Cazzullo AG, Fabio G, Canger R. Immunogenetics of the lennox-gastaut syndrome: frequency of HL-A antigens and haplotypes in patients and first-degree relatives. *Epilepsia.* 1975;16(5):699–703.

117. van Engelen BGM, de Waal LP, Weemaes CMR, Renier WO. Serologie HLA typing in cryptogenic Lennox-Gastaut syndrome. *Epilepsy Res.* 1994;17(1):43–47.

118. van Rijckevorsel-Harmant K, Delire M, Rucquoy-Ponsar M. Treatment of idiopathic West and Lennox-Gastaut syndromes by intravenous administration of human polyvalent immunoglobulins. *Eur Arch Psychiatry Neurol Sci.* 1986;236(2):119–122.

119. van Engelen BGM, Renier WO, Weemaes CMR, Strengers PFW. Treatment of idiopathic West- and Lennox epilepsy with intravenous immunoglobulin. *Clin Neurol Neurosurg.* 1991;93(1):82.

120. Smith KA, Bierkamper GG. Paradoxical role of GABA in a chronic model of petit mal (absence)-like epilepsy in the rat. *Eur J Pharmacol.* 1990;176(1):45–55.

121. Cortez MA, McKerlie C, Snead 3rd OC. A model of atypical absence seizures: EEG, pharmacology, and developmental characterization. *Neurology*. 2001;56(3):341–349.

122. van Luijtelaar G, Onat FY, Gallagher MJ. Animal models of absence epilepsies: what do they model and do sex and sex hormones matter? *Neurobiol Dis*. 2014;(72 Pt B):167–179.

123. Chan KFY, Jia ZP, Murphy PA, Burnham WM, Cortez MA, Snead OC. Learning and memory impairment in rats with chronic atypical absence seizures. *Exp Neurol*. 2004;190(2):328–336.

124. Chan KF, Burnham WM, Jia Z, Cortez MA, Snead 3rd OC. GABAB receptor antagonism abolishes the learning impairments in rats with chronic atypical absence seizures. *Eur J Pharmacol*. 2006;541(1–2):64–72.

125. Buzatu M, Bulteau C, Altuzarra C, Dulac O, Van Bogaert P. Corticosteroids as treatment of epileptic syndromes with continuous spike-waves during slow-wave sleep. *Epilepsia*. 2009;50:68–72.

126. Lesca G, Rudolf G, Bruneau N, et al. GRIN2A mutations in acquired epileptic aphasia and related childhood focal epilepsies and encephalopathies with speech and language dysfunction. *Nat Genet*. 2013;45(9):1061–1066.

127. Nevsimalova S, Tauberova A, Doutlik S, Kucera V, Dlouha O. A role of autoimmunity in the etiopathogenesis of Landau-Kleffner syndrome? *Brain Dev*. 1992;14(5): 342–345.

128. Connolly AM, Chez MG, Pestronk A, Arnold ST, Mehta S, Deuel RK. Serum autoantibodies to brain in Landau-Kleffner variant, autism, and other neurologic disorders. *J Pediatr*. 1999;134(5):607–613.

129. Boscolo S, Baldas V, Gobbi G, et al. Anti-brain but not celiac disease antibodies in Landau-Kleffner syndrome and related epilepsies. *J Neuroimmunol*. 2005;160(1–2): 228–232.

130. Dravet C. Dravet syndrome history. *Dev Med Child Neurol*. 2011;(53 suppl 2):1–6.

131. Berkovic SF, Harkin L, McMahon JM, et al. De-novo mutations of the sodium channel gene SCN1A in alleged vaccine encephalopathy: a retrospective study. *Lancet Neurol*. 2006;5(6):488–492.

132. Verbeek NE, van der Maas NA, Sonsma AC, et al. Effect of vaccinations on seizure risk and disease course in Dravet syndrome. *Neurology*. 2015;85(7):596–603.

133. Rubio M, Valdeolivas S, Piscitelli F, et al. Analysis of endocannabinoid signaling elements and related proteins in lymphocytes of patients with Dravet syndrome. *Pharmacol Res Perspect*. 2016;4(2):e00220.

134. Baraban SC, Dinday MT, Hortopan GA. Drug screening in Scn1a zebrafish mutant identifies clemizole as a potential Dravet syndrome treatment. *Nat Commun*. 2013;4:2410.

135. Kumar MG, Rowley S, Fulton R, et al. Respiration in a zebrafish model of Dravet syndrome. *eNeuro*. 2016;3(2).

136. Berg AT, Darefsky AS, Holford TR, Shinnar S. Seizures with fever after unprovoked seizures: an analysis in children followed from the time of a first febrile seizure. *Epilepsia*. 1998;39(1):77–80.

137. Baulac S, Gourfinkel-An I, Nabbout R, et al. Fever, genes, and epilepsy. *Lancet Neurol*. 2004;3(7):421–430.

138. Heida JG, Pittman QJ. Causal links between brain cytokines and experimental febrile convulsions in the rat. *Epilepsia*. 2005;46(12):1906–1913.

139. Dube CM, Brewster AL, Richichi C, Zha Q, Baram TZ. Fever, febrile seizures and epilepsy. *Trends Neurosci*. 2007;30(10):490–496.

140. Cao D, Ohtani H, Ogiwara I, et al. Efficacy of stiripentol in hyperthermia-induced seizures in a mouse model of Dravet syndrome. *Epilepsia*. 2012;53(7):1140–1145.

141. Han S, Tai C, Westenbroek RE, et al. Autistic-like behaviour in Scn1a+/- mice and rescue by enhanced GABA-mediated neurotransmission. *Nature*. 2012;489(7416):385–390.

142. Oakley JC, Cho AR, Cheah CS, Scheuer T, Catterall WA. Synergistic GABA-enhancing therapy against seizures in a mouse model of Dravet syndrome. *J Pharmacol Exp Ther*. 2013;345(2):215–224.

143. Ohmori I, Kawakami N, Liu S, et al. Methylphenidate improves learning impairments and hyperthermia-induced seizures caused by an Scn1a mutation. *Epilepsia*. 2014;55(10):1558–1567.

144. Auvin S, Cilio MR, Vezzani A. Current understanding and neurobiology of epileptic encephalopathies. *Neurobiol Dis*. 2016;92(Pt A):72–89.

145. Riikonen R. Long-term outcome of patients with West syndrome. *Brain Dev*. 2001;23(7):683–687.

146. Riikonen RS. Favourable prognostic factors with infantile spasms. *Eur J Paediatr Neurol*. 2010;14(1):13–18.

147. Landau WM, Kleffner FR. Syndrome of acquired aphasia with convulsive disorder in children. *Neurology*. 1957;7(8):523–530.

148. Patry G, Lyagoubi S, Tassinari CA. Subclinical "electrical status epilepticus" induced by sleep in children. A clinical and electroencephalographic study of six cases. *Arch Neurol*. 1971;24(3):242–252.

CHAPTER 6

Genetic Background of Encephalopathy

ATSUSHI ISHII, MD, PHD • SHINICHI HIROSE, MD, PHD

INTRODUCTION

The molecular pathomechanisms of acute encephalopathy (AE) remain largely unknown. The incidence of AE in Japanese children is estimated at 1 out of 1700–3400 per year. This high incidence of AE in Japan and among individuals of East Asian ethnicity suggests an underlying genetic background. AE, however, consists of multiple disorders, and hence its heterogeneity and rarity hinder molecular genetic analyses. Nevertheless, several recent studies have been implemented to identify the genetic background of AE. In particular, the discoveries that monogenic familial or recurrent acute necrotizing encephalitis (ANE) may be caused by *RANBP2* mutations have provided evidence that genetic factors contribute to the pathogenesis of AE.[1] This review covers the current understanding of the genetic background of AE as ascertained through recent reports regarding genetic information related to the immunologic, neurologic, and metabolic aspects of AE (Fig. 6.1).

IMMUNOLOGIC GENETIC BACKGROUND

The genetic background underlying the immune response seems to be closely associated with AE. Febrile illnesses and specifically infections caused by viruses such as influenza, human herpesvirus 6, and herpes simplex virus (HSV) are well known as a cause or initiating factor of AE. It is therefore reasonable to consider that the genetic backgrounds underpinning the immune response to such pathogens may be related to the pathomechanisms of AE.

Human leukocyte antigen (HLA) is a key molecule in the immune response and therefore has become a primary target for investigations into the genetic background of AE. In particular, it has been found that HLA-DRB1*1401, HLA- DRB3*0202, and HLA-DQB1*0502 are associated with AE in Korean children.[2,3] In contrast, HLA-DRB1*0901 and DQB1*0303 have been found to be associated with AE in a Japanese cohort.[4] Although

there are differences between the studies themselves, the results support that the genetic background associated with HLA may also contribute to AE risk, given that these ethnicities have been shown to be genetically distinct.[4]

In addition, mutations in the genes encoding two molecules that play an important role in the innate immune response have been identified in AE and acute encephalitis. Specifically, a heterozygous missense mutation of the Toll-like receptor 3 (*TLR3*) gene was first found in a single case of influenza-associated encephalopathy,[5] followed by another heterozygous *TLR3* missense mutation identified in two unrelated, otherwise healthy children with HSV encephalitis.[6] Additionally, a homozygous missense mutation of the gene encoding UNC-93B has been found in two unrelated, otherwise healthy children with HSV encephalitis.[7]

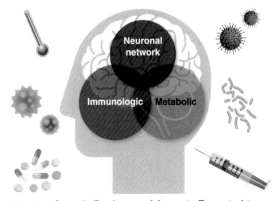

FIG. 6.1 **Genetic Background Aspects Expected to Play a Role in Acute Encephalopathy and/or Encephalitis (AE).** Many exogenous factors or pathogens, such as microorganisms including influenza virus, human herpesvirus 6, mycoplasma, and bacteria, high fever induced by febrile illnesses, and some medicines including vaccines may cause or initiate AE. Three major aspects of the genetic background of the host should be taken into consideration with respect to AE susceptibility: immunologic, neuronal network, and metabolic.

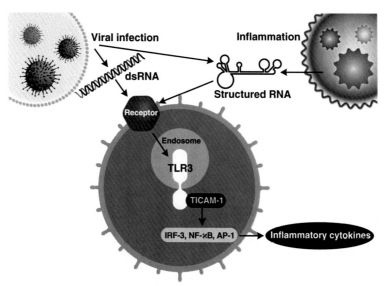

FIG. 6.2 **Toll-Like Receptor 3 (TLR3) in Innate Immunity on Viral Infection.** TLR3 resides in the endo-some in a wide variety of cells. TRL3 binds double-stranded and structured RNAs, both of which are pro-duced during viral infections and inflammation. On activation by RNA binding, it stimulates its downstream cytokine production cascade through TCAM-1-mediated initiation of IRF-3, NF-kb, and AP-A expression followed by release of type 1 interferon and inflammatory cytokines.

TLR3 resides in the endosome in a wide variety of cells ranging from dendritic cells to neurons and glia. TRL3 binds double-stranded and structured RNAs, both of which are produced during viral infections, whereupon the expression of TRL3 is upregulated. TRL3 activated by binding to RNA then stimulates its downstream cytokine production cascade via TCAM-1 to initiate expression of IRF-3, NF-kb, and AP-A, fol-lowed by type 1 interferon and inflammatory cytokine release as well as dendritic cell maturation[8] (Fig. 6.2). UNC-93B is thought to bind to TRL3, contributing to their trafficking and hence playing a similar role to that of TRL3 in innate immunity during viral infection. As the identified mutations in both TRL3 and UNC-93B have been shown to lead to functional deficiencies in these proteins, the genetic background underlying innate immunity, especially with respect to cytokine production, thus seems to be closely associated with the pathomechanisms of AE.[9]

Furthermore, in a Japanese cohort of patients with febrile infection–related epilepsy syndrome (FIRES) or acute encephalitis with refractory, repetitive partial sei-zures (AERRPS), the frequency of a variable number of tandem repeat allele, RN2, of the interleukin 1 receptor antagonist (*IL1RN*) gene was found to be significantly higher in patients than in controls. In addition, the A allele at rs4251981 in the 5′ upstream region of *IL1RN*

was also reportedly more frequent in patients. Accord-ingly, the haplotype containing RN2 appeared to rep-resent a risk factor for FIRES or AERRPS.[10] Recently, a direct association between genetic polymorphism of *IL10* and AE has also been demonstrated. Specifically, ANE is associated with the diplotype (CC/CC), which has been shown to result in lower IL-10 production than other haplotypes.[11]

Taken together, these findings suggest that an indi-vidual with an attenuated immune response, in partic-ular in innate immunity that plays a pivotal role in viral infection, may have increased susceptibility to AE. The genetic background for this altered immune response is therefore likely to contribute to the development of AE, at least in conjunction with infection.

NEURONAL NETWORK GENETIC BACKGROUND

The significance of the genetic background that modu-lates the neuronal network in the pathogenesis of AE has been supported by numerous recent reports. One such finding is that mutations of *SCN1A* and *SCN2A*, which encode the α1 and α2 subunits of the neuronal voltage-gated sodium channel, respectively (Fig. 6.3), have been found in cases of AE. *SCN1A* is well known as the gene responsible for Dravet syndrome, a devastating epileptic

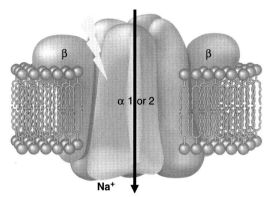

FIG. 6.3 Neuronal Voltage-Gated Sodium Channels, Na$_v$1.1 and Na$_v$1.2. Neuronal voltage-gated sodium channels, Na$_v$1.1 and Na$_v$1.2, are mainly expressed in neurons in the central nerve system and function as the generators of action potential. Na$_v$1.1 has an α1 subunit that has an ion pore, whereas Nav1.2 has an α2 subunit. The α1 and α2 subunit is encoded by *SCN1A* and *SCN2A*, respectively.

encephalopathy. To date, over 700 types of mutations including missense, truncation, indel, and microdeletion mutations of this gene have been found in individuals with Dravet syndrome, primarily as de novo mutations.[12,13] Missense mutations of *SCN1A*, both de novo and inherited, may result in a much milder form of epilepsy, termed genetic epilepsy with febrile seizure plus (GEFS+). Notably, one of the characteristics of both Dravet syndrome and GEFS+ is fever sensitivity, which may be of particular interest when considering the association between *SCN1A* and AE, as febrile illnesses can serve as a trigger for AE. Mutations of *SCN2A* have been reported as the cause of benign familial neonatal infantile epilepsy and were subsequently found to be associated with early-onset neonatal epileptic encephalopathy.[14]

Although the clinical phenotypes of both Dravet syndrome and early-onset epileptic encephalopathy (caused by *SCN1A* and *SCN2A*, respectively) are distinguishable from those of AE, some mutations of these genes have also been found to occur in AE. Whereas initially only a few studies initially reported that some patients with Dravet syndrome had developed AE,[15–17] a cohort study subsequently found that the incidence of AE among individuals with Dravet syndrome was as high as 15/170, suggesting that patients with Dravet syndrome are prone to AE.[18] Moreover, the same study found that 9 of the 15 cases that had developed AE carried *SCN1A* mutations,[18] further supporting the strong relationship between these disorders.

Conversely, mutations of *SCN1A* and *SCN2A* have also been found in apparently healthy children. The first such report examined 14 individuals with alleged vaccine encephalopathy, of which 11 carried *SCN1A* mutations.[19] However, several subsequent reports demonstrated the presence of SCN subunit mutations in individuals with AE, and these mutations were unrelated with vaccination. For example, in a cohort of 87 individuals with ANE, acute encephalopathy with biphasic seizures and reduced diffusion (AESD), and unclassified AE, 3 were found to harbor *SCN1A* mutations.[20]

With respect to *SCN2A*, the minor allele frequency of the G allele at rs1864885 was found to be higher in patients with AERRPS than in controls.[10] Furthermore, three mutations of *SCN2A* were found among 25 individuals with AERRPS, AESD, and ANE.[21] Another cohort study on 92 individuals with AESD identified a single *SCN2A* mutation in addition to three *SCN1A* mutations.[22] These findings suggest that *SCN1A* and *SCN2A*, which encode neuronal sodium channels, are some of the main drivers of the neuronal networks that are associated the pathomechanisms of AE through their mutation or other genetic effects. Notably, all of the *SCN1A* and *SCN2A* mutations that were found in AE were missense mutations except for a few nonsense mutations that were reported in alleged vaccine encephalopathy, whereas approximately half of the mutations causing Dravet syndrome are nonsense *SCN1A* mutations (Figs. 6.4 and 6.5).

Furthermore, a similar result was found in theophylline-related AE.[23] Specifically, 16 patients developed AE during theophylline treatment, of which 12 presented with an AESD phenotype, carrying one *SCN1A* and one *SCN2A* mutation.[23] Theophylline along with caffeine is one of several xanthitane derivatives and is known as a proconvulsant. An association with AE in particular has been suspected based on clinical observations of children taking theophylline. Theophylline and caffeine inhibit both the adenosine A1 and A2a receptors, which exert inhibitory and excitatory functions to produce cAMP on binding to adenosine, their physiologic ligand. As theophylline and caffeine inhibit the adenosine A1 receptor to a greater extent than the adenosine A2a receptor, both compounds lead to a hyperexcitatory state of the neuronal network, which may result in convulsions[24,25] (Fig 6.6).

There is also evidence that the adenosine A2a receptor itself is involved in AE development. In particular, a higher frequency of a haplotype (A) of the gene encoding the adenosine A2a receptor (*ADORA2A*) was found in patients with AESD than in controls. As the presence of the diplotype (AA) was found to result in

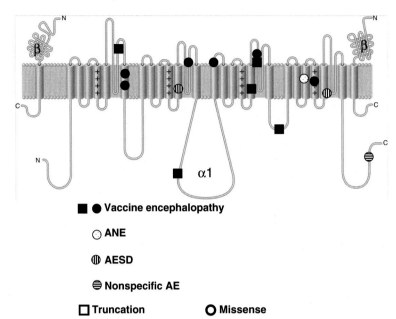

■ ● Vaccine encephalopathy

○ ANE

⦿ AESD

⊜ Nonspecific AE

□ Truncation   ○ Missense

FIG. 6.4 **Mutations of *SCN1A* That Have Been Reported in Acute Encephalopathy and/or Encephalitis (AE).** Several mutations of *SCN1A*, the gene encoding the α1 subunit of the neuronal voltage-gated sodium channel, Na$_v$1.1, have been reported in certain types of AE. The locations of the reported mutations are shown. *AESD*, acute encephalopathy with biphasic seizures and reduced diffusion; *ANE*, acute necrotizing encephalitis.

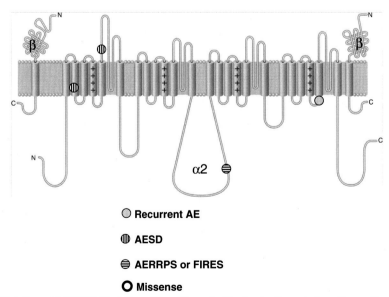

◉ Recurrent AE

⦿ AESD

⊜ AERRPS or FIRES

○ Missense

FIG. 6.5 **Mutations of *SCN2A* That Have Been Reported in Acute Encephalopathy and/or Encephalitis (AE).** Several mutations of *SCN2A*, the gene encoding the α2 subunit of the neuronal voltage-gated sodium channel, Na$_v$1.2, have been reported in certain types of AE. The locations of the reported mutations are shown. *AERRPS*, acute encephalitis with refractory, repetitive partial seizures; *AESD*, acute encephalopathy with biphasic seizures and reduced diffusion; *FIRES*, febrile infection–related epilepsy syndrome.

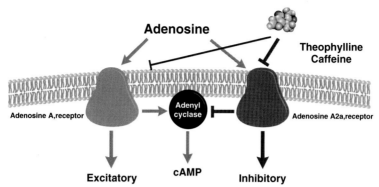

FIG. 6.6 **Adenosine A1 and A2a Receptors.** The adenosine A1 and A2a receptors exert inhibitory and excitatory effects on the production of cAMP, respectively, on their binding to adenosine. Theophylline and caffeine inhibit both receptors. As theophylline and caffeine inhibit the adenosine A1 receptor to a greater extent than the adenosine A2a receptor, both compounds lead to a hyperexcitatory state of the neuronal network, which may result in convulsions.

higher expression of the adenosine A2a, cAMP production increased accordingly in association with the AA diplotype.[23] This may explain the involvement of theophylline in the pathogenesis of AE and suggests that polymorphisms of *ADORA2A*, potentially in addition to some other genetic factors related to the adenosine receptors, are also related to AE.

METABOLIC GENETIC BACKGROUND

Effective metabolism in the central nervous system is crucial as evinced by the neurologic manifestations manifested in many metabolic diseases, some of which mimic the course and outcome of AE. In particular, the metabolic pathways contributing to energy production should be of great importance in maintaining the activity of the brain, considering it is one of the most energy- or ATP-consuming organs in the human body. Insufficient energy production due to metabolic dysfunction for any reason may therefore be associated with the pathomechanisms of AE. Accordingly, it is logical to anticipate genetic propensities in the metabolic systems of individuals with AE.

In particular, the mutations of *RANBP2* found in familial AE provide direct evidence that monogenic abnormality may cause AE as previously discussed. The exact pathomechanisms involved, i.e., why and how *RANBP2* mutations cause AE, remain to be elucidated. *RANBP2* encodes Ran binding protein 2, which is a component of the nuclear pore. It has been suggested that RANBP2 functions as a modulator of neuronal glucose catabolism; RANBP2 is thus considered to be involved in energy homeostasis.[26] Mutations of *RANBP2* may therefore cause AE by impacting energy production.

Furthermore, intriguing reports regarding the metabolism of energy production in relation to AE have recently emerged. These reports relate to variants of carnitine palmitoyltransferase II (CPTII), which is a key enzyme in the process of ATP production from lipids. Specifically, CPTII at the inner membrane of the mitochondria catabolizes acylcarnitine (CAR) and produces acyl-CoA, which in turn is catabolized during β-oxidation to produce ATP. In particular, two variants of CPTII, F352C and V368I, have been reported as being thermolabile, because the enzyme activity of CPTII and its variants was susceptible to high temperatures such as 41°C.[27,28] Notably, these thermolabile variants were identified at higher frequency in individuals with AE compared with those without AE.[23,27,29] Furthermore, databases of genetic variants show that these two variants are more common in East Asians, which agrees with the findings of a higher incidence of AE among individuals of Asian ethnicity. In support of this ethnic bias, both variants were found to be associated with AE in a Chinese cohort as well.[30]

Direct evidence for a direct link between thermolability and AE remains to be revealed. However, the underlying theory of the likely relationship between thermolabile variants and AE is of potential relevance, because it extends the therapeutic implications for AE.[28,31–35] For example, energy production primarily occurs through glycolysis in addition to lipolysis, in which CPTII plays a pivotal role as previously discussed. During influenza infection, the influenza virus is known to attenuate the activity of pyruvate dehydrogenase, which catalyzes pyruvate and provides acetyl-CoA to the TCA cycle to produce ATP. Influenza infection thus hampers glucose-dependent energy production (glycolysis).

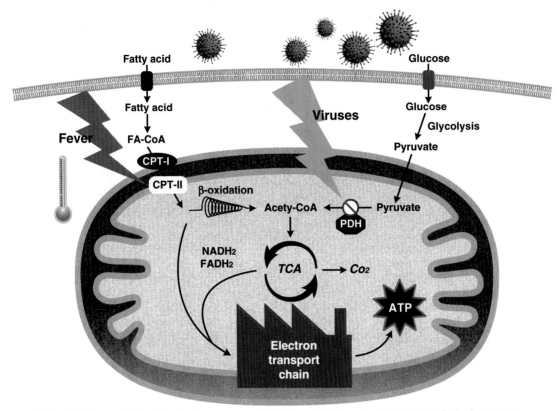

FIG. 6.7 Thermolabile Palmitoyltransferase II (CPTII) and Attenuation of Pyruvate Dehydrogenase May Cause Energy Crisis on Influenza Infection. During influenza infection, the influenza virus is known to attenuate the activity of pyruvate dehydrogenase (PDH), which catalyzes pyruvate and provides acetyl-CoA to the TCA cycle to produce ATP. Influenza infection thereby hampers glucose-dependent energy production. Under such conditions, fatty acid–dependent energy production is relied on as the main ATP source; the presence of thermolabile CPTII would aggravate the insufficiency of the energy supply, because influenza infection causes high fever.

Under such conditions, fatty acid–dependent energy production (lipolysis) is relied on as the main ATP source; however, a thermolabile CPTII would further aggravate the insufficient energy supply because influenza infection causes high fever. It is further convincing that some thermolabile variants of CPTII comprise a genetic background prone to AE (Fig. 6.7).

This theory allows the suggestion of several therapeutic implications for AE. For example, bezafibrate may be effective in ameliorating the enzyme activity of thermolabile CPTII. Bezafibrate is a lipid-lowering agent that is readily available and has been found to be safe through long experience of its use. Bezafibrate may therefore be beneficial to prevent the development of AE during febrile illnesses.[31] The attenuation of pyruvate carboxylase in influenza infection may be also ameliorated with another old drug, diisopropylamine dichloroacetate (DADA),[34] which has long been commercially marketed, albeit in only a few countries such as Japan and Italy. DADA also may be beneficial when used during influenza infection to prevent AE. Together, these findings suggest that genetic backgrounds underlying metabolism are critical for the development of AE and that a better understanding of these backgrounds may provide clues for the development of therapeutic and preventive measures for AE.

CONCLUSIONS

This chapter covers the current understanding of the genetic backgrounds that may be associated with the development of AE. These backgrounds are divided into three aspects: immunologic, neuronal network, and metabolic.

The innate immunity against viral infection may govern a pivotal immune reaction in AE, and the related genetic backgrounds seem to play important roles accordingly. Some ion channels and receptors serving as important components in the neuronal network have been found to be associated with seizures as well as AE. Genetic factors contributing to the neuronal network, therefore, may constitute a component of the underlying background of AE. Viral infection and the associated high fever undermine the energy production of the brain, also potentially leading to the development of AE. Genetic factors that are involved in energy production might thus also be critical in the development of AE. Concomitantly, the restoration of such insufficient energy synthesis through the use of certain drugs may now be suggested.

These genetic identifiers should provide new insights into the genetic background of AE and indicate the necessity of future massive genetic analyses on larger cohorts of patients with AE using next-generation sequencing. The resulting increased understanding of AE at the molecular level will likely facilitate the development of both therapeutic and preventive measures for AE.

ACKNOWLEDGMENTS

This work was supported by a Grant-in-Aid for Scientific Research (A) (24249060 and 151402548) (to S.H.), a Grant-in-Aid for Challenging Exploratory Research (25670481) (to S.H.), and Bilateral Joint Research Projects (to S.H.) from the Japan Society for the Promotion of Science (JSPS); Grants for Scientific Research on Innovative Areas (221S0002 and 25129708) (to A.I and S.H.) from the Ministry of Education, Culture, Sports, Science and Technology (MEXT); the MEXT-supported Program for the Strategic Research Foundation at Private Universities 2013–17 (to S.H.); a grant for Practical Research Project for Rare/Intractable Diseases (15ek0109038a) from the Japan Agency for Medical Research and Development (AMED); a Grant-in-Aid for the Research on Measures for Intractable Diseases (H26-Nanji-Ippan-051 and 049) (to S.H.) from the Ministry of Health, Labor and Welfare; an Intramural Research Grant (24-7 and 27-5) for Neurological and Psychiatric Disorders of NCNP (to S.H.); the Joint Usage/Research Program of Medical Research Institute, Tokyo Medical and Dental University (to S.H.); and grants from the Mitsubishi Foundation (to S.H.) and Takeda Scientific Foundation (to S.H.), the Kobayashi Magobei Foundation (to A.I.), and the Kurozumi Medical Foundation (to A.I.); and a Japan Epilepsy Research Foundation Grant (to A.I.).

REFERENCES

1. Neilson DE, Adams MD, Orr CM, et al. Infection-triggered familial or recurrent cases of acute necrotizing encephalopathy caused by mutations in a component of the nuclear pore, RANBP2. *Am J Human Genet.* 2009;84(1): 44–51.
2. Seo HE, Hwang SK, Choe BH, Cho MH, Park SP, Kwon S. Clinical spectrum and prognostic factors of acute necrotizing encephalopathy in children. *J Korean Med Sci.* 2010;25(3):449–453.
3. Oh HH, Kwon SH, Kim CW, et al. Molecular analysis of HLA class II-associated susceptibility to neuroinflammatory diseases in Korean children. *J Korean Med Sci.* 2004;19(3):426–430.
4. Hoshino A, Saitoh M, Miyagawa T, et al. Specific HLA genotypes confer susceptibility to acute necrotizing encephalopathy. *Genes Immun.* 2016;17(6):367–369.
5. Hidaka F, Matsuo S, Muta T, Takeshige K, Mizukami T, Nunoi H. A missense mutation of the Toll-like receptor 3 gene in a patient with influenza-associated encephalopathy. *Clin Immunol.* 2006;119(2):188–194.
6. Zhang SY, Jouanguy E, Ugolini S, et al. TLR3 deficiency in patients with herpes simplex encephalitis. *Science.* 2007; 317(5844):1522–1527.
7. Casrouge A, Zhang SY, Eidenschenk C, et al. Herpes simplex virus encephalitis in human UNC-93B deficiency. *Science.* 2006;314(5797):308–312.
8. Akira S, Takeda K. Toll-like receptor signalling. *Nat Rev Immunol.* 2004;4(7):499–511.
9. Kim YM, Brinkmann MM, Paquet ME, Ploegh HL. UNC93B1 delivers nucleotide-sensing toll-like receptors to endolysosomes. *Nature.* 2008;452(7184):234–238.
10. Saitoh M, Kobayashi K, Ohmori I, et al. Cytokine-related and sodium channel polymorphism as candidate predisposing factors for childhood encephalopathy FIRES/AERRPS. *J Neurol Sci.* 2016;368:272–276.
11. Hoshino A, Saitoh M, Kubota M, et al. HLA variants and cytokine gene polymorphisms confer susceptibility to acute necrotizing encephalopathy. G-06 at International Symposium on Acute Encephalopathy in Infancy and Its Related Diorders (ISAE2016) in Tokyo, Jul 1-3, 2016.
12. Ishii A, Watkins JC, Chen D, Hirose S, Hammer MF. Clinical implications of *SCN1A* missense and truncation variants in a large Japanese cohort with Dravet syndrome. *Epilepsia,* 2017;58(2):282–290.
13. Lossin C. A catalog of *SCN1A* variants. *Brain Dev.* 2009; 31(2):114–130.
14. Shi X, Yasumoto S, Kurahashi H, et al. Clinical spectrum of *SCN2A* mutations. *Brain Dev.* 2012;34(7):541–545.
15. Chipaux M, Villeneuve N, Sabouraud P, et al. Unusual consequences of status epilepticus in Dravet syndrome. *Seizure.* 2010;19(3):190–194.
16. Takayanagi M, Haginoya K, Umehara N, et al. Acute encephalopathy with a truncation mutation in the *SCN1A* gene: a case report. *Epilepsia.* 2010;51(9):1886–1888.

17. Tang S, Lin JP, Hughes E, Siddiqui A, Lim M, Lascelles K. Encephalopathy and *SCN1A* mutations. *Epilepsia.* 2011; 52(4):e26–e30.
18. Okumura A, Uematsu M, Imataka G, et al. Acute encephalopathy in children with Dravet syndrome. *Epilepsia.* 2012; 53(1):79–86.
19. Berkovic SF, Harkin L, McMahon JM, et al. De-novo mutations of the sodium channel gene *SCN1A* in alleged vaccine encephalopathy: a retrospective study. *The Lancet Neurol.* 2006;5(6):488–492.
20. Saitoh M, Shinohara M, Hoshino H, et al. Mutations of the *SCN1A* gene in acute encephalopathy. *Epilepsia.* 2012;53(3):558–564.
21. Kobayashi K, Ohzono H, Shinohara M, et al. Acute encephalopathy with a novel point mutation in the *SCN2A* gene. *Epilepsy Res.* 2012;102(1–2):109–112.
22. Saitoh M, Ishii A, Ihara Y, et al. Missense mutations in sodium channel *SCN1A* and *SCN2A* predispose children to encephalopathy with severe febrile seizures. *Epilepsy Res.* 2015;117:1–6.
23. Saitoh M, Shinohara M, Ishii A, et al. Clinical and genetic features of acute encephalopathy in children taking theophylline. *Brain Dev.* 2015;37(5):463–470.
24. Persson CG, Andersson KE, Kjellin G. Effects of enprofylline and theophylline may show the role of adenosine. *Life Sci.* 1986;38(12):1057–1072.
25. Jacobson KA, von Lubitz DK, Daly JW, Fredholm BB. Adenosine receptor ligands: differences with acute versus chronic treatment. *Trends Pharmacol Sci.* 1996;17(3): 108–113.
26. Aslanukov A, Bhowmick R, Guruju M, et al. RanBP2 modulates Cox11 and hexokinase I activities and haploinsufficiency of RanBP2 causes deficits in glucose metabolism. *PLoS Genet.* 2006;2(10):e177.
27. Chen Y, Wang Y, Yu H, Wang F, Xu W. The cross talk between protein kinase A- and RhoA-mediated signaling in cancer cells. *Exp Biol Med (maywood).* 2005;230(10): 731–741.
28. Yao D, Mizuguchi H, Yamaguchi M, et al. Thermal instability of compound variants of carnitine palmitoyltransferase II and impaired mitochondrial fuel utilization in influenza-associated encephalopathy. *Hum Mutation.* 2008;29(5):718–727.
29. Shinohara M, Saitoh M, Takanashi J, et al. Carnitine palmitoyl transferase II polymorphism is associated with multiple syndromes of acute encephalopathy with various infectious diseases. *Brain Dev.* 2011;33(6):512–517.
30. Mak CM, Lam CW, Fong NC, et al. Fatal viral infection-associated encephalopathy in two Chinese boys: a genetically determined risk factor of thermolabile carnitine palmitoyltransferase II variants. *J Human Genet.* 2011;56(8):617–621.
31. Yao M, Yao D, Yamaguchi M, Chida J, Yao D, Kido H. Bezafibrate upregulates carnitine palmitoyltransferase II expression and promotes mitochondrial energy crisis dissipation in fibroblasts of patients with influenza-associated encephalopathy. *Mol Genet Metab.* 2011;104(3):265–272.
32. Yao M, Cai M, Yao D, et al. Abbreviated half-lives and impaired fuel utilization in carnitine palmitoyltransferase II variant fibroblasts. *PLoS One.* 2015;10(3):e0119936.
33. Yao D, Yao M, Yamaguchi M, Chida J, Kido H. Characterization of compound missense mutation and deletion of carnitine palmitoyltransferase II in a patient with adenovirus-associated encephalopathy. *J Med Invest.* 2011;58(3–4):210–218.
34. Yamane K, Indalao IL, Chida J, Yamamoto Y, Hanawa M, Kido H. Diisopropylamine dichloroacetate, a novel pyruvate dehydrogenase kinase 4 inhibitor, as a potential therapeutic agent for metabolic disorders and multiorgan failure in severe influenza. *PLoS One.* 2014;9(5):e98032.
35. Kubota M, Chida J, Hoshino H, et al. Thermolabile CPT II variants and low blood ATP levels are closely related to severity of acute encephalopathy in Japanese children. *Brain Dev.* 2012;34(1):20–27.

CHAPTER 7

Neuroimaging on Pediatric Encephalopathy in Japan

JUN-ICHI TAKANASHI, MD, PHD

INTRODUCTION

Encephalitis, defined as inflammation of the brain, has a wide range of central nervous system (CNS) manifestations, i.e., consciousness disturbance, seizures, and delirious behavior. Some viruses, such as herpes simplex virus or Japanese encephalitis virus, directly invade the CNS, and cause encephalitis. Acute encephalopathy is the generic term for acute CNS dysfunction caused by various agents, such as infection, metabolic disease, and hepatic or renal dysfunction. The pathologic substrate of acute encephalopathy is diffuse or widespread, noninflammatory brain edema. Thus, inflammatory cells are not usually found in the brain or cerebrospinal fluid (CSF).[1] In Japan, acute encephalopathy in children is usually preceded by infection, most often by influenza virus (27%), or human herpesviruses (HHV) 6 and 7 (18%).[1,2]

Magnetic resonance imaging (MRI) is a sensitive and nonradiological technique for the diagnosis of encephalitis/encephalopathy; diffusion-weighted imaging (DWI) is particularly useful for detecting early changes. In this paper, I review three infectious encephalitis/encephalopathy syndromes, in which neuroimaging, especially MRI, is essential for the diagnosis.

ACUTE ENCEPHALOPATHY WITH BIPHASIC SEIZURES AND LATE REDUCED DIFFUSION

Clinical Features of Acute Encephalopathy With Biphasic Seizures and Late Reduced Diffusion (Fig. 7.1)

The details of AESD have been given in another chapter (Section 4; Shiomi M. et al.); therefore, I summarize here the clinical features of AESD.

AESD is the most common subtype of infectious encephalopathy in Japan (29%),[2] occurring in about 200 Japanese children (most often around 1 year of age) per year. HHV 6 and 7 (40%) and influenza virus (10%) are the most common pathogens for AESD. Patients with AESD have never been reported from countries other than Japan, including South Korea and Taiwan. AESD is clinically characterized by a biphasic course, that is, a prolonged febrile seizure (early seizure) on days 1–2, followed by late seizures (most often in clusters of complex partial seizures) associated with deterioration of the consciousness level on days 4–6.[3,4] Between the biphasic seizures, most patients exhibit continuous disturbance of the consciousness level, but some patients (around 20%) exhibit normal, clear consciousness with no neurologic symptoms. These findings may lead to an initial misdiagnosis of the febrile seizure status and a delay in initiating therapy. The overall outcome of patients with AESD has been reported to be almost normal (29%), mild to moderately disabled (41%), and severe disabled (25%), which includes intellectual and motor disability, and epilepsy (sometimes intractable). The mortality rate is relatively low (<2%) for AESD.[1]

Radiologic Features of Acute Encephalopathy With Biphasic Seizures and Late Reduced Diffusion (Box 7.1)

MRI reveals delayed reduced diffusion in the subcortical white matter, which is one of the diagnostic criteria of AESD.[3,4] The initial MRI performed within 2 days usually shows no abnormal lesion, including on DWI (Fig. 7.2A). Subcortical white matter lesions are observed between days 3 and 9 and are most obvious on DWI (Fig. 7.2B), which is called the bright tree appearance. The apparent diffusion coefficient (ADC) map shows reduced diffusion of the subcortical lesions (Fig. 7.2C). T2-weighted imaging (T2WI) or fluid-attenuated inversion recovery (FLAIR) imaging show linear high intensity along the U-fibers (Fig. 7.2D), and

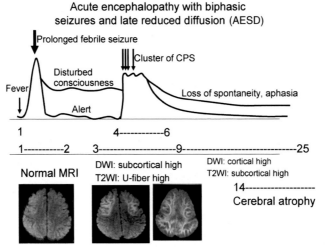

FIG. 7.1 Clinical and radiologic schema of acute encephalopathy with biphasic seizures and late reduced diffusion (AESD). This figure shows the temporal relationship among the seizures, the level of consciousness, and the magnetic resonance imaging (MRI) findings. *CPS*, complex partial seizures; *T2WI*, T2-weighted imaging. (From Takanashi J. Two newly proposed encephalitis/encephalopathy syndromes. *Brain Dev.* 2009;31:521–528 with permission.)

BOX 7.1
Neuroimaging Findings Characteristic of Encephalopathy Syndromes

1. Acute encephalopathy with biphasic seizures and late reduced diffusion (AESD).

   a. No abnormal lesion within 2 days.

   b. Subcortical white matter lesions between days 3 and 9, which is most obvious on DWI (bright tree appearance). The lesions are predominantly frontal or frontoparietal in location with sparing of the peri-Rolandic region (central sparing).

   c. After 9 days, the bright tree appearance on DWI has disappeared, and T2WI or FLAIR imaging show high-intensity lesions with central sparing, and cerebral atrophy.

   d. MRS shows acute Glu elevation (days 1–4), changing to subacute Gln elevation (days 4–12).

2. Clinically mild encephalitis/encephalopathy with a reversible splenial lesion (MERS).

   a. A reversible lesion in the corpus callosum, at least in the splenium, with homogenously reduced diffusion (type 1 MERS).

   b. A splenial lesion is sometimes associated with ones in the symmetrical white matter (usually close to the central sulcus), both of which are also reversible (type 2 MERS).

3. Acute necrotizing encephalopathy (ANE).

   a. Diffuse cerebral edema and symmetric and multifocal lesions in the thalamus and other CNS regions, including the posterior limb of the internal capsule, posterior putamen, cerebral and cerebellar deep white matter, and upper brainstem tegmentum.

   b. The thalamic lesions often show hemorrhagic degeneration and cystic change after 3 days, showing a high signal on T1WI and a low signal on T2WI or T2 star-weighted imaging.

---

cortical hyperintensity is less prominent than U-fiber abnormality. The lesions are predominantly frontal or frontoparietal in location with sparing of the peri-Rolandic region (central sparing); they are usually symmetric, but sometimes asymmetric (a clinical diagnosis

of hemiconvulsion hemiplegia epilepsy [HHE] syndrome is often given for these patients).

The subcortical white matter lesions (the bright tree appearance) are not observed on follow-up after 9 days (Fig. 7.2E).[3,4] High signal intensity in the cortex

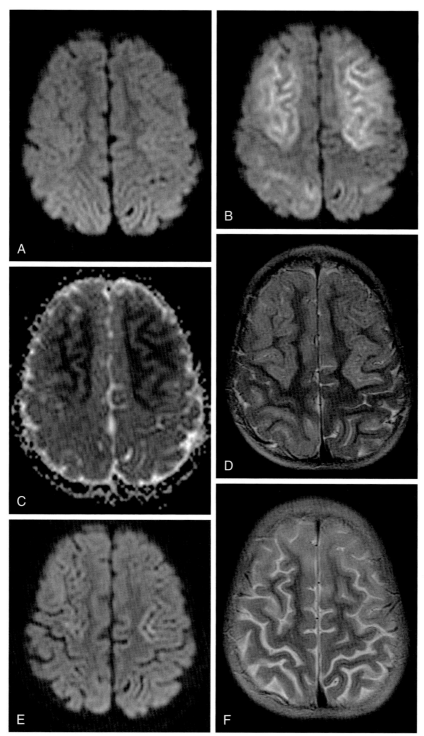

FIG. 7.2 Magnetic resonance imaging (MRI) of a 1-year-old girl with acute encephalopathy with biphasic seizures and late reduced diffusion (AESD). Diffusion-weighted imaging (DWI) on day 1 shows no acute lesion **(A)**, but shows high intensity lesions in the bilateral frontal subcortical white matter **(B)** with homogenously reduced diffusion **(C)** on day 4, so-called bright tree appearance. T2-weighted imaging (T2WI) **(D)** shows cortical swelling and high-intensity lesions in the cortex and U-fibers. DWI on day 20 **(E)** shows no bright tree appearance with cerebral atrophy on T2WI **(F)**.

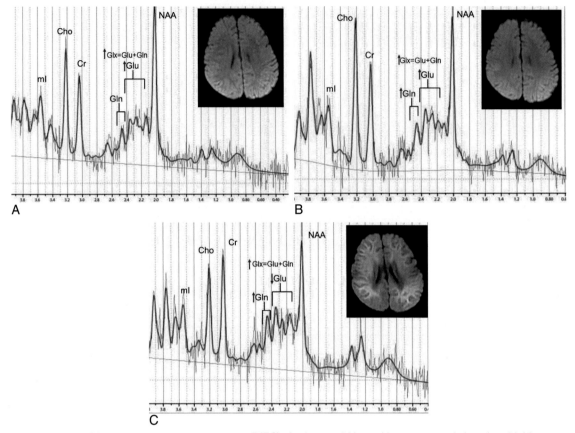

FIG. 7.3 Magnetic resonance spectroscopy (MRS) of a 1-year-old boy with acute encephalopathy with bi-phasic seizures and late reduced diffusion (AESD). MRS of the frontal white matter shows increased Glx on day 1 (**A**, increased glutamate [Glu] and normal glutamine [Gln]), on day 4 (**B**, both increased Glu and Gln), and on day 8 (**C**, decreased Glu and increased Gln). (From Takanashi J, Mizuguchi M, Terai M, Barkovich AJ. Disrupted glutamate-glutamine cycle in acute encephalopathy with biphasic seizures and late reduced diffusion. *Neuroradiology*. 2015;57:1163–1168 with permission.)

overlying the affected subcortical white matter can be observed on DWI on days 9–25. The ADC maps show increased diffusion within the subcortical white matter at this time. T2WI or FLAIR imaging at this stage show the subcortical white matter lesions with central sparing and cerebral atrophy (Fig. 7.2F).

Magnetic Resonance Spectroscopy Findings and Hypothesis for the Pathogenesis of Acute Encephalopathy With Biphasic Seizures and Late Reduced Diffusion

The exact pathogenesis of AESD is uncertain; however, excitotoxic injury with delayed neuronal death is hypothesized as a possible mechanism based on MR spectroscopy (MRS).[5,6] MRS shows glutamate (Glu) and glutamine (Gln) complex (Glx) elevation on days

1–8, i.e., from the acute stage before the bright tree appearance on DWI, and normal or low levels afterward. The elevation of Glx consists of two phases, that is, acute Glu elevation (days 1–4) (Fig. 7.3A) changing to subacute Gln elevation (days 4–12) (Fig. 7.3B and C).[6] The acute Glu elevation corresponds to the clinical stage of the early seizure and consciousness disturbance between biphasic seizures, and the subacute Gln elevation almost corresponds to the clinical stage of late seizures and secondary deterioration of the consciousness level with the bright tree appearance on DWI.

Glutamatergic neurons in the human cerebral cortex release Glu (excitatory neurotransmitter) into the synaptic cleft, where it is taken up by surrounding astrocytes through glutamate transporters to maintain a proper Glu concentration in synapses.[7] Glu taken up by nearby astrocytes is amidated to a harmless compound, Gln, by glutamine synthetase (located only in astrocytes), and returned to the neurons for reuse as Glu, completing the Glu (in neuron)-Gln (in astrocyte) cycle. Astrocytes are, therefore, thought to be neuroprotective because of their ability to convert extracellular Glu into Gln.[8] The MRS finding in AESD patients of acute Glu elevation changing to subacute Gln elevation may reflect the process, in which excessive Glu changes into Gln in astrocytes, and strengthen the hypothesis of hyperexcitotoxicity as a pathogenesis of AESD.

MRS in patients with AESD also reveals decreased *N*-acetylaspartate (NAA), a marker for neuroaxonal function, within a week after the onset of AESD. Afterward, NAA remains low in patients with neurologic sequelae but becomes nearly normalized in those without neurologic sequelae. This suggests that MRS might be predictive of the outcome of AESD. Elevated Glx and decreased NAA observed on MRS may be useful for an early diagnosis of AESD, because AESD is sometimes difficult to distinguish from the febrile seizure status.

CLINICALLY MILD ENCEPHALITIS/ ENCEPHALOPATHY WITH A REVERSIBLE SPLENIAL LESION

Clinical Features of Clinically Mild Encephalitis/Encephalopathy With a Reversible Splenial Lesion

Because MERS is not described in other chapters of this book, I will present the clinical and radiologic features of MERS.

A reversible splenial lesion with homogenously reduced diffusion is observed in some conditions, including high-altitude cerebral edema, patients taking antiepileptic drugs (AEDs), most often when AEDs are being reduced rapidly, and patients with Kawasaki disease, X-linked Charcot-Marie-Tooth disease, etc.[4,9] MERS is an infectious mild encephalitis/encephalopathy, characterized by a reversible lesion of the corpus callosum involving at least the splenium (type 1 MERS), sometimes associated with symmetrical white matter lesions (type 2 MERS).[4,9–12] MERS is the second most common subtype of encephalopathy syndrome (16%), occurring in about 120 children per year.[2] The mean age for MERS is 5 years, which is later than those for ANE (2 years) and AESD (1 year).[2]

Among 54 Japanese patients with MERS (26 males and 28 females; mean age at onset, 9 years), collected from multiple centers, the most common neurologic symptom was delirious behavior in 54%, followed by consciousness disturbance in 35%, and seizures in

33%, all patients showing complete recovery within a month.[4] The onset of neurologic symptoms occurred between days 1 and 3 after the prodromal symptoms in 71%. Influenza viruses A and B (34%) were the most common pathogens, followed by rotavirus (12%) and mumps virus (4%), although the pathogen for MERS was unknown in 33%. As a treatment for MERS, steroids were the most frequently used in 16 of the 54 patients (10 with methylprednisolone pulse therapy, 6 with dexamethasone), followed by antiepileptic drugs in 12 patients, acyclovir in 11, and intravenous immunoglobulin in 8.[4] On the other hand, 19 patients receive no specific treatment; however, all patients with MERS clinically recovered completely within a month, irrespective of the treatment. It is, therefore, difficult to conclude the necessity of treatment for MERS. According to an epidemiologic study of acute encephalopathy in Japan,[2] the prognosis of MERS is complete recovery in 90%, and mild to moderate disability in 10% of patients.

The CSF cell count is increased (cell count >10/ mm³) in 13 of 43 patients so examined,[4] leading to a diagnosis of encephalitis rather than encephalopathy. This is why MERS includes encephalitis in addition to encephalopathy. Hyponatremia is more often observed in patients with MERS (28 patients, 131.8 ± 4.1 mmol/L) than in ones with upper respiratory infection (138.3 ± 2.7 mmol/L), other types of encephalopathy (136.6 ± 2.5 mmol/L), and febrile seizures (136.2 ± 2.6 mmol/L).[13] EEG abnormality is found in around half of the patients with MERS (21/39 patients), including diffuse slow waves in 17 patients, occipital slow waves in 4, and focal spikes in 2.[4] EEG abnormalities are usually normalized on follow-up.

Radiologic Features of Clinically Mild Encephalitis/Encephalopathy With a Reversible Splenial Lesion (Box 7.1)

Among 54 patients with MERS, 45 were classified as type 1 with the lesion in the corpus callosum, at least in the splenium, including 40 patients with an isolated lesion in the splenium (Fig. 7.4), 3 with ones in the splenium plus genu, and another 2 with an entire callosal lesion.[4] The other 9 patients were classified as type 2, having lesions in both the corpus callosum and symmetrical white matter, usually located close to the central sulcus.[4,12] Type 2 MERS with reduced diffusion in the diffuse white matter and entire carpus callosum has been otherwise reported as "transient encephalopathy with reversible white matter lesions in children."[14] All these lesions show homogenously reduced diffusion (high signal on DWI) (Fig. 7.4A) with no contrast

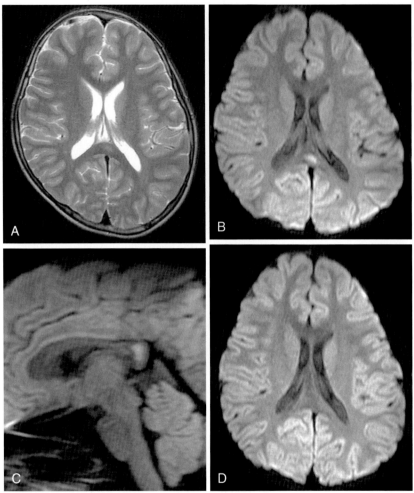

FIG. 7.4 Magnetic resonance imaging (MRI) of a 10-year-old boy with clinically mild encephalitis/encephalopathy with a reversible splenial lesion (MERS) associated with influenza A. A splenial lesion is more obvious on diffusion-weighted imaging (DWI) than T2-weighted imaging (T2WI) on day 4, which has disappeared completely on day 30 (D).

enhancement and have completely disappeared on follow-up MRI (between 3 days and 2 months) (Fig. 7.4D). The time course differed between the splenial and white matter lesions; the latter disappeared earlier than the former.[15] These findings suggest that type 2 MERS resolves completely through MERS type 1 with an isolated splenial lesion.

A reversible splenial lesion is sometimes observed in patients with rotavirus gastroenteritis (Fig. 7.5). Most patients show complete clinical and radiologic recovery; however, some patients have following cerebellitis and finally neurologic sequelae, and MRI findings of cerebellar involvement in spite of complete resolution

of the splenial lesion[16] (Fig. 7.5B–D). It is, therefore, important to recognize that a splenial lesion in patients with gastroenteritis is not always a benign indicator predicting complete recovery.

Hypothesis for the Pathogenesis of Clinically Mild Encephalitis/Encephalopathy With a Reversible Splenial Lesion

The reason for the transiently reduced diffusion within the lesions is unknown; we have proposed some pathomechanisms, including transient development of intramyelinic edema due to separation of myelin layers.[10] Increased choline in a splenial lesion observed on

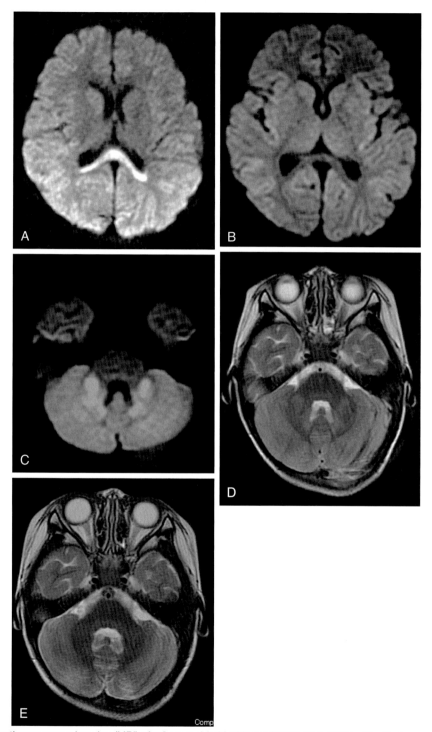

FIG. 7.5 Magnetic resonance imaging (MRI) of a 3-year-old girl with cerebellitis associated with rotavirus gastroenteritis. Diffusion-weighted imaging (DWI) on day 4 **(A)** shows a splenium lesion, compatible with type 1 clinically mild encephalitis/encephalopathy with a reversible splenial lesion (MERS), which has disappeared on day 6 **(B)**. DWI shows abnormally reduced diffusion in the bilateral middle cerebellar peduncles and cerebellar nuclei **(C)**. T2-weighted imaging (T2WI) also shows mild hyperintensity in the cerebellar cortex, in addition to the middle cerebellar peduncle and nuclear lesions **(D)**. MRI on day 65 shows an almost normal cerebellum other than mild atrophy **(E)**. (From Takanashi J, Miyamoto T, Ando N, et al. Clinical and radiological features of rotavirus cerebellitis. *AJNR Am J Neuroradiol*. 2010;31:1591–1295 with permission.)

MRS may support this hypothesis (unpublished data). A reversible splenial lesion, however, has been reported in a 12-day-old neonate.[17] At that age, the splenium is still completely unmyelinated; therefore, another mechanism must be responsible for the reduced diffusion, at least in some patients. As the axons in the splenium are so tightly packed, it is possible that interstitial edema (water between the unmyelinated axons) could have reduced diffusion. Another possible explanation is the development of a transient inflammatory infiltrate, which might cause reduced diffusion, as observed in the active lesion in multiple sclerosis.

RADIOLOGIC FEATURES OF ACUTE NECROTIZING ENCEPHALOPATHY (BOX 7.1)

ANE is described in detail in Section 4; therefore, I will briefly present the radiologic aspects of ANE. ANE was the first encephalopathy syndrome in which the neuroimaging findings in the thalamus are essential for a diagnosis.[1] In the acute stage, CT or MRI shows diffuse cerebral edema and symmetric and multifocal lesions (low density on CT, T1 low/T2 high on MRI) (Fig. 7.6A and B) in the thalamus and other CNS regions, including the posterior limb of the internal capsule, posterior putamen, cerebral and cerebellar deep white matter, and upper brainstem tegmentum. DWI shows reduced diffusion of the acute thalamic lesions (Fig. 7.6C), which is useful for the differential diagnosis of acute disseminating encephalomyelitis, often involving the bilateral thalamus. The thalamic lesions often show hemorrhagic degeneration and a cystic change in the course of ANE. Reflecting petechial hemorrhage, T1WI shows high signal ringlike or circular high signal lesions in the thalamus after 3 days (Fig. 7.6D), some of which show a low signal on T2WI (Fig. 7.6E). The MRI score (positive number of the presence of hemorrhage, cavitation, brainstem lesion, and white matter lesion) has been reported to exhibit a positive correlation to the clinical outcome.[18]

ABBREVIATIONS

ANE   Acute necrotizing encephalopathy
AESD Acute encephalopathy with biphasic seizures and late reduced diffusion
MERS Clinically mild encephalitis/encephalopathy with a reversible splenial lesion
MRI   Magnetic resonance imaging
DWI   Diffusion-weighted imaging
MRS   Magnetic resonance spectroscopy

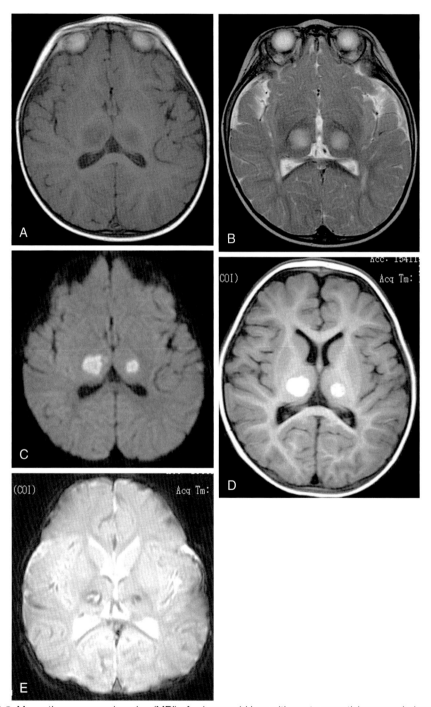

FIG. 7.6 Magnetic resonance imaging (MRI) of a 1-year-old boy with acute necrotizing encephalopathy (ANE). MRI on day 4 shows bilateral symmetric thalamic lesions (low on T1-weighted imaging [T1WI] **(A)**, high on T2-weighted imaging [T2WI] **(B)**) with reduced diffusion **(C)**. MRI on day 14 shows high intensity on T1WI **(D)** with partly low intensity on T2 star-weighted imaging **(E)**, suggesting hemorrhagic degeneration.

REFERENCES

1. Mizuguchi M, Yamanouchi H, Ichiyama T, Shiomi A. Acute encephalopathy associated with influenza and other viral infections. *Acta Neurol Scand.* 2007;115:45–56.
2. Hoshino A, Saitoh M, Oka A, et al. Epidemiology of acute encephalopathy in Japan, with emphasis on the association of viruses and syndrome. *Brain Dev.* 2012;34:337–343.
3. Takanashi J, Oba H, Barkovich AJ, et al. Diffusion MRI abnormalities after prolonged febrile seizures with encephalopathy. *Neurology.* 2006;66:1304–1309.
4. Takanashi J. Two newly proposed encephalitis/encephalopathy syndromes. *Brain Dev.* 2009;31:521–528.
5. Takanashi J, Tada H, Terada H, Barkovich AJ. Excitotoxicity in acute encephalopathy with biphasic seizures and late reduced diffusion. Report of 3 cases. *AJNR Am J Neuroradiol.* 2009;30:132–135.
6. Takanashi J, Mizuguchi M, Terai M, Barkovich AJ. Disrupted glutamate-glutamine cycle in acute encephalopathy with biphasic seizures and late reduced diffusion. *Neuroradiology.* 2015;57:1163–1168.
7. Zhou Y, Danbolt C. Glutamate as a neurotransmitter in the healthy brain. *J Neurol Transm.* 2014;121:799–817.
8. Agarwal N, Renshaw PF. Proton MR spectroscopy-detectable major neurotransmitters of the brain: biology and possible clinical applications. *Am J Neuroradiol AJNR.* 2012;33:595–602.
9. Takanashi J, Shirai K, Sugawara Y, Okamoto Y, Obonai T, Terada H. Kawasaki disease complicated by mild encephalopathy with a reversible splenial lesion (MERS). *J Neurol Sci.* 2012;315:167–169.
10. Tada H, Takanashi J, Barkovich AJ, et al. Clinically mild encephalitis/encephalopathy with a reversible splenial lesion. *Neurology.* 2004;63:1854–1858.
11. Takanashi J, Barkovich AJ, Yamaguchi K, Kohno Y. Influenza-associated encephalitis/encephalopathy with a reversible lesion in the splenium of the corpus callosum: a case report and literature review. *AJNR Am J Neuroradiol.* 2004;25:798–802.
12. Takanashi J, Barkovich AJ, Shiihara T, et al. Widening spectrum of a reversible splenial lesion with transiently reduced diffusion. *AJNR Am J Neuroradiol.* 2006;27:836–838.
13. Takanashi J, Tada H, Maeda M, Suzuki M, Terada H, Barkovich AJ. Encephalopathy with a reversible splenial lesion is associated with hyponatremia. *Brain Dev.* 2009;31:217–220.
14. Okumura A, Noda E, Ikuta T, et al. Transient encephalopathy with reversible white matter lesions in children. *Neuropediatrics.* 2006;37:159–162.
15. Takanashi J, Imamura A, Hayakawa F, Terada H. Differences in the time course of splenial and white matter lesions in clinically mild encephalitis/encephalopathy with a reversible splenial lesion (MERS). *J Neurol Sci.* 2010;292:24–27.
16. Takanashi J, Miyamoto T, Ando N, et al. Clinical and radiological features of rotavirus cerebellitis. *AJNR Am J Neuroradiol.* 2010;31:1591–1595.
17. Takanashi J, Maeda M, Hayashi M. A neonate showing a reversible splenial lesion. *Arch Neurol.* 2005;62:1481–1482.
18. Wong AM, Simon EM, Zimmerman RA, Wang HS, Toh CH, Ng SH. Acute necrotizing encephalopathy of childhood: correlation of MR findings and clinical outcome. *AJNR Am J Neuroradiol.* 2006;27:1919–1923.

Electroencephalography in Children With Acute Encephalitis/Encephalopathy

AKIHISA OKUMURA, MD, PHD

INTRODUCTION

Electroencephalography (EEG) has been widely accepted as one of the useful methods for diagnosis and monitoring for children with acute encephalitis/encephalopathy (AE). One of the advantages of EEG is to evaluate real-time brain function by recording electrical activities of the brain. In this view, there are no alternative methods. Electroencephalograph has become digitized, compact, and paperless according to technical advance. This has made long-time bedside EEG monitoring much easier. In some children with AE, general condition can be seriously ill and unstable. EEG monitoring can be performed even in such cases. Recently, several authors have published reports on the long-term EEG monitoring in seriously ill children with impaired consciousness including those with AE. The usefulness of long-term EEG monitoring is being elucidated. In addition, quantitative EEG such as amplitude-integrated EEG (aEEG) has been applied to continuous brain function monitoring in children. Easy recording and interpretation are a prominent advantage of quantitative EEG. In this review, usefulness of various types of EEG is described.

CONVENTIONAL ELECTROENCEPHALOGRAPHY IN CHILDREN WITH ACUTE ENCEPHALOPATHY

There have been many reports on conventional EEG findings in children with AE.[1–12] These studies have invariably shown that EEG abnormalities are very frequent in children with AE. Therefore, EEG is considered to be useful for the diagnosis of AE. Several different types of EEG abnormalities have been reported, including generalized/unilateral/focal slowing, low voltage, periodic lateralized epileptiform discharges (PLEDs), and paroxysmal discharges.

Generalized Slowing

Generalized slowing will be the most frequent EEG abnormalities in children with AE (Fig. 8.1). Mohammad et al. studied EEG findings in children with various types of AE and stated that 69 of 119 children had generalized slowing in their first EEG with some additional focal dominance in 16.[1] Among children with acute necrotizing encephalopathy (ANE), EEG during the acute stage was dominated by diffuse 1–6 Hz slow waves except in brain dead patients.[2] In children with acute encephalopathy with biphasic seizures and late reduced diffusion (AESD), EEG within 24 h after onset demonstrated continuous delta activities in two of four children.[3] In children with acute encephalitis with refractory, repetitive partial seizures (AERRPS), EEG before the initiation of treatment showed high-voltage slow background activity in 7 of 9 children.[4] Seven of eleven children with acute encephalitis due to *Mycoplasma pneumoniae* had generalized slowing.[5] Six of eleven children with Epstein-Barr virus encephalitis had generalized slowing on EEG.[6] These results indicate that generalized slowing is very frequent in children with acute encephalopathy caused by several different infections and showing different clinical phenotypes. Generalized slowing may be useful for the diagnosis of AE, whereas it is nonspecific abnormalities that can be observed in children with other types of brain injury such as hypoxic-ischemic encephalopathy, drug intoxication, and metabolic derangement.

Unilateral or Focal Slowing

Some children with AE can have focal or hemispheric lesions. In such cases, EEG often shows unilateral or focal slowing (Fig. 8.2). Some children with AESD show unilateral involvement on neuroimaging studies.[7] EEG recorded during the acute phase in six children with unilateral AESD demonstrated marked slowing in the

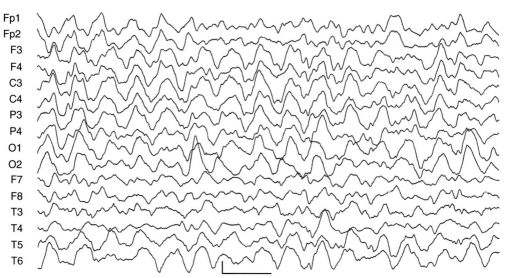

FIG. 8.1 Generalized slowing. Electroencephalography at the first day of illness of a 1-year-old child with severe acute encephalopathy with biphasic seizures and late reduced diffusion. High-voltage irregular slow waves are continuously observed. Calibration 100 µV, 1 s.

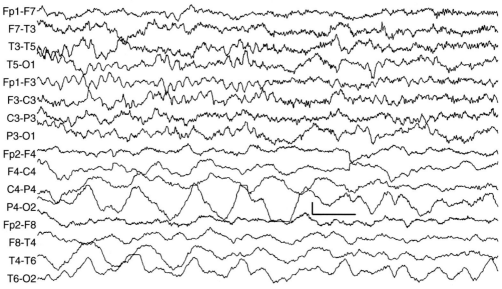

FIG. 8.2 Unilateral slowing. Electroencephalography at the second day of illness of a 1-year-old child with unilateral acute encephalopathy with biphasic seizures and late reduced diffusion. Slowing and decrease in fact activities are seen in the right hemisphere. Calibration 100 µV, 1 s.

affected hemisphere in one patient and mild slowing in the affected hemisphere in four patients. Focal slowing is not uncommon in children with herpes simplex encephalitis.[8] In the study by Mohammad et al., focal slowing in the first EEG was observed in 7 children, hemispheric slowing in 3, and bilateral focal slowing in 13.[1]

Low Voltage

Low-voltage background EEG activities are sometimes observed in children with AE (Fig. 8.3). In most severely affected children, extremely low-voltage or isoelectric EEG can be observed.[2,9] Neuroimaging studies often show severe brain edema with herniation in such children and their outcome is poor. Most children

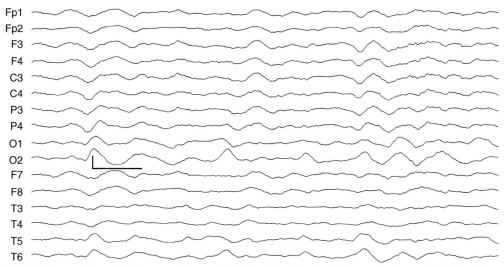

FIG. 8.3 Low voltage. Electroencephalography (EEG) at the first day of illness of a 1-year-old child with acute encephalopathy with acute brain edema. EEG showed intermittent low voltage slow waves alone. Calibration 100 μV, 1 s.

die or survive with severe neurologic sequelae. Some children with severe AE can show rapid deterioration of EEG findings along with that of neurologic symptoms. In our experience, EEG became flat within a few hours after the first presentation in some children, who visited hospitals with complicating delirious behavior or mildly altered consciousness. The outcome is poor even in surviving children who had low-voltage EEG. Hosoya et al. reported that low-voltage EEG activities were seen in 5 of 19 children with AE and all of them had epilepsy within a year after discharge.[10] In children with unilateral AESD, low voltage is sometimes observed in the affected hemisphere.[7]

Abnormalities in Fast Activities
Increased fast activities
Extreme delta brush, characterized by a nearly continuous combination of delta activity with superimposed fast activity, usually in the β range, has been reported as a unique EEG abnormality in adults with anti-NMDA receptor encephalitis.[13] The reports on extreme delta brush in children have been limited, and typical extreme delta brush is presumed to be infrequent in children with anti-NMDA receptor encephalitis.[14] Instead, Gitiaux et al. reported that high-amplitude diffuse α-theta rhythms were seen during non-REM sleep associated with a decrease in normal slow waves in some children with anti-NMDA receptor encephalitis.[14] It is well known that fast activities are increased by an administration of benzodiazepines such as diazepam and midazolam. A differentiation between increase in

fast activities due to benzodiazepines and that caused by brain dysfunction is not always easy.

Decreased fast activities
A decrease in fast activities is sometimes observed in children with AE during the acute period (Fig. 8.4). In our preliminary survey, decreased spindles during non-REM sleep were observed in 6 of 9 children with AESD within 48 h after the onset (unpublished data). Oguri et al. reported a decrease in α and β band powers in EEGs of children with AESD within 24 h after the onset using power spectrum analysis.[15]

Periodic Discharges
PLEDs were first described as a characteristic EEG finding in patients with herpes simplex encephalitis. At present, PLEDs have been reported in children and adults with various types of AE.[1,16] Periodic discharges can be observed in both hemispheres. Akman et al. reported generalized periodic epileptiform discharges in critically ill children including those with AE.[17] They reported that the outcome of children with generalized periodic epileptiform discharges was poor.

Paroxysmal Discharges
Paroxysmal discharges have been described in children with AE. In children with AERRPS, paroxysmal discharges were frequently observed.[4,11,12] Lin et al. reported that the initial EEG patterns in children with AERRPS included focal epileptiform discharges in 11.1%, multifocal in 22.2%, and primary multifocal

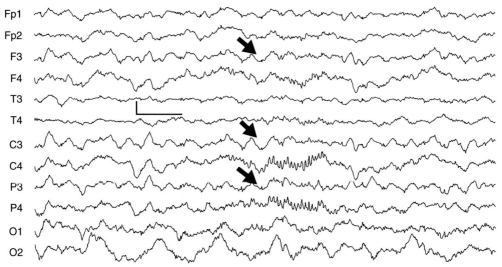

FIG. 8.4 Decreased fast activities. Electroencephalography at the first day of illness of a 1-year-old child with unilateral acute encephalopathy with biphasic seizures and late reduced diffusion. Spindles were not observed in the left hemisphere (*arrows*). Calibration 100 μV, 1 s.

with secondary generalization in 22.2% of the subjects.[11] Mohammad et al. reported that interictal paroxysmal discharges on the initial EEG were frequent in children with febrile infection–related encephalopathy syndrome, but were not observed in children with autoimmune basal ganglia encephalitis or influenza-associated encephalopathy.[1]

Episodic Transients

Intermittent generalized rhythmic delta activity (GRDA) with frontal predominance, formerly called frontal intermittent rhythmic delta activity, is defined as a repetitive appearance of up to 2 s of frontal rhythmic slow wave activity at 4 Hz.[18] Although early studies suggested that intermittent GRDA with frontal predominance is associated with raised intracranial pressure, recent studies indicated that this EEG pattern is observed in a wider range of brain lesions and its relation to AE is unclear.[19] Intermittent GRDA with occipital predominance was also reported in association with AE. This EEG pattern is also considered to be nonspecific at present.[20]

Ictal Changes

Ictal changes can be observed in children with AE. Principally, ictal changes in children with AE are always of focal onset. AERRPS is characterized by frequent repetitive seizures,[4] and ictal changes are almost always observed during the acute period. Electrical storm was reported in children with hemorrhagic shock and encephalopathy syndrome (HSES).[9] Electrical storm is characterized by runs of spike, sharp waves, or often rhythmic activities sometimes gradually increasing or decreasing in rate and frequency associated with changes in morphology with waxing and waning of amplitude. These features are consistent with ictal changes of focal seizures, and electrical storm is presumed to be repetitive focal seizures.

The diagnostic and prognostic values of EEG in children with AE have not been established at present. It is unclear whether or not the diagnosis of AE became more accurate or earlier in relation to EEG recordings. The sensitivity and specificity of EEG for the diagnosis of AE have not been determined until now. It is also unclear whether or not EEG recordings can improve the outcome of children with AE. Although EEG has been considered to be necessary for diagnosis and management of children with AE, its clinical evidence has been insufficient.

EEG findings in children with AE can change according to the timing of the recording, the types and the severity of AE, and causative pathogens. However, no studies have been conducted to clarify the differences in EEG findings according to the timing of the recording or types of AE.

EEG abnormalities are presumed to be more distinct during the acute period when a child had severely impaired consciousness and will become less severe during the convalescent phase. Therefore, EEG abnormalities should be interpreted considering the timing of recording. At present, appropriate timing of EEG recordings has not been elucidated in children with AE. For the purpose of early diagnosis, early EEG recordings are necessary. However, generalized or focal slowing has been reported in children with delirious behavior without AE,[21] immediately after febrile seizures, especially prolonged ones,[22] or other neurologic disorders. The relation between the timing of EEG recordings and their diagnostic value has been unknown in children with AE.

EEG findings will be different according to the types of AE. Markedly low voltage is not infrequent in children with ANE, HSES, or other types of AE with poor outcome. Such EEG findings are not seen in milder types of AE such as clinically mild encephalopathy with reversible splenium lesion. Increased fast activities are often seen in children with anti-NMDA receptor encephalitis. Repetitive ictal activities are distinct in AERRPS or FIRES. However, these characteristic EEG findings are not always to some specific type of AE and can be observed in several different types. The relation between EEG features and the type of AE remains unclear.

These facts indicate that further studies on EEG are necessary to establish its value in children with AE. An accumulation of EEG findings in a large cohort of children with AE and analyses of the relation between EEG findings and clinical, laboratory, neuroimaging, and outcome data will solve several problems. The role that is expected to EEG includes earlier diagnosis of AE, differentiation between AE and febrile seizure and delirious behavior, detection of ictal changes, especially of seizures without obvious clinical symptoms, and prognostication. Prospective multicenter studies will be desirable to establish the diagnostic and prognostic values of EEG in children with AE.

CONTINUOUS ELECTROENCEPHALOGRAPHY MONITORING IN CHILDREN

Continuous multichannel VTR-EEG monitoring has recently been introduced into pediatric intensive care units in North American and European countries. Continuous EEG monitoring is mainly performed in critically ill children with impaired consciousness such as those with brain trauma, stroke, hypoxic-ischemic encephalopathy, and AE. There have been several reports on continuous EEG monitoring findings in critically ill children.[23–26] These reports imply that seizures, especially those without clinical symptoms, are often observed when continuous EEG monitoring is

performed and that a majority of seizures can be overlooked if continuous EEG monitoring is not performed. This is the most important rationale why continuous EEG monitoring is necessary in critically ill children.

Schreiber et al. reported continuous EEG monitoring findings in 94 critically ill children including 4 children with encephalitis.[23] Out of 94 children 28 had seizures captured on continuous VTR-EEG monitoring including 17 patients with nonconvulsive status epilepticus. Variables associated with electrographic seizures were age <24 months and clinical seizures before EEG recordings. Another study demonstrated that electrographic seizures occurred in 46% of critically ill children, and electrographic status epilepticus occurred in 19%.[24] Younger age was associated with an increased risk for seizure occurrence in that study. Topjian et al. investigated whether electrographic seizures and electrographic status epilepticus are associated with higher mortality or worse short-term neurologic outcome of critically ill children.[25] Among 200 children who underwent continuous EEG monitoring including 22 children with encephalitis, 84 had seizures: electrographic seizures in 41 and electrographic status epilepticus in 43. Multivariable analysis showed that electrographic status epilepticus was associated with an increased risk of mortality with an odds ratio of 5.1 (95% confidence interval 1.4–18) and pediatric cerebral performance category worsening with an odds ratio of 17.3 (95% confidence interval 3.7–80), whereas electrographic seizures were not associated with an increased risk of mortality or pediatric cerebral performance category worsening. Abend et al. prospectively studied the impact of continuous EEG monitoring on clinical management in 100 critically ill children including 10 children with central nervous system infection.[26] Continuous EEG monitoring influenced clinical management in 59 of 100 subjects: Antiepileptic drugs were initiated in 28, antiepileptic drugs were escalated in 15, antiepileptic drugs were discontinued in 4, abnormal movements were determined not to be seizures in 16, vital sign fluctuations were determined not to be seizures in 5, and urgent neuroimaging that impacted clinical management in 3.

Background EEG activities can be evaluated in critically ill children using continuous EEG monitoring as well as seizure activities. Kirkham et al. reported continuous EEG monitoring findings in 204 comatose children including 9 children with meningitis, 11 with encephalitis, and 3 with Reyelike syndrome.[27] A large majority of the subjects had background EEG abnormalities such as slowing, low amplitude, burst suppression, and isoelectric. Each type of background EEG

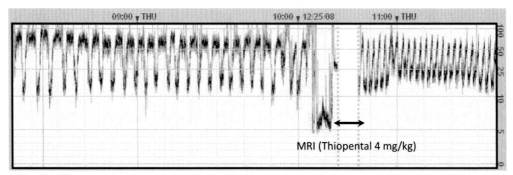

FIG. 8.5 Nonconvulsive status epilepticus on amplitude-integrated electroencephalography (aFEG). aFEG at the fifth day of illness of a 1-year-old child with unilateral acute encephalopathy with biphasic seizures and late reduced diffusion. Repetitive rise-and-falls of aEEG trace indicated clustering seizures, whereas clinical symptoms were not recognized except for reduced responsiveness. (Adapted from Komatsu M, Okumura A, Matsui K, et al. Clustered subclinical seizures in a patient with acute encephalopathy with biphasic seizures and late reduced diffusion. *Brain Dev.* 2010;32:472–6.)

abnormalities correlated with a mortality rate on multivariable analyses. Two other studies also indicated that background EEG abnormalities on continuous EEG monitoring including slowing, discontinuation, burst suppression, and attenuation were associated with an increased mortality risk.[25,28] As to short-term neurologic outcome, Payne et al. described that slow and disorganized background and discontinuous or burst suppression were associated with a worsening of Pediatric Cerebral Performance Category score at hospital discharge on univariable analysis in 259 critically ill children including 30 with central nervous system inflammation or infection.[29] These results suggest that continuous EEG monitoring will be useful for prognostication of critically ill children including those with AE. Although a large majority of the subjects of previous studies on continuous EEG monitoring were children with head trauma, hypoxic-ischemic encephalopathy, stroke, or other acute brain injury other than AE, the results of these studies can be applied to children with AE to some extent.

The limitation of continuous EEG monitoring is resource requirements. To perform continuous EEG monitoring, electroencephalographs and technicians to record EEG are necessary even in holidays and nighttime. EEG should be interpreted by well-trained pediatric neurologists without delay and the results of interpretation should be informed to attending intensivists. These requirements are not easy to be fulfilled in Japan and even in North American and European countries. However, continuous EEG monitoring will provide useful information that may alter management and improve the outcome in children with AE, when it can be performed.

QUANTITATIVE ELECTROENCEPHALOGRAPHY IN CHILDREN

Quantitative EEG techniques separate complex EEG signals into some components such as amplitude and frequency and compress time, permitting display of several hours of data on one image. Quantitative EEG has been applied in critically ill children including those with AE.

aEEG is the most commonly used type of quantitative EEG, especially in neonatal intensive care units. aEEG is a processed electroencephalogram that is filtered and time-compressed. Time is displayed on the x-axis and amplitude on the y-axis. Lower border of y-axis is correlated with minimal amplitude and continuity of EEG activities during an EEG epoch, and upper border with maximal amplitude. Seizures are usually shown as transient rises of lower border of aEEG trace. Application and maintenance of electrodes, and interpretation of aEEG findings are easier than conventional EEG. Therefore, aEEG can allow early recognition of seizures by nonexperts. In term neonates, the relation between aEEG findings and the outcome has been established, whereas it is unclear in older children. We reported aEEG findings in children with AESD[30] and AERRPS.[31] In a child with AESD, aEEG revealed an unexpected cluster of subclinical seizures before an occurrence of clinical seizures during the late clinical phase (Fig. 8.5). aEEG monitoring allowed us to evaluate efficacy of antiepileptic drugs; intravenous diazepam did not alter clustering seizures, and drip infusion of phenytoin stopped the seizures and improved responsiveness. In children with AERRPS, aEEG revealed frequent subclinical seizures that were missed by clinical observation. Efficacy of high-dose phenobarbital was also evaluated objectively by continuous aEEG monitoring.

On color density spectral array (CDSA), time is displayed on the x-axis, frequency on the y-axis. Power of EEG activities is analyzed by fast Fourier transform, determined by amplitude and frequency, and displayed in the color dimension. Seizures are usually displayed as upward arches indicating increased frequency on the y-axis with warmer colors indicating an increase in power of EEG activities. Stewart et al. reported that the median sensitivity for seizure identification was 83% with CDSA in critically ill children and that the sensitivity varied from 0% to 100% according to individual tracings.[32] Pensirikul et al. reported that sensitivity and specificity of CDSA was 65% and 95%, respectively.[33] This suggests that some electrographic seizures were missed and that some nonictal events such as artifacts were misdiagnosed as seizures.

FUTURE DIRECTIONS

Most pediatric neurologists seem to believe conventional EEG will be useful for diagnosis and prognostication of children with AE. However, firm evidence is lacking at present. An evaluation of real-time brain function is difficult without EEG. The diagnostic and prognostic value of EEG should be confirmed by prospective multicenter studies using a uniform protocol in near future. Continuous EEG monitoring is necessary to detect electrographic seizures that are presumed to be common in children with AE. Moreover, chronologic changes in background EEG activity may possibly add useful information regarding management of children with AE. Solution for resource requirements is desirable to spread an application of continuous EEG monitoring. Quantitative EEG may partly solve this issue, because application and interpretation of aEEG and CDSA are much easier than those of continuous multichannel EEG monitoring. A proper combination of conventional EEG, continuous EEG monitoring, and quantitative EEG may be realistic in clinical settings. Another important problem to be solved will be interrater variability of EEG interpretation. Automated EEG interpretation and quantification may be developed by using artificial intelligence technique in the future.

REFERENCES

1. Mohammad SS, Soe SM, Pillai SC, et al. Etiological associations and outcome predictors of acute electroencephalography in childhood encephalitis. *Clin Neurophysiol.* 2016;127:3217–3224.
2. Mizuguchi M, Abe J, Mikkaichi K, et al. Acute necrotising encephalopathy of childhood: a new syndrome presenting with focal, symmetric brain lesions. *J Neurol Neurosurg Psychiatry.* 1995;58:555–561.
3. Maegaki Y, Kondo A, Okamoto R, et al. Clinical characteristics of acute encephalopathy of obscure origin: a biphasic clinical course is a common feature. *Neuropediatrics.* 2006;37:269–277.
4. Sakuma H, Awaya Y, Shiomi M, et al. Acute encephalitis with refractory, repetitive partial seizures (AERRPS): a peculiar form of childhood encephalitis. *Acta Neurol Scand.* 2010;121:251–256.
5. Bitnun A, Ford-Jones EL, Petric M, et al. Acute childhood encephalitis and *Mycoplasma pneumoniae. Clin Infect Dis.* 2001;32:1674–1684.
6. Domachowske JB, Cunningham CK, Cummings DL, Crosley CJ, Hannan WP, Weiner LB. Acute manifestations and neurologic sequelae of Epstein-Barr virus encephalitis in children. *Pediatr Infect Dis J.* 1996;15: 871–875.
7. Okumura A, Suzuki M, Kidokoro H, et al. The spectrum of acute encephalopathy with reduced diffusion in the unilateral hemisphere. *Eur J Paediatr Neurol.* 2009;13:154–159.
8. Kohl S. Herpes simplex virus encephalitis in children. *Pediatr Clin North Am.* 1988;35:465–483.
9. Harden A, Boyd SG, Cole G, Levin M. EEG features and their evolution in the acute phase of haemorrhagic shock and encephalopathy syndrome. *Neuropediatrics.* 1991;22:194–197.
10. Hosoya M, Ushiku H, Arakawa H, Morikawa A. Low-voltage activity in EEG during acute phase of encephalitis predicts unfavorable neurological outcome. *Brain Dev.* 2002;24:161–165.
11. Lin JJ, Lin KL, Wang HS, Hsia SH, Wu CT. Effect of topiramate, in combination with lidocaine, and phenobarbital, in acute encephalitis with refractory repetitive partial seizures. *Brain Dev.* 2009;31:605–611.
12. Shyu CS, Lee HF, Chi CS, Chen CH. Acute encephalitis with refractory, repetitive partial seizures. *Brain Dev.* 2008;30:356–361.
13. Schmitt SE, Pargeon K, Frechette ES, Hirsch LJ, Dalmau J, Friedman D. Extreme delta brush: a unique EEG pattern in adults with anti-NMDA receptor encephalitis. *Neurology.* 2012;79:1094–1100.
14. Gitiaux C, Simonnet H, Eisermann M, et al. Early electro-clinical features may contribute to diagnosis of the anti-NMDA receptor encephalitis in children. *Clin Neurophysiol.* 2013;124:2354–2361.
15. Oguri M, Saito Y, Fukuda C, et al. Distinguishing acute encephalopathy with biphasic seizures and late reduced diffusion from prolonged febrile seizures by acute phase EEG spectrum analysis. *Yonago Acta Med.* 2016;59:1–14.
16. Yoshikawa H, Abe T. Periodic lateralized epileptiform discharges in children. *J Child Neurol.* 2003;18:803–805.
17. Akman CI, Abou Khaled KJ, Segal E, Micic V, Riviello JJ. Generalized periodic epileptiform discharges in critically ill children: clinical features, and outcome. *Epilepsy Res.* 2013;106:378–385.
18. Sutter R, Kaplan PW, Valença M, De Marchis GM. EEG for diagnosis and prognosis of acute nonhypoxic encephalopathy: history and current evidence. *J Clin Neurophysiol.* 2015;32:456–464.

19. Accolla EA, Kaplan PW, Maeder-Ingvar M, Jukopila S, Rossetti AO. Clinical correlates of frontal intermittent rhythmic delta activity (FIRDA). *Clin Neurophysiol.* 2011;122:27–31.

20. Watemberg N, Linder I, Dabby R, Blumkin L, Lerman-Sagie T. Clinical correlates of occipital intermittent rhythmic delta activity (OIRDA) in children. *Epilepsia.* 2007;48:330–334.

21. Okumura A, Nakano T, Fukumoto Y, et al. Delirious behavior in children with influenza: its clinical features and EEG findings. *Brain Dev.* 2005;27:271–274.

22. Nordli Jr DR, Moshé SL, Shinnar S, et al. Acute EEG findings in children with febrile status epilepticus: results of the FEBSTAT study. *Neurology.* 2012;79:2180–2186.

23. Schreiber JM, Zelleke T, Gaillard WD, Kaulas H, Dean N, Carpenter JL. Continuous video EEG for patients with acute encephalopathy in a pediatric intensive care unit. *Neurocrit Care.* 2012;17:31–38.

24. Abend NS, Gutierrez-Colina AM, Topjian AA, et al. Nonconvulsive seizures are common in critically ill children. *Neurology.* 2011;76:1071–1077.

25. Topjian AA, Gutierrez-Colina AM, Sanchez SM, et al. Electrographic status epilepticus is associated with mortality and worse short-term outcome in critically ill children. *Crit Care Med.* 2013;41:215–223.

26. Abend NS, Topjian AA, Gutierrez-Colina AM, Donnelly M, Clancy RR, Dlugos DJ. Impact of continuous EEG monitoring on clinical management in critically ill children. *Neurocrit Care.* 2011;15:70–75.

27. Kirkham FJ, Wade AM, McElduff F, et al. Seizures in 204 comatose children: incidence and outcome. *Intensive Care Med.* 2012;38:853–862.

28. Abend NS, Arndt DH, Carpenter JL, et al. Electrographic seizures in pediatric ICU patients: cohort study of risk factors and mortality. *Neurology.* 2013;81:383–391.

29. Payne ET, Zhao XY, Frndova H, et al. Seizure burden is independently associated with short term outcome in critically ill children. *Brain.* 2014;137:1429–1438.

30. Komatsu M, Okumura A, Matsui K, et al. Clustered subclinical seizures in a patient with acute encephalopathy with biphasic seizures and late reduced diffusion. *Brain Dev.* 2010;32:472–476.

31. Okumura A, Komatsu M, Abe S, et al. Amplitude-integrated electroencephalography in patients with acute encephalopathy with refractory, repetitive partial seizures. *Brain Dev.* 2011;33:77–82.

32. Stewart CP, Otsubo H, Ochi A, Sharma R, Hutchison JS, Hahn CD. Seizure identification in the ICU using quantitative EEG displays. *Neurology.* 2010;75:1501–1508.

33. Pensirikul AD, Beslow LA, Kessler SK, et al. Density spectral array for seizure identification in critically ill children. *J Clin Neurophysiol.* 2013;30:371–375.

CHAPTER 9

Electroencephalographic Approach for Early Diagnosis of Acute Encephalopathy and Encephalitis

SOOYOUNG LEE, MD

BACKGROUND

Acute pediatric encephalopathy and encephalitis are severe neurologic syndromes associated with significant mortality and long-term morbidity in survivors. In the emergency setting, stabilization of the vital functions and prompt diagnosis and treatment are required to minimize neurologic impairments. Because of their similar clinical manifestations, it is sometimes difficult to differentiate pediatric acute encephalopathy from prolonged febrile seizure in emergency rooms. Underestimation of the disease severity and treatment delay may lead to severe impairments.

Electroencephalography (EEG) has been one of the most widely used laboratory tests for the clinical evaluation of neurologic disorders. EEG is helpful to assess the brain function and seizure activity, including nonconvulsive status epilepticus.

In this chapter, the usefulness/limitation of EEG during the acute phase of encephalopathy and encephalitis is described and its value, especially for differentiating pediatric encephalopathy from prolonged febrile seizure, is highlighted.

ELECTROENCEPHALOGRAPHY FINDINGS OF PEDIATRIC ACUTE ENCEPHALITIS AND ENCEPHALOPATHY

General Electroencephalography Findings During Acute Phase of Pediatric Acute Encephalitis

EEG plays an important role in evaluating pediatric encephalitis. It typically demonstrates progressive slowing as the level of consciousness decreases. The degree of slowing usually parallels the severity of clinical findings.[1] Focal and lateralizing findings may be noted in primary encephalitis. Because of the advances of computerized tomography and magnetic resonance imaging (MRI), the utilization of EEG as a diagnostic tool has decreased. However, it is still used to evaluate the epileptogenic potentials and process of diffuse or focal cerebral dysfunction, and it remains an essential tool to evaluate and treat seizures.

Some EEG features can suggest the underlying etiology, such as periodic discharges in herpes simplex encephalitis (HSE),[2] extreme delta brush in anti-N-methyl-D-aspartate receptor encephalitis,[3,4] and temporal slowing and epileptic discharges in limbic encephalitis.[5] Kalita reported EEG findings in 90 patients with HSE and Japanese encephalitis (JE).[6] Epileptiform discharges were seen in only 10% of HSE patients. Generalized delta slowing was more common in JE. Shekeeb reviewed 354 EEGs from 119 pediatric patients with acute encephalitis to examine EEG features, etiologic associations, and outcome predictors of acute encephalitis.[7] Eighty-six percent of children had an abnormal initial EEG and eighty-nine percent had at least one abnormal EEG. Abnormal slowing of the EEG background (92/119); abnormal fast activity that included extreme spindle, persistent alpha activity, continuous spindle coma, and drug-induced beta activity (29/119); and epileptiform discharges (28/119) were noted in their initial EEGs. A nonreactive EEG background (48% of the initial EEG) was a predictor of a poor outcome (OR: 3.8, $P<.001$). A shifting focal seizure pattern was seen in those with febrile infection–related epilepsy syndrome (4/5), antivoltage-gated potassium channel encephalitis (2/3), mycoplasma (1/10), other viral infections (1/10), and other unknown encephalitis (1/28), and the EEG findings were predictors of an unfavorable outcome and drug-resistant epilepsy. Kim reported the prognostic value of initial standard EEG and MRI in patients with HSE.[8] The presence of severe EEG abnormalities (dominant widespread delta activity, nonreactive pattern, burst suppression pattern; epileptiform discharges, low-output activity; alpha coma pattern, theta coma pattern, and isoelectric activity) and epileptic seizures at the initial presentation was significantly correlated with a poor clinical outcome at 6 months. Thus, the various EEG findings during the acute phase of encephalitis can be prognostic markers. Of note, EEG findings are generally nonspecific and cannot be used to distinguish between different etiologies. The main contribution of EEG during the acute phase is that it provides an objective measure of the brain function and detects seizure activity.

In the emergency setting, pediatric acute encephalitis is diagnosed based on neurodiagnostic evaluation that includes a cerebrospinal fluid (CSF) examination and an imaging study of the brain or spinal cord, accompanied by electrophysiologic studies. It is relatively straightforward to distinguish encephalitis from prolonged febrile seizure because CSF pleocytosis is typically identified in pediatric acute encephalitis and meningitis. The risk of herniation by performing lumbar puncture must always be considered.

General Electroencephalography Findings During Acute Phase of Pediatric Acute Encephalopathy

Pediatric acute encephalopathy frequently develops with common infections. The less specific term "encephalopathy" is used when neurologic manifestations suggest encephalitis but inflammation is not identified in the brain or CSF. Acute encephalopathy encompasses various etiologies with acute insult to the brain and clinical manifestations of seizures, impaired consciousness, and other neurologic symptoms.[9] It is difficult to distinguish between pediatric acute encephalopathy and prolonged febrile seizure because many pediatric acute encephalopathies show no abnormality in the initial neuroimaging and CSF study. EEG abnormalities of pediatric acute encephalopathy have been reported as follows: background slowing, paroxysms, diffuse slow waves in acute necrotizing encephalopathy (ANE),[10] electrical storm, low amplitude activity, nonelectrical activity, diffuse slow waves in hemorrhagic shock and encephalopathy syndrome (HSES),[11] focal attenuation, focal slowing, diffuse slowing, diffuse attenuation, paroxysms in acute encephalopathy with biphasic seizures and late reduced diffusion (AESD),[12-14] background slowing, and frontal/occipital dominance rhythmic delta activity in clinically mild encephalopathy with reversible splenial lesions (MERS).[13,14] In general, the most prominent features of EEG during the acute phase in acute encephalopathy are background slowing and epileptic activity, similar to those in pediatric acute encephalitis. These findings are often nonspecific.

ELECTROENCEPHALOGRAPHY FINDINGS DURING ACUTE PHASE IN FEBRILE COMATOSE CHILDREN

Case Presentation

Case 1

A 2-year-old girl, who had shown normal growth and development, had a fever lasting for 1 day and was transferred to the hospital because of a convulsive seizure lasting for 1 h. In the emergency room, the seizure appeared to stop and she did not show cyanosis, but she was in a comatose state with increased limb tonus, tonic posture, and left-deviated eyes, suggesting that the seizure had not ceased. Immediate EEG, however, did not show epileptic discharges at that time (Fig. 9.1), and her consciousness fully recovered in 2 h. Her final diagnosis was complex febrile seizure. Her condition may have been a prolonged nonepileptic twilight state.[15]

Case 2

A previously healthy 1-year-old boy, who had fever and cough for 1 day, was brought to the hospital because of a seizure lasting for 40 min. He was comatose and flaccid, with closed eyes and shallow breathing. He was not convulsive, but immediate EEG disclosed an ictal pattern (Fig. 9.2). He was immediately treated with intravenous midazolam and his seizure activity stopped. His consciousness fully recovered in 4 h. His final diagnosis was complex febrile seizure.

Discussion of Case Presentation

EEG is essential to detect seizure activities including nonconvulsive status epilepticus in febrile comatose patients.

A prolonged nonepileptic twilight state with convulsive manifestations (case 1) was proposed by Yamamoto.[15] He reviewed EEG recordings of 14 infants resembling complex partial seizures with a convulsive manifestation, which showed nonepileptiform discharge. EEG revealed continuous diffuse delta waves or diffuse rhythmic theta waves, which showed no response to intravenous diazepam. The duration of the condition could be from 30 min to 4 h. It is difficult to distinguish an ongoing seizure from the twilight state without immediate EEG.

Nonconvulsive status epilepticus can be seen in prolonged febrile seizure (case 2). Nonconvulsive seizures

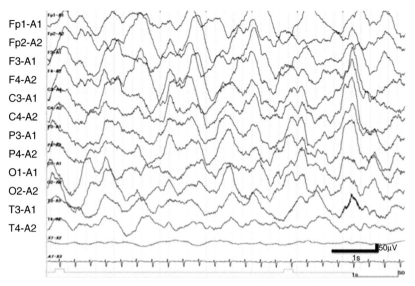

FIG. 9.1 Electroencephalography (EEG) screenshot of case 1. The acute EEG shows diffuse high-voltage slow waves. Epileptic seizure was excluded.

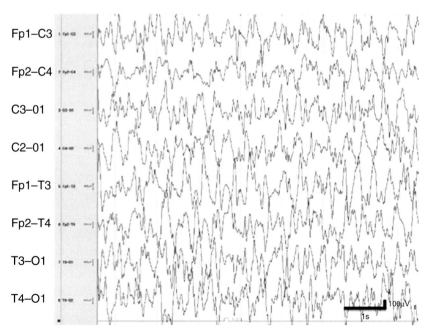

FIG. 9.2 Electroencephalography (EEG) screenshot of case 2. The EEG shows high-voltage rhythmic spikes and a wave burst considered to be ictal discharges.

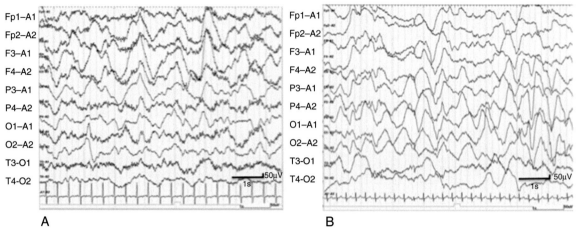

FIG. 9.3 Critical difference in acute-phase electroencephalography (EEG): prolonged febrile seizure (FS) versus acute encephalopathy. **(A)** The acute EEG findings in a 1-year-old boy 1 h after seizure cessation. The final diagnosis was prolonged FS. The patient showed a favorable outcome. **(B)** The acute EEG findings in an 11-month-old girl 5 h after seizure cessation. The final diagnosis was hemorrhagic shock and encephalopathy syndrome. The patient showed a poor outcome.

in children with an infection-related altered mental status have been reported.[16] Approximately one-third of children infected with influenza with an altered mental status showed nonconvulsive seizures. Although there is no definitive evidence supporting how vigorously and aggressively we should identify and treat nonconvulsive status epilepticus, the misdiagnosis of this condition and its delayed treatment might lead to further brain damage and severe neurologic sequelae.[17,18]

WHAT ARE ACUTE-PHASE ELECTROENCEPHALOGRAPHY FINDINGS IN PROLONGED FEBRILE SEIZURE AND PEDIATRIC ENCEPHALOPATHY?

Diffuse high-voltage slow waves are seen in both acute encephalopathy and prolonged febrile seizure. Acute EEG findings in children with febrile status epilepticus were reported in the FEBSTAT study.[19] Of the 199 EEGs, 90 (45.2%) were abnormal: diffuse slowing in 22 (11.1%), focal slowing in 47 (29.1%), focal attenuation in 25 (12.6%), epileptiform abnormality in 13 (6.5%), focal spike in 13 (6.5%), and generalized spike and wave in 1 (0.5%). The study suggests that it may be difficult to distinguish pediatric acute encephalopathy from prolonged febrile seizure based on acute-phase EEG findings such as diffuse slowing, focal slowing, and seizure activity. A limitation of the study is that EEG data were collected within 72 h. In the emergency setting, patients with a prolonged febrile seizure are

typically awake within half a day after onset. Sequential EEGs of prolonged febrile seizures reflecting the natural clinical course may gradually improve within several hours. The EEG of pediatric acute encephalopathy may not improve. Continuous diffuse background slowing might be a notable finding to diagnose pediatric acute encephalopathy in febrile comatose children (Fig. 9.3). Further studies are needed to investigate this.

On the other hand, severe EEG patterns (isovoltage, persistent low voltage [<20 μV], burst suppression, and generalized periodic discharges) have been reported to indicate a poor outcome for comatose patients after cardiac arrest.[20,21] To our knowledge, there has been no report of these severe patterns seen in patients with prolonged febrile seizures. In the acute setting, these severe patterns of EEG abnormalities may suggest acute encephalopathy, which requires specific and immediate treatment (Fig. 9.4).

POSSIBLE USEFULNESS OF QUANTITATIVE ELECTROENCEPHALOGRAPHY ANALYSIS TO DISTINGUISH PROLONGED FEBRILE SEIZURE AND PEDIATRIC ACUTE ENCEPHALOPATHY

Quantitative EEG is commonly used for the detection of seizures and brain ischemia.[22,23] Quantitative EEG for detecting brain ischemia highlights the EEG changes that occur with decreased cerebral follow: the loss of fast activity and increase in slow activity. Frequency-based

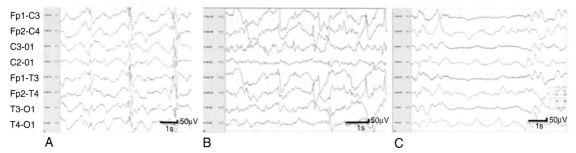

FIG. 9.4 Severe electroencephalography (EEG) patterns accompanied by pediatric acute encephalopathy. **(A)** Generalized periodic discharge seen in an acute encephalopathy patient with biphasic seizure and late reduced diffusion (8-month-old boy, 5 h after onset). **(B)** High-voltage slow wave with multifocal epileptiform discharges in a patient with hemorrhagic shock and encephalopathy syndrome (4-year-old boy, 6 h after onset). **(C)** Burst suppression pattern in a patient with hemorrhagic shock and encephalopathy syndrome (4-year-old girl, 7 h after onset).

trends using fast Fourier transform (FFT) reveal the power spectrum at various frequencies. Oguri reported the usefulness of acute quantitative EEG analysis to differentiate prolonged febrile seizure and pediatric acute encephalopathy to facilitate an early diagnosis.[24] Sixty-eight children who had status epilepticus underwent recording within 120 h after the onset of seizures. Final diagnoses were febrile seizures (FS; n = 20), epilepsy (n = 10), AESD (n = 18), and MERS (n = 7). Quantitative EEG revealed that the MERS group showed the highest theta band power. The ratios of delta/alpha and delta + theta/ alpha + beta band powers were significantly higher in the AESD group than in other groups. The alpha and beta band powers in EEGs within 24 h after the onset were significantly lower in the AESD group. The band powers and ratios showed earlier improvement toward 24 h in febrile seizures than in AESD. The results suggest that sequential quantitative EEG using Fourier analysis might be useful to differentiate pediatric acute encephalopathy from prolonged febrile seizure. Further studies should be conducted.

SUMMARY

- Some EEG findings suggest etiologies in pediatric acute encephalitis.
- Acute-phase EEG is useful to detect the presence of seizure activity in febrile comatose patients.
- Diffuse high-voltage slow waves are seen in both acute encephalopathy and prolonged febrile seizure.
- Severe patterns of EEG abnormalities suggest the development of acute encephalopathy.
- Sequential studies of acute-phase EEG may provide clues to distinguish prolonged febrile seizure from acute encephalopathy in childhood.

REFERENCES

1. Swaiman KF, Ashwal S, Ferriero DM, ed. Pediatric Neurology, 4th ed. Scher MS;2005:203–254.
2. Whitley RJ, Soong SJ, Alford CA, et al. Herpes simplex encephalitis. Clinical Assessment *JAMA*. 1982;247(3):317–320.
3. Schmitt SE, Pargeon K, Friedman D, et al. Extreme delta brush: a unique EEG pattern in adults with anti-NMDA receptor encephalitis. *Neurology*. 2012;79(11):1094–1100.
4. Abbas A, Garg A, Jain R, Jacob S, et al. Extreme delta brushes and BIRDs in the EEG of anti-NMDA-receptor encephalitis. *Pract Neurol*. 2016;16(4):326–327.
5. Steriade C, Mirsattari SM, Wennberg R, et al. Subclinical temporal EEG seizure pattern in LGI1-antibody-mediated encephalitis. *Epilepsia*. 2016;57(8):e155–e160.
6. Kalita J, Misra UK, Bhoi SK, et al. Can we differentiate between herpes simplex encephalitis and Japanese encephalitis? *J Neurol Sci*. 2016;366:110–115.
7. Mohammad SS, Soe SM, Dale RC, et al. Etiological associations and outcome predictors of acute electroencephalography in childhood encephalitis. *Clin Neurophysiol*. 2016;127:3217–3224.
8. Kim YS, Jung KH, Chu K, et al. Prognostic value of initial standard EEG and MRI in patients with herpes simplex encephalitis. *J Clin Neurol*. 2016;12(2):224–229.
9. Mizuguchi M, Yamanouchi H, Shiomi M, et al. Acute encephalopathy associated with influenza and other viral infections. *Acta Neurologica Scand Suppl*. 2007;186:45–56.
10. Mizuguchi M. Acute necrotizing encephalopathy. *Nihon Rinsho*. 2011;69(3):465–470.
11. Harden A, Boyd SG, Levin M, et al. EEG features and their evolution in the acute phase of haemorrhagic shock and encephalopathy syndrome. *Neuropediatrics*. 1991;22(4):194–197.
12. Takanashi J, Oba H, Koyasu Y, et al. Diffusion MRI abnormalities after prolonged febrile seizures with encephalopathy. *Neurology*. 2006;66(9):1304–1309.
13. Takanashi J. Two newly proposed infectious encephalitis/encephalopathy syndromes. *Brain Dev*. 2009;31(7):521–528.

14. Takanashi J. [Radiological and EEG findings in acute encephalopathy syndromes in children]. *Nihon Rinsho.* 2011;69(3):490–498. Japanese.

15. Yamamoto N. Prolonged nonepileptic twilight state with convulsive manifestations after febrile convulsions: a clinical and electroencephalographic study. *Epilepsia.* 1996;37(1):31–35.

16. Fujita K, Nagase H, Uetani Y, et al. Non-convulsive seizures in children with infection-related altered mental status. *Pediatr Int.* 2015;57(4):659–664.

17. Tay SK, Hirsch LJ, Akman CI, et al. Nonconvulsive status epilepticus in children: clinical and EEG characteristics. *Epilepsia.* 2006;47(9):1504–1509.

18. Jafarpour S, Loddenkemper T. Outcomes in pediatric patients with nonconvulsive status epilepticus. *Epilepsy Behav.* 2015;49:98–103.

19. Nordli Jr DR, Moshé SL, Sun S, et al. Acute EEG findings in children with febrile status epilepticus: results of the FEBSTAT study. *Neurology.* 2012;79(22):2180–2186.

20. Kessler SK, Topjian AA, Gutierrez-Colina AM, et al. Short-term outcome prediction by electroencephalographic features in children treated with therapeutic hypothermia after cardiac arrest. *Neurocrit Care.* 2011;14(1):37–43.

21. Hofmeijer J, van Putten MJ. *Clin Neurophysiol.* 2016;127(4): 2047–2055.

22. Finnigan S, Wong A, Read S. Defining abnormal slow EEG activity in acute ischaemic stroke: delta/alpha ratio as an optimal QEEG index. *Clin Neurophysiol.* 2016;127(2):1452–1459.

23. Haider HA, Esteller R, LaRoche SM, et al. Critical Care EEG Monitoring Research Consortium. Sensitivity of quantitative EEG for seizure identification in the intensive care unit. *Neurology.* 2016;87(9):935–944.

24. Oguri M, Saito Y, Maegaki Y, et al. Distinguishing acute encephalopathy with biphasic seizures and late reduced diffusion from prolonged febrile seizures by acute phase EEG spectrum analysis. *Yonago Acta Med.* 2016;59(1):1–14.

CHAPTER 10

Biomarkers for the Diagnosis and Evaluation in Acute Encephalopathy

TAKASHI ICHIYAMA, MD

INTRODUCTION

Acute encephalopathy in childhood is an acute progressive and life-threatening disease that can result in death or the development of neurologic sequelae.[1] Therefore it is important to diagnose it and evaluate the severity as soon as possible. However, the pathophysiology of acute encephalopathy is not homogeneous. Acute encephalopathies could be induced by cytokine storm, excitotoxicity, metabolic errors, or other causes.[2] Biomarkers for diagnosis and evaluating the severity vary according to types of acute encephalopathy (Table 10.1).

ACUTE ENCEPHALOPATHY DUE TO CYTOKINE STORM

In the end of the 20th century, influenza-associated encephalopathy has been identified as an important subtype of acute encephalopathy in childhood.[1,3,4] Most of patients with the encephalopathy had multiple organ failures and hypercytokinemia.[5–8] The patients with acute encephalopathy due to cytokine storm often have systemic inflammatory response syndrome (SIRS). Therefore it is likely that patients with acute encephalopathy who have SIRS will have hypercytokinemia. The diagnosis of SIRS in the childhood has been previously demonstrated.[9]

Several prognostic factors in influenza-associated encephalopathy, which will be cytokine storm type, have been reported. The elevation of aspartate aminotransferase, hyperglycemia, the presence of hematuria or proteinuria, and use of diclofenac sodium were associated with poor prognosis.[10] Serum tumor necrosis factor-α (TNF-α) and cytochrome c concentration were elevated in the affected patients with poor prognosis.[11] We reported that the serum interleukin-6 (IL-6), soluble tumor necrosis factor receptor 1 (sTNFR1), and IL-10 levels in the patients with a poor prognosis were significantly higher than those in those without sequelae.[8] In particular, the serum levels of IL-6, sTNFR1, and IL-10 in dead patients were significantly higher than those in other patients with a poor

prognosis.[8] The serum concentrations of tissue inhibitors of metalloproteinases 1 (TIMP-1) as a protective factor of the blood-brain barrier in the patients with poor prognosis were significantly higher than those without sequelae.[12] The CD163 is a marker of the activation of peripheral monocytes/macrophages, and the serum soluble CD163 concentrations of the patients with poor prognosis were significantly higher than those without sequelae.[13] The serum levels of high mobility group box 1 (HMGB1) were significantly higher in the patients with poor outcomes compared with those without neurologic sequelae.[14] The HMGB1 is a ubiquitous nuclear protein that induces the production of proinflammatory cytokines.[14,15]

ACUTE ENCEPHALOPATHY DUE TO EXCITOTOXICITY

About 10 years ago, acute encephalopathy with biphasic seizures and late reduced diffusion (AESD) has been identified as a subtype of acute encephalopathy.[16] The acute encephalopathy due to excitotoxicity has frequently neurologic sequelae, although the mortality rate due to it is not high.[1] The initial symptom is characterized by a seizure or a cluster of seizures lasting for >30 min within 1 day after the onset of fever.[1,2,16] Therefore it is hard to distinguish AESD from prolonged febrile seizures without neurologic sequelae during the initial stage. Several studies have reported about biomarkers for diagnosing AESD during the early stage. The CSF levels of tau protein as a marker of axonal damage in patients with AESD were elevated during the early stage.[17] It has been reported that CSF S100B and tau protein were good diagnostic markers for AESD.[18] We measured serum and CSF visinin-like protein-1 (VILIP-1) levels in patients with AESD and those with prolonged febrile seizures during the early stage.[19] It is known that VILIP-1 is one of prognostic peripheral biomarker in Alzheimer's disease.[20] CSF VILIP-1 was elevated in 7 of 13 patients with AESD, but in none of patients with prolonged febrile seizures.

TABLE 10.1
Markers for Diagnosis and Indicating Poor Outcomes of Acute Encephalopathy

	Diagnostic Markers	Markers Indicating Poor Outcomes

Acute encephalopathy due to cytokine storm	Factors for diagnosing SIRS
	    Body temperature
	    Heart rate
	    Respiratory rate
	    White blood cell counts
		Serum elevated aspartate aminotransferase
		Hyperglycemia
		Serum elevated TNF-α, cytochrome *c*
		Serum elevated IL-6, sTNFR1, IL-10
		Serum elevated TIMP-1
		Serum elevated soluble CD163
		Serum elevated HMGB1
		Hematuria or proteinuria

Acute encephalopathy due to excitotoxicity	CSF tau protein CSF S100B CSF VILIP-1 CSF IL-6	Serum elevated MMP-9 Serum elevated MMP-9/TIMP-1 ratio

HMGB1, high mobility group box 1; *IL-6*, interleukin-6; *MMP-9*, matrix metalloproteinase-9; *SIRS*, systemic inflammatory response syndrome; *sTNFR1*, soluble TNF receptor 1; *TIMP-1*, tissue inhibitors of metalloproteinases 1; *TNF-α*, tumor necrosis factor-α; *VILIP-1*, visinin-like protein.

We suggested that patients with elevated CSF VILIP-1 levels during the early stage have AESD. Moreover, we revealed that CSF IL-6 levels in patients with AESD were significantly higher than those with prolonged febrile seizures.[21] However, there were no significant differences in serum IL-6, sTNFR1, IL-10, CSF sTNFR1, or IL-10 concentrations between the AESD groups and the prolonged febrile seizures ones.

The reports on biomarkers for the severity of AESD are few. We have previously measured serum matrix metalloproteinase-9 (MMP-9) levels, TIMP-1 levels, and MMP-9/TIMP-1 ratios in AESD patients.[22] Serum MMP-9 levels and MMP-9/TIMP-1 ratios in patients with motor paralysis were significantly higher than in those without motor paralysis. MMP-9 is a member of this family that degrades collagen IV, a major component of the basement membrane of the cerebral epithelium, which is also responsible for the integrity of the blood-brain barrier.[23] We suggested that the severity of AESD was related to the balance of MMP-9 and TIMP-1 and the function of the blood-brain barrier.

REFERENCES

1. Ichiyama T. Acute encephalopathy/encephalitis in childhood: a relatively common and potentially devastating clinical syndrome. *Brain Dev.* 2010;32:433–434.
2. Mizuguchi M, Yamanouchi H, Ichiyama T, et al. Acute encephalopathy associated with influenza and other viral infections. *Acta Neurol Scand.* 2007;115:45–56.
3. Kasai T, Togashi T, Morishima T. Encephalopathy associated with influenza epidemics. *Lancet.* 2000;355:1558–1559.
4. Morishima T, Togashi T, Yokota S, et al. Encephalitis and encephalopathy associated with an influenza epidemic in Japan. *Clin Infect Dis.* 2002;35:512–517.
5. Aiba H, Mochizuki M, Kimura M, et al. Predictive value of serum interleukin-6 level in influenza virus-associated encephalopathy. *Neurology.* 2001;57:295–299.
6. Ichiyama T, Endo S, Kaneko M, et al. Serum cytokine concentrations of influenza-associated acute necrotizing encephalopathy. *Pediatr Int.* 2003;45:734–736.
7. Ichiyama T, Isumi H, Ozawa H, et al. Cerebrospinal fluid and serum levels of cytokines and soluble tumor necrosis factor receptor in influenza virus-associated encephalopathy. *Scand J Infect Dis.* 2003;35:59–61.
8. Ichiyama T, Morishima T, Isumi H, et al. Analysis of cytokine levels and NF-κB activation in peripheral blood mononuclear cells in influenza virus-associated encephalopathy. *Cytokine.* 2004;27:31–37.
9. Goldstein B, Giroir B, Randolph A. International Consensus Conference on Pediatric Sepsis. International pediatric sepsis consensus conference: definitions for sepsis and organ dysfunction in pediatrics. *Pediatr Crit Care Med.* 2005;6:2–8.
10. Nagao T, Morishima T, Kimura H, et al. Prognostic factors in influenza-associated encephalopathy. *Pediatr Infect Dis J.* 2008;27:384–389.
11. Hosoya M, Nunoi H, Aoyama M, et al. Cytochrome c and tumor necrosis factor-alpha values in serum and cerebrospinal fluid of patients with influenza-associated encephalopathy. *Pediatr Infect Dis J.* 2005;24:467–470.
12. Ichiyama T, Morishima T, Kajimoto M, Matsushige T, Matsubara T, Furukawa S. Matrix metalloproteinase-9 and tissue inhibitors of metalloproteinases 1 in influenza-associated encephalopathy. *Pediatr Infect Dis J.* 2007;26:542–544.

13. Hasegawa S, Matsushige T, Inoue H, et al. Serum soluble CD163 levels in patients with influenza-associated encephalopathy. *Brain Dev.* 2013;35:626–629.
14. Momonaka H, Hasegawa S, Matsushige T, et al. High mobility group box 1 in patients with 2009 pandemic H1N1 influenza-associated encephalopathy. *Brain Dev.* 2014;36:484–488.
15. Yamada S, Maruyama I. HMGB1, a novel inflammatory cytokine. *Clin Chim Acta.* 2007;375:36–42.
16. Takanashi J, Oba H, Barkovich AJ, et al. Diffusion MRI abnormalities after prolonged febrile seizures with encephalopathy. *Neurology.* 2006;66:1304–1309.
17. Tanuma N, Miyata R, Kumada S, et al. The axonal damage marker tau protein in the cerebrospinal fluid is increased in patients with acute encephalopathy with biphasic seizures and late reduced diffusion. *Brain Dev.* 2010;32:435–439.
18. Shiihara T, Miyake T, Izumi S, et al. Serum and cerebrospinal fluid S100B, neuron-specific enolase, and total tau protein in acute encephalopathy with biphasic seizures and late reduced diffusion: a diagnostic validity. *Pediatr Int.* 2012;54:52–55.
19. Hasegawa S, Matsushige T, Inoue H, et al. Serum and cerebrospinal fluid levels of visinin-like protein-1 in acute encephalopathy with biphasic seizures and late reduced diffusion. *Brain Dev.* 2014;36:608–612.
20. Tarawneh R, D'Angelo G, Macy E, et al. Visinin-like protein-1: diagnostic and prognostic biomarker in Alzheimer disease. *Ann Neurol.* 2011;70:274–285.
21. Ichiyama T, Suenaga N, Kajimoto M, et al. Serum and CSF levels of cytokines in acute encephalopathy following prolonged febrile seizures. *Brain Dev.* 2008;30:47–52.
22. Suenaga N, Ichiyama T, Kubota M, et al. Roles of matrix metalloproteinase-9 and tissue inhibitors of metalloproteinases 1 in acute encephalopathy following prolonged febrile seizures. *J Neurol Sci.* 2008;266:126–130.
23. Lukes A, Mun-Bryce S, Lukes M, et al. Extracellular matrix degradation by metalloproteinases and central nervous system diseases. *Mol Neurobiol.* 1999;19:267–284.

CHAPTER 11

Differential Diagnosis

FEDERICO VIGEVANO, MD • PAOLA DE LISO, MD

INTRODUCTION

Pediatric encephalitis and encephalopathy are severe neurologic conditions associated with significant mortality and long-term morbidity in survivors. Some of them are potentially treatable if a correct diagnosis and an appropriate management are put in place early. We are facing a lot of conditions with few clinical elements in common, but with different etiologies and different therapeutic approaches. Therefore, having acknowledged guidelines for the investigation and management of encephalitis and mainly a diagnostic algorithm could be very useful in the clinical practice.

In addition, there is some confusion between the term *encephalitis* and *encephalopathy*, sometimes used interchangeably. Although their definitions have been already treated in other chapters of this book, we will stress again the difference between these two entities.

DEFINITIONS

Encephalitis is defined as *inflammation of the brain parenchyma associated with neurologic dysfunction*. Based on this definition, the "gold standard" of its diagnostic test is considered to be the histologic examination of brain tissue rarely performed in vivo. Therefore, the diagnosis is defined on the basis of clinical, laboratory, electroencephalogram (EEG), and neuroimaging features.

From a clinical point of view, there is an overlap between *encephalitis* and *encephalopathy*, but actually they represent two distinct pathophysiologic entities.

Encephalopathy refers to a clinical state of altered mental status, manifesting as confusion, disorientation, behavioral changes, or other cognitive impairments, with or without inflammation of brain tissue. For example, FIRES, a severe condition in which a brain inflammation is suspected but not confirmed by CNF/blood examinations or by neuroimaging, is considered an "encephalopathy." Encephalopathy without inflammation can be triggered by a number of metabolic or toxic conditions but may also be associated with specific infectious agents (such as influenza virus).

In contrast, *encephalitis* is characterized by brain inflammation due to a direct infection of the brain parenchyma, to a postinfectious process, or to a noninfectious condition such as anti-*N*-methyl-D-aspartate receptor (NMDAR) encephalitis. In the absence of pathologic evidence of brain inflammation, an inflammatory response in the cerebrospinal fluid (CSF) or the presence of parenchymal abnormalities on neuroimaging is often used as a surrogate marker of brain inflammation. However, some encephalitis can occur without significant CSF pleocytosis or demonstrable neuroimaging abnormalities.

DIAGNOSTIC TOOLS

The diagnosis of encephalitis or encephalopathy is based on clinical criteria, not always very specific, and on instrumental examinations, particularly neuroimages and LCR examination. We will try to provide a diagnostic algorithm, stressing how a cluster of clinical elements and instrumental examinations features can be strongly indicative of a specific cause.

Regarding the differential diagnosis, first, pathologies possibly linked to encephalitis with similar clinical presentation, such as vascular disease, cerebral abscess or tumor, PRESS encephalopathy, metabolic encephalopathies, and psychosis, should be taken into account.

Moreover, in pediatric age, the diagnosis of encephalitis and encephalopathy, as recommended by the International Encephalitis Consortium,[1,3] is based on the following criteria:

Major criterion (always required):
- **Altered mental status** (defined as decreased or altered level of consciousness, lethargy, or personality change) lasting >24 h with no alternative cause identified

Minor criteria (two criteria required for possible encephalitis; three or more criteria required for probable or confirmed encephalitis):
- Documented fever ≥38°C (100.4°F) within the 72 h before or after presentation
- Generalized or partial seizures not fully attributable to a preexisting seizure disorder

- New onset of focal neurologic findings
- CSF WBC count ≥5/cubic mm
- Abnormality of brain parenchyma on neuroimaging suggestive of encephalitis that is either new from prior studies or appears acute in onset
- Abnormality on electroencephalography that is consistent with encephalitis and not attributable to another cause

Clinical Features

It is challenging to identify encephalitis in children because features are nonspecific (lethargy, excessive irritability, poor feeding) and often not easy to detect in young age. We recommend obtaining a comprehensive case history, including recent and remote travel, animal contacts, and insect exposure.

Physical examination should include an objective assessment of the level of consciousness and look for subtle seizure activity, meningism, abnormal movements (e.g., chorea, parkinsonism), weakness, sensory loss, and cranial nerve involvement (including deafness and anosmia), noting any focal findings, and for features suggesting other diagnoses. Temperature and other vital signs should be assessed for features of raised intracranial pressure or autonomic dysfunction. Mental status should be performed, particularly if there are psychotic features (e.g., hallucinations). A rash or other skin lesions (e.g., bite marks, eschar) or respiratory or gastrointestinal signs may give clues to etiology. Fever is a common finding in patients with acute encephalitis, but it is nonspecific.

Few hypotheses about correlations between clinical features and etiologies are proposed in Table 11.1. If the main symptoms are psychiatric associated with extrapyramidal manifestations, it is reasonable to hypothesize an autoimmune-mediated encephalitis (particularly anti-NMDAR). In case of focal seizures, an HSV infection should be taken into account; if you face with parkinsonian symptoms, a

---

TABLE 11.1
Clinical Features

1.	Psychosis, movement disorder, hypoventilation, coprolalia: anti-NMDAR
2.	Cognitive dysfunction, seizures: anti-VGKC, anti-NMDAR, HSV, HHV6, anti-GAD, anti-Hu, anti-Ma
3.	Subacute behavioral/personality change: HSV, anti-NMDAR, anti-VGKC, HIV, *Treponema pallidum*, Whipple disease, trypanosomiasis, SSPE, anti-GAD, anti-Hu, anti-Ma
4.	Hydrophobia, hypersalivation, delerium: rabies virus, ABLV
5.	Parkinsonian features: flaviviruses (especially JEV), anti-DR2 (basal ganglia encephalitis)
6.	Brainstem dysfunction: enteroviruses (especially Ev71), flaviviruses (especially MVEV, JEV, KUNV), Nipah, *Listeria monocytogenes*, *Burkholderia pseudomallei*, MTB, anti-Hu, anti-Ma
7.	Associated limb weakness (flaccid paralysis) or tremor: enteroviruses (especially Ev71, poliovirus), flaviviruses, rabies virus, arbovirus
8.	Rash: enteroviruses, VZV, HHV6, measles, dengue, rickettsiae, *Neisseria meningitidis* (meningococcus)
9.	Associated pneumonia: *Mycoplasma pneumoniae*, influenza, Nipah, Hendra, *Coxiella burnetii* (Q fever)
10.	Parotitis, testicular pain: mumps
11.	Cervical lymphadenopathy: EBV, CMV
12.	SIADH: anti-VGKC, SLEV
13.	Chronic symptoms: HIV, JCV, BKV, trypanosomiasis, SSPE, *Treponema pallidum*, Whipple disease
14.	Cranial nerve palsy: neuroborreliosis

Data from Venkatesan A, Tunkel AR, Bloch KC, et al. Case definitions, diagnostic algorithms, and priorities in encephalitis: consensus statement of the International Encephalitis Consortium. *Clin Infect Dis*. 2013;57(8):1114–1128 and Britton A, Ben-Shlomo Y, Benzeval M, et al. Life course trajectories of alcohol consumption in the United Kingdom using longitudinal data from nine cohort studies. *BMC Medicine* 2015;13:47. http://dx.doi.org/10.1186/s12916-015-0273-z.

ABLV, Australian bat lyssavirus; *CMV*, cytomegalovirus; *EBV*, Epstein–Barr virus; *HHV*, human herpes virus; *HIV*, human immunodeficiency virus; *HSV*, herpes simplex virus; *JEV*, Japanese encephalitis virus; *MTB*, *Mycobacterium tuberculosis*; *MVEV*, Murray valley encephalitis virus; *NMDAR*, N-methyl-ᴅ-aspartate receptor; *SLEV*, St Louis encephalitis virus; *SSPE*, subacute sclerosing panencephalitis; *VGKC*, voltage-gated potassium channel; *VZV*, varicella-zoster virus.

basal ganglia encephalitis (anti-DR2) should be suspected, whereas when a brainstem dysfunction is documented an encephalitis caused by enterovirus should be considered.[2]

Seizures and Electroencephalogram Features

Seizures associated with encephalitis may be generalized, suggestive of global CNS dysfunction, or focal, indicating a localized process. Subclinical seizures may also occur and can be a cause of altered sensorium. Seizures associated with high temperature are relatively common in young children and, if occurring in isolation, do not mandate evaluation for encephalitis.

When movement disorders coexist, the differential diagnosis between seizures and dystonia could be hard and a video EEG monitoring is needed.

Sometimes seizures can be the first symptom of the encephalitis, associated just with a minimal temperature increase, as in the case of HSV encephalitis. In this condition interictal EEG focal periodic discharges in the temporal area can suggest the underlying etiology.

The presence of bilateral, synchronous, periodic, sharp, and slow waves associated with myoclonic jerks is still diagnostic in the subacute sclerosing panencephalitis.

The interictal EEG can be useful for the diagnosis in the anti-NMDAR encephalitis, showing extreme delta brush, or in limbic encephalitis, showing temporal slowing and epileptic discharges (Table 11.2). All these aspects are presented in detail in Chapter 9, Electroencephalographic Approach for Early Diagnosis of Acute Encephalopathy and Encephalitis, by Sooyoung Lee.

Laboratory Features

A confirmed laboratory diagnosis is not frequently obtained; however, CSF analysis is needed to confirm encephalitis and confirm a cause. CSF pleocytosis is suggestive of an inflammatory process of the brain parenchyma, meninges, or both (meningoencephalitis). The absence of CSF, however, does not exclude encephalitis. In the majority of cases of encephalitis, the absolute number of leukocytes is <1000/mm³ and lymphocytes typically predominate. Antibody testing are of utmost importance, but it must be taken into account that the absence of autoantibodies does not exclude the possibility that a disorder is immune-mediated and a positive test does not always imply an accurate diagnosis (Tables 11.3 and 11.4). The laboratory features of encephalitis due to cytokine storm or to excitotoxicity are reported in Chapter 10, Biomarkers for the Diagnosis and Evaluation in Acute Encephalopathy, by Takashi Ichiyama.

Radiologic Features

Neuroimaging plays a crucial role in the evaluation of patients with suspected encephalitis, because it may support diagnosis of a specific etiology or identify

---

TABLE 11.2
Electroencephalogram Features

1. Focal periodic discharges in the temporal area: HSV
2. Bilateral, synchronous, periodic, sharp, and slow waves associated with myoclonic jerks: subacute sclerosing panencephalitis
3. Extreme delta brush: anti-NMDAR encephalitis
4. Temporal slowing and epileptic discharges: limbic encephalitis

HSV, herpes simplex virus; *NMDAR*, N-methyl-D-aspartate receptor.

TABLE 11.3
Laboratory Features

1. EBV serology suggestive of acute infection: EBV PCR (CSF)
2. Elevated transaminases: rickettsia serology, tick-borne disease testing
3. CSF protein >100 mg/dL or CSF glucose <2/3 peripheral glucose or lymphocytic pleocytosis with subacute symptom onset: MTB testing, fungal testing, *Balamuthia mandrillaris* testing
4. CSF protein >100 mg/dL or CSF glucose <2/3 peripheral glucose and neutrophilic predominance with acute symptom onset and recent antibiotic use: CSF PCR for *Streptococcus pneumoniae* and *Neisseria meningitidis*
5. CSF eosinophilia: MTB testing, fungal testing, *Baylisascaris procyonis* antibody (serum and CSF); *Angiostrongylus cantonensis*, *Gnathostoma* sp. testing
6. Hyponatremia: MTB testing
7. *Mycoplasma pneumoniae* serology or throat PCR positive: *M. pneumoniae* PCR (CSF)

Data from Venkatesan A, Tunkel AR, Bloch KC, et al. Case definitions, diagnostic algorithms, and priorities in encephalitis: consensus statement of the International Encephalitis Consortium. *Clin Infect Dis.* 2013;57(8):1114–1128 and Britton A, Ben-Shlomo Y, Benzeval M, et al. Life course trajectories of alcohol consumption in the United Kingdom using longitudinal data from nine cohort studies. *BMC Medicine.* 2015;13:47. http://dx.doi.org/10.1186/s12916-015-0273-z.
CSF, cerebrospinal fluid; *EBV*, Epstein-Barr virus; *MTB*, Mycobacterium tuberculosis.

TABLE 11.4
Antibodies in the Diagnosis of Autoimmune Encephalitis

ANTIBODIES AGAINST INTRACELLULAR ANTIGENS

Hu (ANNA1)	Limbic encephalitis
Ma2	Limbic encephalitis
Glutamic acid decarboxylase—GAD	Limbic encephalitis

ANTIBODIES AGAINST SYNAPTIC RECEPTORS

NMDA receptor	Anti-NMDA receptor encephalitis
AMPA receptor	Limbic encephalitis
GABA-B receptor	Limbic encephalitis
GABA-A receptor	Limbic encephalitis
mGluR5	Encephalitis
Dopamine 2 receptor	Basal ganglia encephalitis

ANTIBODIES AGAINST ION CHANNELS AND OTHER CELL-SURFACE PROTEINS

Leucine-rich glioma-inactivated 1—LGI1	Limbic encephalitis
Contactin-associated protein 2—CASPR2	Morvan's syndrome or limbic encephalitis
Dipeptidyl-peptidase-like protein-6—DPPX	Encephalitis
Myelin oligodendrocyte glycoprotein—MOG	Acute disseminated encephalomyelitis
Aquaporin 4	Encephalitis
GQ1b	Bickerstaff's brainstem encephalitis

Adapted from Graus F, Titulaer MJ, Balu R, et al. A clinical approach to diagnosis of autoimmune encephalitis. *Lancet Neurol.* 2016;15(4):391–404. http://dx.doi.org/10.1016/S1474-4422(150040 1-9). Epub February 20, 2016.

TABLE 11.5
Radiologic Features

1. Brainstem: respiratory virus, arbovirus, MTB, *Listeria monocytogenes, Brucella,* enteroviruses (especially Ev71), MVEV, JEV, WNV, Nipah, *Burkholderia pseudomallei,* anti-NMO (anti-AQP4), anti-Hu, anti-Ma
2. Limbic: HSV, HHV6, anti-NMDAR, anti-VGKC, anti-GAD, anti-Hu, anti-Ma
3. Cerebellum: EBV, VZV, enteroviruses, *Mycoplasma pneumoniae*
4. Subcortical gray matter (basal ganglia, thalami): respiratory virus, arbovirus, MTB, EBV, flaviviruses (especially JEV, MVEV), influenza, poststreptococcal, *M. pneumoniae,* anti-DR2
5. Temporal lobe: HHV6/7, HSV
6. Vasculitis: VZV, systemic lupus erythematosus (SLE) and other cerebral vasculitides
7. White matter lesions: ADEM, JCV-PML, Lyme, *Brucella*
8. Diffuse cerebral edema: respiratory virus
9. Space occupying and/or ring-enhancing lesions: MTB, Balamuthia mandrillaris, Toxoplasma gondii, Cryptococcus neoformans, Aspergillus, Acanthamoeba

Data from Venkatesan A, Tunkel AR, Bloch KC, et al. Case definitions, diagnostic algorithms, and priorities in encephalitis: consensus statement of the International Encephalitis Consortium. *Clin Infect Dis.* 2013;57(8):1114–1128 and Britton A, Ben-Shlomo Y, Benzeval M, et al. Life course trajectories of alcohol consumption in the United Kingdom using longitudinal data from nine cohort studies. *BMC Medicine.* 2015;13:47. http://dx.doi.org/10.1186/s12916-015-0273-z.
ADEM, acute disseminated encephalomyelitis; *EBV,* epstein-Barr virus; *HHV,* herpesvirus; *HSV,* herpes simplex virus; *JCV,* John Cunningham virus; *JEV,* Japanese encephalitis virus; *MTB, Mycobacterium tuberculosis; MVEV,* murray valley encephalitis virus; *NMDAR,* N-methyl-D-aspartate receptor; *VGKC,* voltage-gated potassium channel; *VZV,* varicella-zoster virus; *WNV,* West Nile virus.

alternate conditions that mimic encephalitis. MRI, demonstrated to be superior to CT scanning for demonstration of CNS abnormalities, may aid in defining an etiology, because localization of inflammation may be suggestive of particular pathogens or an autoimmune phenomenon (Table 11.5). The neuroradiological features of the most frequent encephalitis/encephalopathy in Japan are presented in detail in Chapter 7, Neuroimaging on Pediatric Encephalopathy in Japan, by Junichi Takanashi.

DIAGNOSTIC ALGORITHM

First of all, in the case of altered state of consciousness in pediatric age, all the pathologies that may have a similar clinical presentation should be excluded, and then an encephalitis can be hypothesized. In particular, pathologic conditions that could be treated in a short time with targeted therapies should be identified earlier as metabolic diseases or those conditions that rise intracranial pressure. As a first step, a comprehensive history, including seizure semiology's description, and

ENCEPHALITIS/ENCEPHALOPATHY

A child who presents:
1. **Encephalopathy:** defined by some or all of the following features: a) altered level of consciousness, b) altered cognition, c) personality/behavioral change, lethargy; lasting > 24 h.
2. **In combination with:** a) Fever or history of fever (>38°C) within 72 h before/after presentation. b) Generalized or partial seizures not fully attributable to a preexisting seizure disorder. c) New onset focal neurologic findings. d) CSF pleocytosis(≥ 5WBC/uL). e) Abnormal results of neuroimaging suggestive of encephalitis. f) EEG abnormality consistent with encephalitis and not attributable to another cause.
3. **AND no alternative cause identified/diagnosis made.**

Comprehensive history and clinical examination (see Table 11.1)

FIRST-LINE INVESTIGATIONS

LABORATORY

✓ *Blood:*
Full count, electrolytes, glucose, urea, creatinine, calcium, liver function tests, blood culture
✓ *CSF:*
Cell count, Gram stain, culture and biochemistry (protein and glucose), HSV, EBV, CMV, HHV6, VZV, parvovirus, adenovirus, and enterovirus PCR (see Table 11.3)

SEIZURES and EEG

✓ *Acute seizures* management according ILAE guidelines
✓ *EEG:* see Table 11.2

NEUROIMAGES

✓ *CT*
CT should be performed prior to lumbar puncture in the following circumstances:
a) impairment of consciousness;
b) signs of raised intracranial pressure (papilloedema, bradycardia with hypertension, oculomotor palsy, or abnormal response);
c) focal neurologic deficits;
d) new onset seizures (until stabilized);
e) immunocompromised state;
f) previous history of CNS lesion (masslesion, stroke, focal infection)

SECOND-LINE INVESTIGATIONS

✓ *MRI* (see Table 5): preferable to CT
✓ *CSF:* autoimmune investigation (see Table 11.5)
✓ *Other laboratory investigations: Mycoplasma pneumoniae* PCR from throat sample in those with pneumonia/pulmonary lesions; biopsy of skin lesions; stool culture in those with diarrhea

TARGETED TREATMENT

FIG. 11.1 Diagnostic algorithm for encephalitis in pediatric age.

a complete clinical examination are mandatory. Then, laboratory examinations on blood and CSF, EEG, and neuroimaging can be performed (Fig. 11.1).

The aim of our diagnostic algorithm is to stress how cluster of clinical and instrumental examination elements can be strongly indicative of a specific cause. This allows a correct diagnosis in the shortest time to start a targeted treatment as soon as possible, such as acyclovir for herpetic encephalitis or immunomodulatory therapy in immune-mediated encephalitis.

REFERENCES

1. Venkatesan A, Tunkel AR, Bloch KC, et al. Case definitions, diagnostic algorithms, and priorities in encephalitis: consensus statement of the international encephalitis consortium. *Clin Infect Dis.* 2013;57(8):1114–1128.
2. Graus F, Titulaer MJ, Balu R, et al. A clinical approach to diagnosis of autoimmune encephalitis. *Neurology.* 2016 Apr; 15(4):391–404.
3. Britton PN, Eastwood K, Paterson B, et al. Consensus guidelines for the investigation and management of encephalitis in adults and children in Australia and New Zealand. *Int Med J.* 2015;45(5):563–576.

CHAPTER 12

Acute Necrotizing Encephalopathy

MASASHI MIZUGUCHI, MD, PHD • AI HOSHINO, MD, PHD •
MAKIKO SAITOH, MD, PHD

In the 1980s, with the introduction of computed tomography (CT) into clinical practice, some pediatricians in Japan recognized a novel type of acute encephalopathy characterized by a peculiar CT finding: symmetric low-density areas in the bilateral thalamus.[1-3] In the 1990s, when this finding was demonstrated pathologically to represent edematous necrosis, the syndrome was named as "acute necrotizing encephalopathy" (ANE).[4,5] To date, hundreds of ANE cases have been reported from many countries in Asia, America, Europe, and Oceania.

ANE is a fulminant type of acute encephalopathy following a febrile infectious disease, presenting with convulsions, coma, and signs of systemic organ involvement and showing the bilateral thalamic lesions on CT (Fig. 12.1) or magnetic resonance imaging (MRI) (Fig. 12.2). This chapter reviews the accumulated data on the clinical, pathologic, and genetic aspects of ANE.

NOSOLOGY

Bilateral symmetric thalamic lesions are the most important finding in the definition and diagnosis of ANE (Box 12.1). Although very characteristic of ANE, this morphologic finding is shared by several types of acute encephalopathy that show other features distinct from authentic ANE. Their nosologic identity with ANE needs to be further discussed and elucidated.

Familial and recurrent ANE, also called ANE1, is an autosomal dominantly inherited disorder occurring in Caucasian ethnics.[6] The genetic cause of ANE1 is a missense mutation in the *RANBP2* gene encoding a component of nuclear pore complex, Ran-binding protein 2.[7] The clinical course of ANE1 is characterized by recurrent episodes of acute encephalopathy, as well as better outcome than that of typical ANE. Between ANE and ANE1, there are many similarities and differences in clinical and radiologic findings[5,8] (Box 12.2). From the viewpoint of pathogenesis, however, the reasons for these similarities and differences remain to be elucidated.

The morphologic feature of bilateral thalamic involvement is shared by another type of acute encephalopathy secondary to enterohemorrhagic *Escherichia coli* (EHEC) infection. Cranial CT and MRI of patients with EHEC-associated encephalopathy often demonstrate bilateral symmetric involvement of the deep cerebral nuclei: the thalami in some and basal ganglia in others.[9] Without clinical information, neuroradiologists may be unable to distinguish the thalamic lesions of EHEC-associated encephalopathy from those of ANE. From a practical viewpoint, however, the diagnosis of EHEC-associated encephalopathy is easily made based on the presence of antecedent hemorrhagic colitis and hemolytic uremic syndrome.

EPIDEMIOLOGY

Except for Japan, there are no data available on the epidemiology of ANE. Judging from the number of cases reported, the prevalence of ANE is apparently much higher in East Asian countries, such as Japan, Taiwan, and Korea, than in the rest of the world.[5,10-12] In Japan, a country with a population of 128 million, a nationwide survey on the epidemiology of acute encephalopathy was conducted in the year 2010 and estimated the incidence of ANE to be 15–30 cases per year. Among the syndromes of acute encephalopathy, ANE ranked the third, following acute encephalopathy with biphasic seizures and late reduced diffusion (AESD) and mild encephalitis/encephalopathy with a reversible splenial lesion (MERS).[13] During the last two decades from 1996 to 2016, the incidence of ANE in Japan has apparently decreased, as reported by several reference hospitals. The reason for this decline remains obscure.

With regard to age at onset and gender, ANE is most prevalent in infants and young children under 5 years of age, with no sex difference. However, it should be also

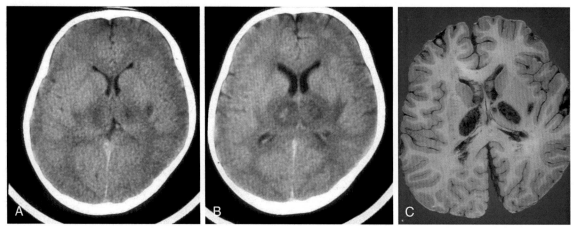

FIG. 12.1 Computed tomography (CT) and autopsy findings of a fatal case of acute necrotizing encephalopathy (ANE). A 3-year-old Japanese boy developed ANE following a febrile infectious disease. **(A)** Initial CT on day 2 showed symmetric low-density areas in the bilateral thalamus. **(B)** Follow-up CT on day 4 revealed high-density areas in the center of thalamic lesions, as well as low-density areas in the periphery of thalamus, posterior part of putamen, and cerebral deep white matter. **(C)** Autopsy on day 5 demonstrated the central lesion of hemorrhage (blackish) and peripheral lesion of softening (pale brown), corresponding to the high-density and low-density areas on CT, respectively.

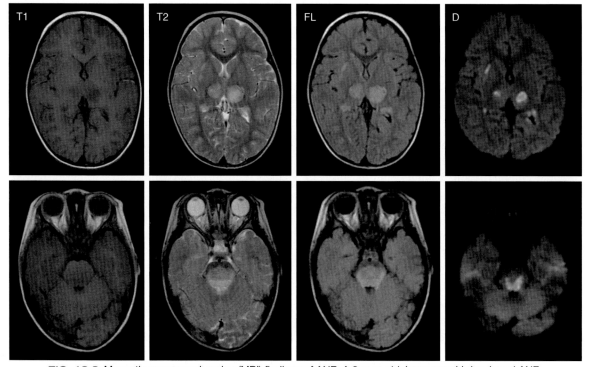

FIG. 12.2 Magnetic resonance imaging (MRI) findings of ANE. A 2-year-old Japanese girl developed ANE following influenza A. Cranial MRI on day 2 demonstrated symmetric lesions in the thalamus and pons. They were slightly hypointense on T1-weighted images (T1), hyperintense on T2-weighted (T2), and fluid attenuated inversion recovery (FL) images. Their central areas showed markedly restricted diffusion on diffusion-weighted images (D).

BOX 12.1
Diagnostic Criteria of Acute Necrotizing Encephalopathy (ANE)

1. Acute encephalopathy following a viral febrile disease. Rapid deterioration in the level of consciousness. Convulsions.

2. No CSF pleocytosis. Increase in CSF protein commonly observed.

3. CT or MRI evidence for symmetric, multifocal brain lesions. Involvement of the bilateral thalami. Lesions also common in the cerebral periventricular white matter, internal capsule, putamen, upper brainstem tegmentum, and cerebellar white matter. No involvement of other CNS lesions.

4. Elevation of serum aminotransferases of variable degrees. No increase in blood ammonia.

5. Exclusion of resembling diseases.

   a. Differential diagnosis from clinical viewpoints.

      i. Overwhelming bacterial and viral infections, and fulminant hepatitis.

      ii. Toxic shock, hemolytic uremic syndrome (acute encephalopathy associated with enterohemorrhagic *Escherichia coli* infection), and other toxin-induced diseases.

      iii. Reye syndrome, hemorrhagic shock and encephalopathy syndrome, and heatstroke.

   b. Differential diagnosis from radiologic (or pathologic) viewpoint.

      i. Leigh encephalopathy and related mitochondrial cytopathies.

      ii. Glutaric aciduria, methylmalonic acidemia, and infantile bilateral striatal necrosis.

      iii. Wernicke encephalopathy and carbon monoxide poisoning.

      iv. Acute disseminated encephalomyelitis, acute hemorrhagic leukoencephalitis, and other types of encephalitis (Japanese encephalitis, cerebral malaria); arterial or venous infarction and the effects of severe hypoxia or head trauma.

---

kept in mind that ANE occasionally occurs in children, adults, and even the elderly.[14,15] As the pathogen of antecedent infection, influenza virus is by far the most common (41%), followed by human herpesvirus-6 (20%), adenovirus (3%), herpes simplex virus (3%), and rotavirus (2%).[13] With regard to prognosis, there was little improvement in the 1990s and 2000s. The outcome remains poor, with death occurring in 28% and neurologic sequelae in 63%.[13] A Japanese research committee on influenza-associated encephalopathy previously demonstrated that the fatality is higher in patients who have been given nonsteroidal antiinflammatory drugs (NSAIDs), such as diclofenac and mefenamic acid.[16]

CLINICAL AND LABORATORY FINDINGS

Despite the term "encephalopathy," ANE affects not only the brain but also many of the systemic organs including the heart, liver, and kidney, as well as the blood cells. The overall clinical picture resembles sepsis or systemic inflammatory response syndrome.[16]

Before the onset of ANE, there is always a febrile infectious disease, being viral in the majority of cases. Influenza is the most common, followed by exanthem subitum.[13] An endemic of influenza is often followed by successive occurrence of multiple ANE cases in the region. Half a day to three days after the onset of fever, there appears the first sign of encephalopathy: impairment of consciousness or convulsion. Some patients initially show a mild disturbance of consciousness, such as somnolence of delirium, but otherwise patients uniformly develop deep coma within 24 h. The vast majority of patients (94%) have convulsions, often being prolonged. More than 60% of patients show signs of increased intracranial pressure: vomiting, hyperventilation, and decorticate or decerebrate posturing. Other common findings on admission include neurologic signs, such as exaggerated tendon jerks (66%) and extensor Babinski responses (66%), and systemic signs, such as vomiting (70%), diarrhea (42%), and hepatomegaly (41%).[4,5]

Laboratory examination at the acute stage shows high levels of serum transaminases and lactic dehydrogenase, the degree of which varies from 50 to 50,000 units. Also common are other blood abnormalities such as high blood urine nitrogen, metabolic acidosis, high C-reactive protein, high creatine kinase, low total protein, low platelet count, low fibrinogen, and high fibrin degradation product. Examination of the cerebrospinal fluid (CSF) reveals high opening pressure and high CSF protein (67%). In some patients, CSF protein was as high as 0.8 g/dL, showing xanthochromia and/or Froin sign, i.e.,

BOX 12.2
Comparison Between Typical, Sporadic Acute Necrotizing Encephalopathy (ANE) and Familial, Recurrent ANE (ANE1)

SIMILARITIES
- Acute encephalopathy with onset in the acute stage of infectious diseases.
- Symmetric lesions in the bilateral thalamus.
- Elevated CSF protein.

DIFFERENCES
- Positive family history is common in ANE1, but not in sporadic ANE.
- Recurrence of encephalopathy is common in ANE1, but rare in sporadic ANE.
- High fever at onset is very common in sporadic ANE, but not in ANE1.
- Physical signs and laboratory data of systemic organ damage are often prominent in sporadic ANE, but not in ANE1.
- Lesions in the cerebral periventricular white matter and cerebellum are common in sporadic ANE, but not in ANE1.
- Lesions in the claustrum, external capsule, insula, medial temporal lobe, amygdala, hippocampus, mammillary bodies, and spinal cord are common in ANE1, but not in sporadic ANE.
- Outcome is likely better in ANE1 than in sporadic ANE, for both survival and neurologic condition.

yellow dyscoloration and coagulation of CSF. Electrophysiologic examinations show slowing of basic rhythms on electroencephalography, as well as diminished or abolished brainstem auditory evoked potentials.[4,5]

During the acute period, some patients die either from brainstem damage or from systemic damage (multiple organ failure). In surviving patients, damage to systemic organs is transient, showing recovery from around the fifth day of illness. However, many of the patients are left with permanent neurologic sequelae. Typical neurologic signs in severely handicapped patients are motor paralysis, intellectual deficits, and epilepsy.[4,5] On the other hand, moderately handicapped patients may show a characteristic combination of focal motor signs, such as hemiparesis, dysarthria, intention tremor, ataxia, abducens nerve palsy, and facial palsy, resulting from the unique topographic distribution of focal lesions in the deep cerebral nuclei and brainstem tegmentum.[17]

RADIOLOGIC AND PATHOLOGIC FINDINGS

Symmetric brain lesions in the bilateral thalamus and some other regions are the hallmark of ANE. Soon after the patients fall into coma, cranial CT and MRI demonstrate these multiple lesions. Some of them primarily involve the gray matter, such as the thalamus, putamen, and brainstem tegmentum, whereas others mainly affect the white matter, such as the cerebral periventricular white matter and cerebellar parenchyma surrounding the dentate nucleus. All these lesions appear hypodense on CT (Fig. 12.1A), and T1-hypointense and T2-hyperintense on MRI (Fig. 12.2).[4,5]

On follow-up CT/MRI one to several days later, the contrast between the lesions and the surrounding tissue becomes clearer. In the center of thalamic and/or brainstem lesions of severe cases, there appear areas of hyperdensity on CT and T1-hyperintensity on MRI, resulting in a concentric appearance (Fig. 12.1B).[18] Neuropathologic examination in the acute stage demonstrates that the concentricity reflects hemorrhage in the center and edema in the periphery of the lesions (Fig. 12.1C). Perivascular hemorrhage and edema apparently resulted from excessive permeability of cerebral blood vessels, the degree of which is more severe in the center than the periphery. Except for aggregation of macrophages and activation of microglial cells,[4,19] there is neither infiltration of inflammatory cells nor presence of viruses such as influenza virus.

After the third day of illness, the brain shows a progressive and diffuse atrophic change. Focal lesions in the thalamus and other regions shrink gradually. They may eventually disappear in mild cases but may remain as multiple cystic lesions in severe cases. Neuropathology in the chronic stage demonstrates the aggregation of fat-laden macrophages in the cavity, as well as gliosis in the wall. Thalamic cysts show deposition of hemosiderin.[4]

PATHOGENESIS

The main pathogenesis of ANE is considered to be cytokine storm, systemic inflammatory response, or exaggerated natural immunity.[16] This notion is supported by multiple pieces of clinical evidence. First, severe cases of ANE often show signs of multiple organ failure, notably shock and disseminated intravascular coagulation. Second, ANE is occasionally complicated by hemophagocytic syndrome. Third, botryoid nuclei (radial segmentation) of neutrophils are seen in ANE, as well as in hemorrhagic shock and encephalopathy syndrome and heatstroke, syndromes characterized by hyperthermia and cytokine storm.[20]

Laboratory studies demonstrate very high levels of inflammatory cytokines, such as interleukin-6 (IL-6) and tumor necrosis factor-α.[16,21] Simultaneous sampling of blood and CSF demonstrates that the levels are higher in the serum than in CSF, suggesting that the inflammatory response is systemic, rather than localized in the brain.

GENETIC BACKGROUND

Except for the cases of ANE1, there is no evidence of Mendelian inheritance for ANE. In the vast majority of patients, neither familial nor past history is positive. Taking the ethnic difference in its incidence into consideration, multiple factors, genetic and environmental, are likely to be involved.

To identify gene variations at risk for ANE, we have conducted a nationwide collaborative study in Japan since 2009, employing a candidate gene approach. We recruited Japanese patients with ANE from all the regions of Japan. The vast majority of patients were sporadic. None of them had clinical features of ANE1. We selected candidate genes on the basis of the suspected pathogenesis and examined whether their mutations and polymorphisms are associated with ANE.

To date, several genes have been demonstrated to be in association with ANE. As expected, there were several genes regulating immune responses: *HLA-DRB1*09:01*, *HLA-DQB1*03:03*,[22] *IL6*, and *IL10* (manuscript in preparation). On the other hand, we found possible association of ANE with other kinds of genes, including a missense mutation of *SCN1A*, encoding a subunit of a voltage-gated sodium ion channel,[23] and thermolabile variations of *CPT2*, encoding a mitochondrial enzyme, carnitine palmitoyl transferase 2.[24] We sequenced all the exons of *RANBP2*, the causative gene for ANE1, but found no pathogenic mutations. Thus, sporadic ANE is genetically distinct from familial and recurrent ANE, or ANE1.

DIAGNOSIS

The diagnosis of ANE is made on the basis of a combination of clinical, laboratory, and radiologic findings. Although symmetric thalamic lesions are quite characteristic of ANE, some conditions also show similar imaging findings and need to be differentiated from ANE[4,5] (Box 12.1).

TREATMENT

The treatment of ANE consists of general supportive treatment and specific treatment (Box 12.3). For the latter, many antiinflammatory therapies, as well as targeted

---

BOX 12.3
Treatment of Acute Necrotizing Encephalopathy (ANE)

GENERAL TREATMENT
- Intensive care
- Monitoring
  - Vital signs, consciousness
  - Intracranial pressure (ICP)
- Systemic supportive treatment
  - Temperature
  - Water, electrolytes
  - Hematologic
- CNS treatment
  - Convulsion
  - Increased ICP

SPECIFIC TREATMENT
- Antiinflammatory therapies
  - Corticosteroids (Level IV/Grade B)
  - Intravenous immunoglobulin (Level V/Grade none)
  - Plasma exchange (Level V/Grade none)
  - Continuous hemodiafiltration (Level V/Grade none)
- Targeted temperature management (Level V/Grade none)
  - Hypothermia
  - Normothermia

---

temperature management, have been proposed and tried. However, there has been little statistic evidence for their efficacy, except for borderline efficacy of corticosteroids administered early in the course (within 24 h from the onset) for patients without brainstem lesions.[25]

REFERENCES

1. Aoki N. Acute toxic encephalopathy with symmetrical low density areas in the thalami and the cerebellum. *Childs Nerv Syst.* 1985;1:62–65.
2. Tateno A, Sakai K, Sakai S, Koya N, Aoki T. Computed tomography of bilateral thalamic hypodensity in acute encephalopathy. *J Comput Assist Tomogr.* 1988;12:637–639.
3. Mizuguchi M. Acute encephalopathy with necrosis of bilateral thalami. Clinical aspects. *Neuropathology.* 1993;13:327–331.
4. Mizuguchi M, Abe J, Mikkaichi K, et al. Acute necrotizing encephalopathy of childhood: a new syndrome presenting with multifocal, symmetric brain lesions. *J Neurol Neurosurg Psychiatry.* 1995;58:555–561.

5. Mizuguchi M. Acute necrotizing encephalopathy of childhood: a novel form of acute encephalopathy prevalent in Japan and Taiwan. *Brain Dev*. 1997;19:81–92.

6. Neilson DE, Eiben RM, Waniewski S, et al. Autosomal dominant acute necrotizing encephalopathy. *Neurology*. 2003;61:226–230.

7. Neilson DE, Adams MD, Orr CM, et al. Infection-triggered familial or recurrent cases of acute necrotizing encephalopathy caused by mutations in a component of the nuclear pore, *RANBP2*. *Am J Hum Genet*. 2009;84:44–51.

8. Singh RR, Sedani S, Lim M, Wassmer E, Absoud M. RANBP2 mutation and acute necrotizing encephalopathy: 2 cases and a literature review of the expanding clinico-radiological phenotype. *Eur J Pediatr Neurol*. 2015;19:106–113.

9. Takanashi JI, Taneichi H, Misaki T, et al. Clinical and radiologic features of encephalopathy during 2011 *E coli* O111 outbreak in Japan. *Neurology*. 2014;82:564–572.

10. Wang HS, Huang SC. Acute necrotizing encephalopathy of childhood. *Chang Gung Med*. 2001;24:1–10.

11. Kim JH, Kim IO, Lim MK, et al. Acute necrotizing encephalopathy in Korean infants and children: imaging findings and diverse clinical outcome. *Korean J Radiol*. 2004;5:171–177.

12. Mastroyianni SD, Gionnis D, Voudris K, Skardoutsou A, Mizuguchi M. Acute necrotizing encephalopathy of childhood in non-Asian patients. Report of three cases and literature review. *J Child Neurol*. 2006;21:872–879.

13. Hoshino A, Saitoh M, Oka A, et al. Epidemiology of acute encephalopathy in Japan, with emphasis on the association of viruses and syndromes. *Brain Dev*. 2012;34:337–343.

14. Jardine DL, Hurrell MA, Anderson TJ. A bad dose of flu. *Lancet*. 2003;362(9391):1198.

15. Ishii N, Mochizuki H, Moriguchi-Goto S, et al. An autopsy case of elderly-onset acute necrotizing encephalopathy secondary to influenza. *J Neurol Sci*. 2015;354:129–130.

16. Mizuguchi M, Yamanouchi H, Ichiyama T, Shiomi M. Acute encephalopathy associated with influenza and other viral infections. *Acta Neurol Scand*. 2007;115:45–56.

17. Mizuguchi M, Iai M, Takashima S. Acute necrotizing encephalopathy of childhood: recent advances and future prospects. *No To Hattatsu*. 1998;30:189–196 (in Japanese).

18. Mizuguchi M, Hayashi M, Nakano I, et al. Concentric structure of thalamic lesions of acute necrotizng encephalopathy. *Neuroradiology*. 2002;44:489–493.

19. Nakai Y, Itoh M, Mizuguchi M, Becker LE, Itoh M, Takashima S. Apoptosis and microglial activation in influenza encephalopathy. *Acta Neuropathol*. 2003;105:233–239.

20. Takasugi H, Ishihara M, Ando Y, Shimanouchi Y. Botryoid nuclei in neutrophils of patient with acute necrotizing encephalopathy. *J Jpn Pediatr Soc*. 2002;106:1470–1473 (in Japanese).

21. Ichiyama T, Endo S, Kaneko M, Isumi H, Matsubara T, Furukawa S. Serum cytokine concentrations of influenza associated acute necrotizing encephalopathy. *Pediatr Int*. 2003;45:734–736.

22. Hoshino A, Saitoh M, Miyagawa T, et al. Specific HLA genotypes confer susceptibility to acute necrotizing encephalopathy. *Genes Immun*. 2016;17:367–369.

23. Saitoh M, Shinohara M, Hoshino H, et al. Mutations of the *SCN1A* gene in acute encephalopathy. *Epilepsia*. 2012;53:558–564.

24. Shinohara M, Saitoh M, Takanashi JI, et al. Carnitine palmitoyl transferase II polymorphism is associated with multiple syndromes of acute encephalopathy with various infectious diseases. *Brain Dev*. 2011;33:512–517.

25. Okumura A, Mizuguchi M, Kidokoro H, et al. Outcome of acute necrotizing encephalopathy in relation to treatment with corticosteroids and gammaglobulin. *Brain Dev*. 2009;31:221–227.

CHAPTER 13

Acute Encephalopathy With Febrile Convulsive Status Epilepticus (AEFCSE)

MASASHI SHIOMI PHD, MD

INTRODUCTION

Aicardi reported that among 402 patients with febrile convulsive status epilepticus who were observed from 1963 to 1971, 113 patients were found to have subsequent neurologic complications, including 37 patients with motor paralysis, 54 patients with mental deficits, and 114 patients with epilepsy. He concluded that neurologic sequelae after febrile convulsive status epilepticus are not uncommon.[1]

Recent reports on febrile convulsive status epilepticus in children from Europe and the United States have shown the following two points: (1) Prognosis is commonly good even if febrile convulsive seizure epilepticus lasts for a long duration; however, in a part of them medial temporal sclerosis develops later. (2) some patients with febrile convulsive status epilepticus develop acute encephalitis and/or acute encephalopathy with poor prognosis.[2] However, some cases of encephalitis and/or encephalopathy are not clearly distinguished from febrile convulsive status epilepticus. Aicardi mentioned that the cause of hemiconvulsion-hemiparesis epilepsy syndrome (HHES) was regarded as sequelae of febrile convulsive status epilepticus, the incidence of which decreased after routine usage of intravenous diazepam to cease the prolonged seizures after the 1960s.[3] In fact, in his study on 73 patients with HH, the duration longer than 24 h was found in 31 patients, between 5 and 24 h in 20 patients, and less than 90 min in no patients.[3] There are various opinions about the cause of HHE.[4] Some reports have suggested that HHE is due to selective neuronal injury disorder following status epilepticus, and that the special distribution of the lesion is consistent with the distribution of neuronal excessive excitation.[5]

I was inspired by Kimura's image classification of acute encephalopathy[6] and, by attempting to classify acute encephalopathy associated with influenza, proposed a novel subtype of acute encephalopathy, "acute encephalopathy with febrile convulsive status epilepticus (AEFCSE)."[7] In 2006, Takanashi summarized multicenter cases and reported[8] them as acute encephalopathy with biphasic seizures and late reduced diffusion (AESD), while Yamanouchi reported a study of patients with bilateral frontal lobe lesions as acute infantile encephalopathy predominantly affecting the frontal lobes (AIEF).[9] AEFCSE is considered the same disorder as AESD and AIEF. The final criteria of this subtype have been shown in the practice guideline for acute encephalopathy in childhood released from the Japanese Society of Child Neurology (JSCN) in 2016.[10] In a nationwide survey in Japan,[11] acute encephalopathy in childhood has been estimated to be 400 to 700 cases per year, AEFCSE being the most common with ~30% with a mean age of onset around 1.7 years (median 1 year old, 41% in boys) and estimated to affect 100 to 200 people per year. The incidence of AEFCSE in febrile convulsive status epilepticus has been estimated around 5%.

ACUTE ENCEPHALOPATHY WITH FEBRILE CONVULSIVE STATUS EPILEPTICUS

Theory

After an early seizure (ES) at the time of fever, and after a recovery of consciousness, late seizure (LS) occurs around 4–5 days after the onset with a decline in the level of consciousness. There are abnormalities such as lobar or multilobar edema on CT of the brain and "bright tree" appearance (BTA) in diffusion weighted image (DWI), indicative of dendritic high signal lesions in the subcortical white matter (BTAs). Subsequently, many children are left with permanent brain damage. Typical examples take the course shown in Table 13.1 and Fig. 13.1.[12] HHE may be considered as unilateral

TABLE 13.1
Progression/Image Features of Acute Encephalopathy With Febrile Status Epilepticus
1. Febrile status epilepticus phase: early seizure (ES)   Seizures that persist for more than 30 min   2. Temporary recovery period: second to fourth day of the disease with improvements in the level of consciousness.   3. Late seizure (LS) appear fourth to fifth day of the disease in clusters.   Repeated focal seizures and cerebral lobar edema. Affected brain lobes are distributed to hemispheric, bi-frontal, temporal regions. "Bright tree" appearance on MRI with DWI, with little changes near the central sulcus and occipital lobes (centrooccipital sparing).   4. There may be permanent damage. Permanent damage affects mental aspects more than motor aspects. There are speech disturbances associated with bilateral frontal lobe lesions.

DWI, diffusion weighted image; *MRI*, magnetic resonance imaging.

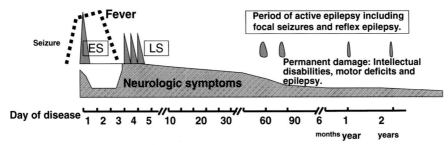

FIG. 13.1 Features of progress in acute encephalopathy with febrile convulsive status epilepticus. *ES*, early seizure; *LS*, late seizure

AEFCSE. Although there are cases affecting only the frontal lobe bilaterally and cases with extensive lesions in the cerebral cortex, lesions in the vicinity of the central sulcus and the occipital lobe are uncommon (centrooccipital sparing). Because status epilepticus occurring in association with a neurologic disorder is a common cause of status epilepticus and is included in the remote symptomatic group in the etiologic classification, these cases were excluded in early studies of AEFCSE, and a case of bacterial meningitis was included in the study when lobar edema followed by status epilepticus was the primary lesion.

Examination of Cases Hospitalized at the Osaka City General Hospital, Japan[12]

Twenty-seven patients admitted between 1997 and 2005 have the features of AEFCSE; eleven patients had a history of theophylline exposure. There was a significant difference ($P<.01$) in the age the symptoms first appear, with the theophylline exposed group (THEO+) being older (33.1 ± 12.7 months old) than the group not exposed to it (THEO–) (15.4 ± 10.7 months old). The male-to-female ratio was 11:5 in the THEO– group and 7:4 in the THEO+ group. As to the cause of fever in THEO– group, nine patients had evidence of HHV-6

infection, 2 had influenza virus and one patient each measles, measles vaccine, haemophilus influenzae type b (Hib)meningitis, human metapneumovirus and adenovirus. The patient with Hib required dialysis because of acute renal failure, and its clinical course was verified by image findings consistent with HH syndrome. In the THEO+ group, there was one patient with HHV-6, two patients with influenza, one patient with Respiratory Syncytial Virus (RSV), and the rest were unknown. The THEO+ case with HHV-6 primary infection was complicated by the emergence of hemophagocytosis syndrome and acute renal failure, as well as extensive white matter lesions, leaving severe permanent neurologic damage including epilepsy. In nine patients in whom the theophylline serum levels were measured at the time of hospitalization, one patient showed a level over 20 µg/L, one patient between 15 and 19 µg/L, four patients between 10 and 14 µg/L, two patients between 5 and 9 µg/L, and one patient below 5 µg/L. There was no history of febrile seizure in the THEO– group, and although four cases were observed in the THEO+ group, this may have been the effect of the difference in age distribution between the two groups. Although AEFCSE seems to be related to exposure of theophylline, our hospital has not seen a case of THEO+ since 2005. This was thought to be due to the revision of the asthma guidelines by Japan Society for Pediatric Allergy and Clinical Immunology in November 2005 and the introduction of restrictions to theophylline use in infants, brought on by the appeals regarding theophylline risks made by the authors at Osaka Pediatric Association, following the three consecutive cases of THEO + AEFCSE that were hospitalized in the second half of 2004.

Nineteen patients with AEFCSE were hospitalized in the ES phase, and only six of them did not require intubation for cease of seizure and all patients developed LSs after 3 days on average. Two of six were then intubated together with barbital treatments (pentobarbital or thiopental) and four patients received large intravenous doses of phenytoin. Thirteen patients required mechanical ventilation, twelve patients received barbital therapy, while one patient received continuous infusion of midazolam (MDZ) under mechanical ventilation. The period of mechanical ventilation varied from 4 to 17 days (median of 10 days). There were severe complications for the cases hospitalized during the ES phase, with one patient with Takotsubo cardiomyopathy and two patients with acute renal failure requiring hemodialysis. Pulmonary edema was seen on chest CT of many cases; there were no patient deaths. Brain CT examinations were repeatedly performed on patients during the ES phase, and when lobar edema appeared during mechanical ventilation, respiratory management continued until it was judged that there was no danger of cerebral herniation due to cerebral edema. In addition, intracranial pressure monitoring was performed in two patients.

On the other hand, seven patients were hospitalized in the LS phase, with ES having been easily controlled by the previous doctors. These patients received barbiturate therapy under mechanical ventilation, because the seizures did not easily stop even with other treatments. The duration of mechanical ventilation was 3–9 days (median of 5.5 days). Repetitive focal seizures of around 1 min were a common manifestation in the LS phase; as there were cases who maintained consciousness, these seizures were sometimes misinterpreted as myoclonus, but the diagnosis was confirmed with EEG recordings. Separately, there was a case that was hospitalized on the ninth day of recovery period.

In the follow-up study, 20 out of 27 patients could walk alone. Three patients with HHE syndrome with lesions on only one side were relatively well in intelligence testing, but the others had motor and/or mental deficits. In addition, in patients with lesions restricted to both frontal lobes, there were severe speech delays. Epileptiform discharges on EEG commonly became evident 1–6 months after the initial event. However, epilepsy developed in 10 of 27 cases, 6 of which were controlled, but 4 patients were refractory, 1 patient had epileptic spasms, and 2 patients were diagnosed as reflex epilepsy (1 patient developed tonic seizures in response to sound, and another when trying to touch faucet water).

In brain imaging, lobar edema was seen on CT 4–5 days after the onset. Although BTA (Fig. 13.2) on

| Day 2 | Day 5 | Day 8 |

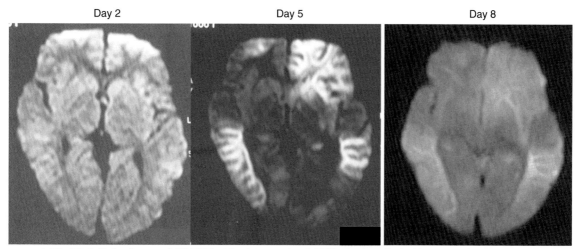

FIG. 13.2 Daily changes (MRI/DWI) of the intense signal (BTA) of subcortical white matter due to acute encephalopathy with febrile status epilepticus. *BTA*, bright tree appearance; *DWI*, diffusion weighted image; *MRI*, magnetic resonance imaging. (Images for Day 2 and Day 5 were provided from Dr. Yasunobu Nakajima of Izumi Municipal Hospital.)

diffusion weighted MR image was typically a linear, intense high signal of subcortical white matter, it was often ambiguous in DWI because of pseudonormalization; however, it was identified as a linear low signal with ADC (apparent diffusion coefficient) map image. The appearance of BTA varies depending on the examination date, and the positive case/examination number is 0/2 on the first to third days of the disease, 3/4 on the fourth day of disease, 3/4 on the fifth day of disease, 2/2 on the seventh day of disease, 3/4 on the eighth day of the disease, and 0/3 after the ninth day of disease. Although BTA on the fourth day of disease was evident in the patient as shown in Fig. 13.2, it becomes less clear by the eighth day of disease.

In routine blood examinations, the median aspartate aminotransferase at the time of hospitalization in the 19 patients admitted during the ES phase was 111 IU/mL, with 2 patients having 50 IU/mL or less, 5 patients between 51 and 100 IU/mL, 5 patients between 101 and 200 IU/mL, 4 patients between 201 and 300 IU/mL, 2 patients with 501 IU/mL or above, with the maximum being 998 IU/mL.

Pathogenesis of Acute Encephalopathy With Febrile Convulsive Status Epilepticus

The frequency of febrile seizures in Japanese children is 6%–10%, which is more than twice as much as the frequency, 2%–4%, in European and US cohorts. According to the epidemiologic survey of pediatric SE studies in Okayama City, Japan, carried out by Nishiyama et al., the frequency is about 40/100,000 people, and among 120 cases studied for 3 years,[13] nearly half of the cases were diagnosed as febrile seizures. In terms of the virus, 10 cases were due to influenza and 16 cases due to exanthema subitum. Out of the 11 patients with acute encephalitis/encephalopathy, 4 patients had influenza and 3 patients had exanthema subitum, suggesting the similarities in agents between febrile convulsions and acute encephalitis/encephalopathy. It has been suggested that around 5% of cases with Febrile Status Epileptics (FSE) develop AEFCSE, thus estimating that there may be 100–200 cases every year. Acute necrotizing encephalopathy (ANE) is also common in Japanese children, but the frequency of AEFCSE is about 10 times that of ANE. Although reports of ANE are seen all over the world, AEFCSE reports are uncommon in Europe, the United States, and also in East Asia. There was a report from Australia recently, in a patient of Asian descent.[14] Many of AEFCSE reports did not fulfill the diagnostic criteria by JSCM.[15-16] There are a few reports of HHE, but most are probably of AEFCSE.[17] In animal experiments, a model by Suchomelova et al. that

adds high fever to the lithium-pilocarpine convulsion model of young rats is considered to have the pathology most similar to AEFCSE. In this model, status epilepticus was stopped with the use of diazepam and the body temperature was kept at 39°C during the status epilepticus lasting for over 50 min. On the following day, the rat ate well and recovered, but developed epilepsy as well as brain atrophy after 4 months. Neuronal necrosis and/or apoptosis was seen 24 h after status epileptics. No biphasic experimental model like AEFCSE was found. Although manifestation of epilepsy was observed in the febrile convulsion model by Dubé et al.,[18] neuronal cell death or brain atrophy was not observed. I suggest that two hits of high fever and status epilepticus are likely to cause brain atrophy like AEFCSE. Attempts have been made to administer antiinflammatory agents, antioxidants, etc. to prevent apoptosis of nerve cells caused by status epileptics, but those which were clinically not proved effective so far.

DIAGNOSTIC CRITERIA OF ACUTE ENCEPHALOPATHY WITH FEBRILE CONVULSIVE STATUS EPILEPTICUS (ACUTE ENCEPHALOPATHY WITH BIPHASIC SEIZURES AND LATE REDUCED DIFFUSION)*

Clinical findings

1. In children, pathologies based on other triggers such as head trauma, other encephalopathy syndromes, and encephalitis that manifests during the thermophilic phase of infectious diseases should be excluded.
2. It manifests as seizure (ES, often status epilepticus) on the day of fever or the next day.
3. Recurrence of seizures (LS, mostly clusters of focal seizure) on third to seventh day of disease, with pronounced changes in the level of consciousness, is found.
4. Diffusion weighted MR images on the 3rd to 14th day of disease show intense high signals in the subcortical white matter ("BTA"; Fig. 13.2). The central sulcus is frequently spared (central sparing).
5. After 2 weeks, there is residual atrophy in the frontal region, or frontal and parietal combined region on CT or MRI, with decreased blood flow as seen with SPECT.

The diagnosis is considered if any of the 3, 4, or 5 criterion is fulfilled in addition to 1 and 2.

---

*JSCN, 2016 personal English translation by the author.

Other findings

i High frequency of HHV-6 and influenza virus being the causative pathogen

ii Commonly temporal improvement of consciousness after the ES

iii Commonly normal brain CT and MRI at the first and second day

iv Variable prognosis (from subtle developmental delay to severe psychomotor disorder)

DISCUSSION

Preventing Acute Encephalopathy With Febrile Convulsive Status Epilepticus

If we consider AEFCSE to be caused by febrile convulsive status epilepticus, it is conceivable that stopping the status epilepticus early will lead to a decrease in AEFCSE. In Japan, febrile convulsions are common, but because of the optimistic estimate of the prognosis as well as the lack of a fully organized emergency medical care system for children, the management for febrile convulsive status epilepticus was suboptimal until around 2000. As AEFCSE became more known, the importance of quick cessation of febrile convulsive status epilepticus became of paramount importance. As shown by RAMPART study,[19] midazolam intramuscular injection by an emergency personnel should be encouraged in the future. In addition, the restrictions to theophylline administration is suspected to have contributed to the decrease in the occurrence of AEFCSE.

Treatment of Acute Encephalopathy With Febrile Convulsive Status Epilepticus

Hypothermia therapy of neonatal hypoxic ischemic encephalopathy (HIE) has been shown to be effective, in both animal experiments and clinical application, and is now highly recommended in applied cases. When moderate to severe cases were selected as the inclusion criteria and hypothermia therapy was performed in neonatal HIE, the cases with poor prognosis fell from 60% to 40%. To investigate the effect of hypothermia, which is invasive in AEFCSE, we propose careful assessment of the diagnosis and treatment of febrile status epilepticus cases, of which more than half advances to AEFCSE. When hypothermia is not used, antiinflammatory therapy and antioxidant treatments can be used, but a large number of cases will need to be enrolled. Efficacy was not demonstrated in a study comparing hypothermia and normothermia therapy for status epileptics requiring mechanical ventilation for adults.[20] With AEFCSE, because ESs commonly

stop, the target of AEFCSE study is different from clinical trials of refractory status epilepticus.

When introducing hypothermia therapy after ES, how long should it be done and whether or not to continue for the 4–5 days after onset of symptoms when LS develop are not known. Furthermore, when LS occur, it is suggested that the lesion is irreversible, especially when the BTA emerges in the MRI. However, in neonatal HIE, nearly half of the cases develop convulsion at the beginning of hypothermia therapy, and convulsions often disappear in a few days. If we consider that late seizures of AEFCSE occur through the same mechanism as the neonatal HIE seizure, hypothermia therapy after the onset of the late phase seizures.

CONCLUSION

AEFCSE is thought to be an acute encephalopathy triggered in some children who experienced febrile status epilepticus. Although this disease concept was established early for HHE syndrome, advancements in image techniques such as diffusion weighted MRI have been instrumental to establish the disease concept of AEFCSE. It is strange that majority of reports is mostly from Japan. Because AEFCSE develops in 100–200 patients per year in Japan, research on prevention and treatment is necessary.

REFERENCES

1. Aicardi J, Chevrie JJ. Febrile convulsions: neurological sequelae and mental retardation. In: Brazier MAB, Ccceani F, eds. *Brain Dysfunction in Infantile Febrile Convulsions.* New York: Raven Press; 1976:247–257.
2. Holland K, Shinnar S. Status epilepticus in children. *Handb Clin Neurol.* 2012;108:795–812.
3. Aicardi J. Consequences and prognosis of convulsive status epilepticus in infants and children. *Jpn J Psychiatry Neurol.* 1986;40:283–290.
4. Auvin S, Bellavoine V, Merdariu D, et al. Hemiconvulsion-hemiplegia-epilepsy syndrome: current understandings. *Eur J Paediatr Neurol.* 2012;16:413–421.
5. Men S, Lee DH, Barron JR, Muñoz DG. Selective neuronal necrosis associated with status epilepticus: MR findings. *AJNR Am J Neuroradiol.* 2000.
6. Kimura S, Nezu A, Ohtsuki N, Tanaka M, Takeshita S. Clinical studies on 35 patients with infection-related acute encephalopathy. *No-to-Hattatsu.* 1998;30:244–249 (in Japanese).
7. Shiomi M. A proposal of the clinical classification of influenza encephalopathy (in Japanese). *Shonika Rinsho.* 2000;53:1739–1746.
8. Takanashi J, Oba H, Barkovich AJ, et al. Diffusion MRI abnormalities after prolonged febrile seizures with encephalopathy. *Neurology.* 2006;66:1304–1309.

9. Yamanouchi H, Mizuguchi M. Acute infantile encephalopathy predominantly affecting the frontal lobes (AIEF): a novel clinical category and its tentative diagnostic criteria. *Epilepsy Res.* 2006;70:S263–S268.

10. Japanese Society of Child Neurology. Practice Guideline for acute encephalopathy in childhood (in Japanese) 2016.

11. Hoshino A, Saitoh M, Oka A, et al. Epidemiology of acute encephalopathy in Japan, with emphasis on the association of viruses and syndromes. *Brain Dev.* 2012;34:337–343.

12. Shiomi M, Ishikawa J, Togawa M, et al. Acute encephalopathy with febrile convulsive status epilepticus and theophylline as its trigger. *No To Hattatsu.* 2008;40:122–127 (In Japanese).

13. Nishiyama I, Ohtsuka Y, Tsuda T, et al. An epidemiological study of children with status epilepticus in Okayama, Japan: incidence, etiologies, and outcomes. *Epilepsy Res.* 2011;96:89–95.

14. Srinivasan D, Gupta S, Prelog K. Acute encephalopathy: when febrile status more than 'fits'. *J Paediatr Child Health.* 2016;52(10):957–960.

15. Goenka A, Michael BD, Ledger E, et al. Neurological manifestations of influenza infection in children and adults: results of a National British Surveillance Study. *Clin Infect Dis.* 2014;58:775–784.

16. Hoffman EM, Ruff MW, Patterson MC. Acute encephalopathy with biphasic seizures and late restricted diffusion. *Pediatr Neurol.* February 2016;55:74–75.

17. Franzoni E, Garone C, Marchiani V, et al. A new case of idiopathic hemiplegia hemiconvulsion syndrome. *Neurol Sci.* 2010;31:799–805.

18. Suchomelova L, Lopez-Meraz ML, Niquet J, Kubova H, Wasterlain CG. Hyperthermia aggravates status epilepticus-induced epileptogenesis and neuronal loss in immature rats. *Neuroscience.* 2015;05:209–224.

19. Dubé CM, Ravizza T, Hamamura M, et al. Epileptogenesis provoked by prolonged experimental febrile seizures: mechanisms and biomarkers. *J Neurosci.* 2010;30:7484–7494.

20. Silbergleit R, Durkalski V, Lowenstein D, et al. Intramuscular versus intravenous therapy for prehospital status epilepticus. *N Engl J Med.* 2012;366:591–600.

21. Legriel S, Lemiale V, Schenck M, et al. Hypothermia for neuroprotection in convulsive status epilepticus. *N Engl J Med.* 2016;375(25):2457–2467.

FURTHER READING

1. Auvin S, Devisme L, Maurage CA, Soto-Ares G, Cuisset JM, Leclerc F. Vallée L Neuropathological and MRI findings in an acute presentation of hemiconvulsion–hemiplegia: a report with pathophysiological implications. *Seizure.* 2007;16:371–376.

CHAPTER 14

Acute Mitochondrial Encephalopathy

HITOSHI OSAKA, MD, PHD

MITOCHONDRIAL DISEASES AND ENCEPHALOPATHY

Mitochondria are small membranous organelles responsible for the production of cellular energy, e.g., adenosine triphosphate (ATP) (Fig. 14.1). Mitochondrial diseases lead to malfunction of organs that depend on mitochondria for their energy supply.[1,2]

Multiple organs manifest with various symptoms: the brain with epilepsy, developmental regression, migraine, and ataxia; eyes with optic atrophy, restriction of extraocular movement, and retinal pigmentation; muscle with increased fatigability and muscle weakness; gastrointestinal tract with symptoms such as constipation and nausea.[3,4]

The mitochondrial genome is derived from ovary and, therefore, maternally transmitted. Each mitochondrion carries 2–10 copies of mitochondrial DNA (mtDNA). Each cell involves significantly different numbers of mitochondria ranging from few to more than 10000. MtDNA consists of 16,569 nucleotides that code 13 subunits of respiratory chain complex, 2 ribosomal RNAs, and 24 transfer RNAs.[5] Mutant mtDNA exists as the mixture of wild-type and mutant mtDNA, which is called heteroplasmy. If the heteroplasmic rate exceeds the limit of compensation level in the cell, energy failure manifests as mitochondrial disease. Mitochondrial tRNAs are responsible for the production of 13 subunits and their mutations can affect each of these subunits encoded by mtDNA. Mutations in the subunit coding region affect the stability and/or activity of the corresponding complex.

Among subgroups of mitochondrial diseases, two subgroups may mimic acute encephalopathy: Leigh syndrome/encephalopathy (LS) and mitochondrial myopathy, encephalopathy, lactic acidosis, and stroke-like episodes (MELAS).

LEIGH SYNDROME/ENCEPHALOPATHY

LS was originally described as a pathologic diagnosis consisting of spongy degeneration in the brainstem tegmentum, basal ganglia, thalamus, cerebellum, and posterior columns of the spinal cord with capillary proliferation and gliosis.[6] Radiologic modalities, specifically CT and MRI, enabled diagnose before death.[7,8] Although LS usually manifests at infancy, adult cases are also reported.[9] Energy failure damages a subset of neuronal cells with a high ATP requirement; this damage results in brainstem and basal ganglia lesions similar to those observed in anoxic encephalopathy.

Diagnostic criteria defined by Rahman et al.[10] are as follows: progressive neurologic disease with motor and intellectual impairment; signs and symptoms of brainstem or basal ganglia disease; raised lactate concentration in blood or cerebrospinal fluid (CSF); neuroradiological or pathologic changes of necrotic lesions in the basal ganglia, thalamus, brainstem, dentate nuclei, and optic nerves. Normal values of serum lactate do not exclude the possibility of high lactate in the CNS, and demonstration of lactate elevation in CSF is more important.[11]

Clinically, brainstem lesions cause symptoms such as oculomotor abnormalities, hearing dysfunction, ataxic respiration, and swallowing difficulty.[11] Cellular dysfunction near the reticular formation in the brainstem distorts consciousness. Basal ganglia lesions may cause hypotonia, rigidity, or dystonia. It usually manifests during infancy.[11] The course of disease is gradual with recurrent episodes of regression during the periods that increase energy demand such as infectious diseases. Chronic insufficient ATP supply in the central nervous system (CNS) typically causes a clinical course of developmental delay before episodes of encephalopathy occur. These lesions can be visualized by brain MRI. Magnetic resonance spectroscopy may reveal elevated lactic acid, a hallmark of LS.[12]

As the oxidation-reduction potential is affected by respiratory chain defects, lactate values are disproportionately elevated and the lactate/pyruvate ratio is increased more than 20-fold. Over 100 nuclear and mitochondrial genes are responsible for LS. Prevalent mutations of LS are m.DNA 8993T>C or T>G in

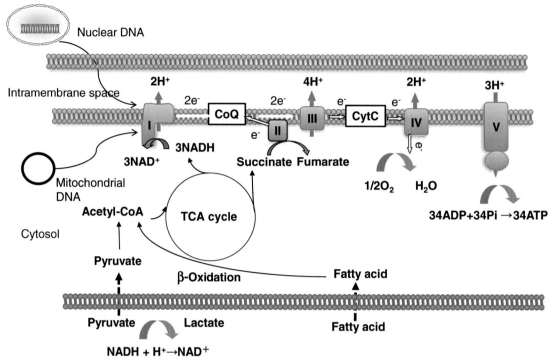

FIG. 14.1 Mitochondrial respiratory chain complex. Respiratory chain complex is composed of complexes I, II, III, IV, and V. For clarity, complexes are separately depicted in this figure. Actually, complexes I, III, and IV associate to generate supercomplexes and cooperatively oxidize these substrates and make proton gradients from intramembranous space to cytosol. This proton gradient is used to produce ATP by complex V, ATP synthase. Any enzyme defect in the system can cause mitochondrial disease. Complex II is composed of only nuclear DNA, whereas the other subunits are coded from both nuclear and mitochondrial DNA.

the *ATPase 6* in complex V of the respiratory chain as well as mutations of pyruvate dehydrogenase complex (PDHC) and pyruvate carboxylase.

Case Presentation

Patient 1 is a 2-year-old male born at term to healthy unrelated parents. At 3 months, he was able to hold his head up. He could sit alone without support at 6 months and walk independently and speak words at 12 months. Around the age of 2 years, he developed gait dysfunction with frequent falls. At the age of 3 years, his mother noticed he could no longer use a spoon. Around the age of 3 years 9 months, he presented with limping on his right foot and leaning forward as he walked. He became lethargic with febrile illnesses and was referred for evaluation at 4 years. Values of lactate and L/P ratio in the CSF (lactate 17.7 mg/dL; pyruvate 1.06 mg/dL; L/P ratio, 16.7) and plasma (lactate 12.6 mg/dL; pyruvate 0.92 mg/dL; L/P ratio, 13.7) were elevated. MRI showed symmetrical hyperintensity on

T2-weighted images in the bilateral putamina, globus pallidi, subthalamic nuclei, and left caudate nuclei (Fig. 14.2). Muscle biopsy showed ragged red fibers. Quantitative muscle respiratory chain analysis yielded decreased complex I/III activity. DNA from muscle revealed a homoplasmic mutation of m.8993T>G (p.L156R) ND6. His current status at age 12 years is that he uses a wheelchair and attends a regular elementary school.

Comment: Complex I is the largest enzyme in the respiratory chain and catalyzes the oxidation of NADH by coenzyme Q. Of 43 subunits, 7 subunits are transcribed from mitochondrial DNA and 36 from nuclear DNA.[13] Complex I is composed of 14 core subunits and 31 accessory subunits and its deficiency is the most frequent cause of LS.[14]

Patient 2 was a 23-year-old male when he suffered from abrupt respiratory distress. He was born at term uneventfully and had no family history of neurologic illness. He was able to hold up his head at 3 months, sit

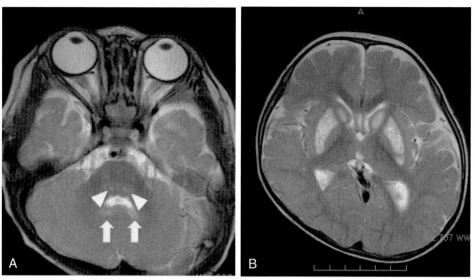

FIG. 14.2 MRI images in patient 1. T2-weighted MRI showed hyperintensity in the bilateral pons (**A**; *arrow heads*), cerebellum (**A**; *arrows*), caudate nuclei, putamina, thalami, and globus pallidi (**B**).

without support at 6 months, speak a meaningful word at 12 months, and walk independently at 30 months of age. He was referred to our clinic at age 6 years because of motor developmental delay. Neurologic examination revealed truncal ataxia, intention tremor, and nystagmus. There was no weakness, and deep tendon reflexes were normal. Laboratory examinations were within normal range including serum lactate, pyruvate, and creatine kinase. Cranial CT scan revealed cerebellar atrophy and nerve conduction velocity measured 26.1 m/s in the peroneal nerve. Tanaka Binet IQ score was 84. A clinical diagnosis was made of cerebellar ataxia and peripheral neuropathy of unknown etiology. His neurologic state was stable thereafter, and he demonstrated satisfactory physical and cognitive development. He suffered sudden respiratory failure without any warning signs at age 23 years and required chronic mechanical ventilatory support. MRI showed hyperintensity on T2-weighted images in the brainstem and thalami, and unchanged cerebellar atrophy (Fig. 14.3). Muscle biopsy showed ragged red fibers. Serum lactate and pyruvate were within normal range although CSF lactate was 26.6 mg/dL. Activities in the respiratory chain showed decreased complex IV in muscle. Compound heterozygous mutations, c.574 C>T. R192W/c.743 C>A (p.A248D), were found.

Comment: SURF1 is an assembly factor of complex IV (cytochrome *c* oxidase) and one of the major causes of LS.[15] Approximately 20% of patients with SURF1 deficiency present with encephalopathy.[16]

Patient 3 is a 17-year-old male born at term to healthy unrelated Japanese parents. His mother had a previous miscarriage. He was able to hold his head up at 3 months, sit independently at 6 months, pull himself to stand and use words at 24 months, and walk by himself at 20 months. After the age of 1 year and 3 months, he had impairment in consciousness associated with a viral upper respiratory infection. Serum lactate and pyruvate were elevated, but the L/P ratio was normal. MRI showed hyperintensity on T2-weighted images in the dorsal pons and cerebellar white matter (Fig. 14.3). Dysarthria, nystagmus on lateral gaze, dystonia, and hypotonia were noted. Deep tendon reflexes were depressed. Babinski signs and ankle clonus were positive. After several episodes of impaired consciousness, he was diagnosed with LS. Now, he goes to a special class. He cannot speak words because of dystonia and is wheelchair bound. We found the mutation of PDHA1 c.121T>C (p.C41R).[17]

Comment: PDHC is one of the common responsible enzymes for LS. It consists of three functional subunits: pyruvate dehydrogenase (E1), dihydrolipoamide transacetylase (E2), and dihydrolipoamide dehydrogenase (E3) and E3-binding protein (E3BP). E1 consists of α/β subunits and the majority of mutations are found in E1α, encoded by the PDHA1 gene on the X chromosome.[18] Some patients with PDHC deficiency show a prominent forehead and large ears, which may provide clues to the diagnosis.[19] As this enzyme is out of the respiratory chain complex, the value of the lactate/ pyruvate ratio is maintained within 20-fold. As some

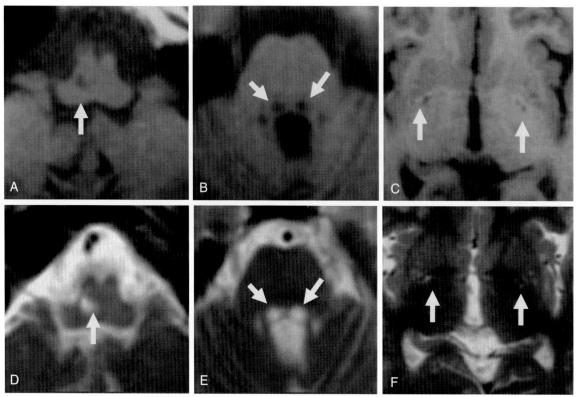

FIG. 14.3 MRI images in patient 2. T1-weighted **(A–C)** and T2-weighted **(D–F)** axial images are shown. In addition to cerebellar atrophy, necrotic lesions are observed at the medulla (**A** and **D**; *arrows*), pons (**B** and **F**; *arrows*), and basal ganglia (**C** and **E**).

mutations are responsive to vitamin B1, a coenzyme of PDHC, high doses of thiamine (10 mg/kg) should be attempted.[20]

MITOCHONDRIAL MYOPATHY, ENCEPHALOPATHY, LACTIC ACIDOSIS, AND STROKELIKE EPISODES

MELAS is the most prevalent clinical entity in mitochondrial diseases.[21] Clinical features are strokelike episodes, encephalopathy (seizures, cognitive dysfunction), and mitochondrial myopathy with lactic acidosis.[22] Other clinical symptoms are short stature, deafness, cortical blindness, and diabetes mellitus.[23,24] Disturbance of consciousness is noticed in ~20% of patients at the first episode. The molecular defect is mtDNA 3243A>G transition in tRNA$^{Leu\ (UUR)}$ (MT-TL1) gene in 80% of cases,[25,26] followed by 3271T>C in 10% of cases. Typically, strokelike episodes consist of headache, vomiting, hemiparesis, and hemianopia. Patient may present with acute encephalopathy. Head MRI shows edematous lesions at the cerebrum cortex,

appearing as hyperintensity on FLAIR and diffusion weighted images.

Case Presentation

Patient 4 is an 18-year-old girl from nonconsanguineous parents. Her mother suffers from migraine. She showed normal development until 10 years when she was diagnosed with short stature. At 11 years of age, she presented with fever, headache, and paresis of the right arm. She was admitted with right arm myoclonus and a generalized tonic-clonic convulsion. On admission, she presented with height of 121.4 cm (−3.6 SD) and weight of 21.9 kg (−2.2 SD). She showed decreased expressive and receptive language. She also presented with mild muscle weakness (MMT: 4/5) of the left upper and lower extremities. Deep tendon reflexes were symmetrical and within normal limits. Pathologic reflexes were not observed. Laboratory studies revealed elevated blood lactate and pyruvic acid (43.1 and 2.20 mg/dL, respectively) and CSF lactate and pyruvate (44.1 and 1.66 mg/dL, respectively). Herpes simplex DNA and titers were both negative in serum and

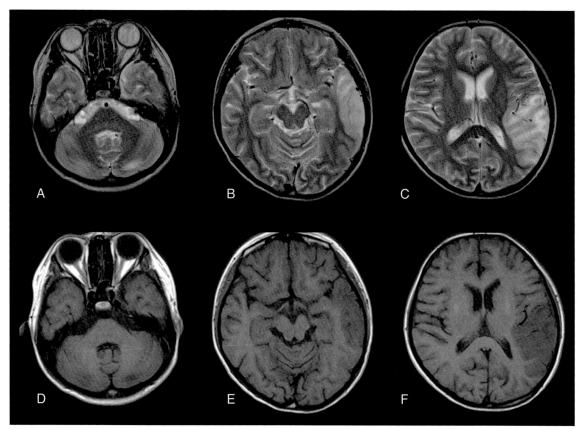

FIG. 14.4 T2-weighted **(A–C)** and T1-weighted **(D–F)** MRIs of patient 4. MRI demonstrated high-intensity areas of small multifocal gray matter regions in the temporal and parietal lobes and cerebellum, and diffuse white matter lesions in the left temporal lobe on T2-weighted images **(A–C)**. These regions are depicted as low-intensity areas and below the border of cortex and white matter **(D–F)**. In addition, the high-intensity region of the pallidum is corresponding calcification **(F)**.

CSF. MRI demonstrated high-intensity T2-weighted areas of small multifocal gray matter regions in the cerebellum and left cerebral temporal and parietal lobes (Fig. 14.4). These areas are visualized as low-intensity areas on T1-weighted images, which blurred the cortical-white matter interface (Fig. 14.4). Intravenous injections of arginine, mannitol, and predonisolone were used. Oral arginine, coenzyme Q10, and vitamin B1 were also initiated. Her hemiparesis and aphasia gradually recovered. Carbamazepine was effective for seizures. Mitochondrial DNA analysis from peripheral white blood cells revealed a heteroplasmic mutation, m.3243A>G.

Comment: The radiologic characteristics of stroke-like episodes are asymmetrical edematous cortical or cortical-subcortical lesions that do not match with arterial distributions. The occipital lobe is the most commonly involved and associated with production of hemianopia. As with this patient, short stature and nonneurologic manifestations, such as hypertrichosis, are usually noticed before encephalopathic episodes.

THERAPY FOR MITOCHONDRIAL ENCEPHALOPATHY

In the acute phase, avoid intravenous fluid including lactate and prefer intravenous sodium bicarbonate. For increased intracranial pressure, mannitol is preferred to glycerol, as the latter may accelerate hepatic steatosis. For stroke in MELAS, L-arginine infusion 5 mL/kg is used, preferably within 3–6 h.[27] Edaravone, a free radical scavenger, is infused two times per day (0.6 mg/kg).[28] Vitamin C, B1, coenzyme Q10, and carnitine are frequently used. There is no proven therapy for mitochondrial disease except idebenone, which was recently approved for Leber's hereditary optic neuropathy.[29,30]

CONCLUSION

Mitochondrial disorders are chronic conditions that affect multiple organs. CNS manifestations range from epilepsy, myoclonus, dystonia, ataxia, and developmental delay to psychiatric symptoms. Although lactate elevation is a key signal for mitochondrial dysfunction, it is not always present. Awareness of different types of organ involvement may lead to correct diagnosis. Therefore, physical and neurodevelopmental assessment, with careful taking of the past and family history, are key to diagnosis and management.

REFERENCES

1. Voet D, Voet JG, Pratt CW. *Fundamentals of Biochemistry: Life at the Molecular Level*; 2016.
2. Swaiman KF, Ashwal S, Ferreiro DM, Schor NF. *Swaiman's Pediatric Neurology*. Saunders: Elsevier; 2012.
3. Chinnery PF. Mitochondrial disorders overview. In: Pagon RA, Adam MP, Ardinger HH, et al., eds. *GeneReviews(R)*. Seattle, WA: University of Washington; 1993. All Rights Reserved.
4. DiMauro S, Hirano M, Schon EA. *Mitochondrial Medicine*. CRC Press; 2006.
5. Andrews RM, Kubacka I, Chinnery PF, Lightowlers RN, Turnbull DM, Howell N. Reanalysis and revision of the Cambridge reference sequence for human mitochondrial DNA. *Nat Genet*. 1999;23(2):147.
6. Leigh D. Subacute necrotizing encephalomyelopathy in an infant. *J Neurol Neurosurg Psychiatry*. 1951;14(3):216–221.
7. Thorburn DR, Rahman S. Mitochondrial DNA-associated Leigh syndrome and NARP. In: Pagon RA, Adam MP, Ardinger HH, et al., eds. *GeneReviews(R)*. Seattle, WA: University of Washington; 1993. All Rights Reserved.
8. Rahman S, Thorburn D. Nuclear gene-encoded Leigh syndrome overview. In: Pagon RA, Adam MP, Ardinger HH, et al., eds. *GeneReviews(R)*. Seattle, WA: University of Washington; 1993.
9. Nagashima T, Mori M, Katayama K, et al. Adult Leigh syndrome with mitochondrial DNA mutation at 8993. *Acta Neuropathol*. 1999;97(4):416–422.
10. Rahman S, Blok RB, Dahl HH, et al. Leigh syndrome: clinical features and biochemical and DNA abnormalities. *Ann Neurol*. 1996;39(3):343–351.
11. Sofou K, De Coo IF, Isohanni P, et al. A multicenter study on Leigh syndrome: disease course and predictors of survival. *Orphanet J Rare Dis*. 2014;9:52.
12. Baertling F, Rodenburg RJ, Schaper J, et al. A guide to diagnosis and treatment of Leigh syndrome. *J Neurol Neurosurg Psychiatry*. 2014;85(3):257–265.
13. Fiedorczuk K, Letts JA, Degliesposti G, Kaszuba K, Skehel M, Sazanov LA. Atomic structure of the entire mammalian mitochondrial complex I. *Nature*. 2016;538(7625):406–410.
14. Stroud DA, Surgenor EE, Formosa LE, et al. Accessory subunits are integral for assembly and function of human mitochondrial complex I. *Nature*. 2016;538(7623):123–126.
15. Zhu Z, Yao J, Johns T, et al. SURF1, encoding a factor involved in the biogenesis of cytochrome c oxidase, is mutated in Leigh syndrome. *Nat Genet*. 1998;20(4):337–343.
16. Wedatilake Y, Brown RM, McFarland R, et al. SURF1 deficiency: a multi-centre natural history study. *Orphanet J Rare Dis*. 2013;8:96.
17. Patel KP, O'Brien TW, Subramony SH, Shuster J, Stacpoole PW. The spectrum of pyruvate dehydrogenase complex deficiency: clinical, biochemical and genetic features in 371 patients. *Mol Genet Metab*. 2012;105(1):34–43.
18. Sperl W, Fleuren L, Freisinger P, et al. The spectrum of pyruvate oxidation defects in the diagnosis of mitochondrial disorders. *J Inherit Metab Dis*. 2015;38(3):391–403.
19. Willemsen M, Rodenburg RJ, Teszas A, van den Heuvel L, Kosztolanyi G, Morava E. Females with PDHA1 gene mutations: a diagnostic challenge. *Mitochondrion*. 2006;6(3):155–159.
20. van Dongen S, Brown RM, Brown GK, Thorburn DR, Boneh A. Thiamine-responsive and non-responsive patients with PDHC-E1 deficiency: a retrospective assessment. *JIMD Rep*. 2015;15:13–27.
21. Pavlakis SG, Phillips PC, DiMauro S, De Vivo DC, Rowland LP. Mitochondrial myopathy, encephalopathy, lactic acidosis, and strokelike episodes: a distinctive clinical syndrome. *Ann Neurol*. 1984;16(4):481–488.
22. DiMauro S, Hirano M. Melas. In: Pagon RA, Adam MP, Ardinger HH, et al., eds. *GeneReviews(R)*. Seattle, WA; 1993.
23. Hirano M, Pavlakis SG. Mitochondrial myopathy, encephalopathy, lactic acidosis, and strokelike episodes (MELAS): current concepts. *J Child Neurol*. 1994;9(1):4–13.
24. Yatsuga S, Povalko N, Nishioka J, et al. MELAS: a nationwide prospective cohort study of 96 patients in Japan. *Biochim Biophys Acta*. 2012;1820(5):619–624.
25. Goto Y, Nonaka I, Horai S. A mutation in the tRNA (Leu)(UUR) gene associated with the MELAS subgroup of mitochondrial encephalomyopathies. *Nature*. 1990;348(6302):651–653.
26. Kobayashi Y, Momoi MY, Tominaga K, et al. A point mutation in the mitochondrial tRNA(Leu)(UUR) gene in MELAS (mitochondrial myopathy, encephalopathy, lactic acidosis and stroke-like episodes). *Biochem Biophys Res Commun*. 1990;173(3):816–822.
27. Koga Y, Akita Y, Nishioka J, et al. L-arginine improves the symptoms of strokelike episodes in MELAS. *Neurology*. 2005;64(4):710–712.
28. Katayama Y, Maeda K, Iizuka T, et al. Accumulation of oxidative stress around the stroke-like lesions of MELAS patients. *Mitochondrion*. 2009;9(5):306–313.
29. Pfeffer G, Majamaa K, Turnbull DM, Thorburn D, Chinnery PF. Treatment for mitochondrial disorders. *Cochrane Database Syst Rev*. 2012;4:CD004426.
30. Gueven N. Idebenone for Leber's hereditary optic neuropathy. *Drugs Today (Barc)*. 2016;52(3):173–181.

CHAPTER 15

Genetic-Metabolic Disorders Presenting as Acute, but Reversible, Severe Epilepsies

MOHAMED ALMUQBIL, MD, FRCP(C) • PHILLIP L. PEARL, MD

INTRODUCTION

Inborn errors of metabolism may have nonspecific phenotypes but targeted therapies. In the case of epilepsy, severe disorders in neonates, infants, or children may be caused by these disorders and require specific intervention aimed at the underlying defect as opposed to intervention with standard antiseizure drugs. Use of the latter may have some antiseizure effects, potentially masking the overall situation, or be deleterious to the underlying disorder. This review emphasizes the phenotypic spectrum of metabolic epilepsies and focuses on those that are amenably treatable but are associated with profound impairment if specific intervention is not implemented.

Phenotypes may include early-onset epileptic encephalopathy including refractory neonatal seizures and early myoclonic encephalopathy, infantile/epileptic spasms, or mixed generalized seizures in addition to focal onset seizures. A typical clinical presentation is a progressively ill infant with development of hypotonia, lethargy, or respiratory distress. EEGs may show discontinuous patterns including burst-suppression as well as intermittent generalized paroxysms of slow, sharp, or spike activity or hypsarrhythmia as well as background abnormalities affecting graphoelements of both awake and sleep states.

VITAMIN-RESPONSIVE EPILEPSIES

Case scenario: A full-term newborn, 3220 g, presented with abnormal eye movements, grunting at 12 h of age, and episodic suppression separated by bilateral sharp waves on EEG. He was treated initially with phenobarbital, levetiracetam, and pyridoxine, and then became seizure-free for 6 weeks. At the age of 3.5 months, he was hospitalized again for stiffening and treated with topiramate. He continued to have myoclonic and tonic-clonic seizures; steroids were ineffective. Pyridoxal-5-phosphate

(PLP) was started, which stopped the seizures with the first dose; breakthrough events occurred as a dose became due. Cerebrospinal fluid (CSF) was studied for neurotransmitters and the PLP level was 23 nmol/L (reference range 23–64), along with elevated threonine and the appearance of an extra peak, suspected as pyridoxine phosphate as the child was on exogenous pyridoxine at the time of the lumbar puncture. Subsequent pyridox(am)ine 5′-phosphate oxidase (PNPO) sequencing showed homozygous mutations in a highly conserved area, leading to conversion of glycine to arginine. The case demonstrated partial pyridoxine responsiveness in PNPO deficiency, i.e., PLP-dependent epilepsy.[1]

Vitamin B6–Related Disorders

The importance of pyridoxine in animal and human nutrition has been a subject of wide interest since its original description as a vitamin B factor in 1934. Unlike the majority of vitamins, no pathologic condition in humans had been described, which occurred spontaneously and was corrected solely by the administration of pyridoxine until the first published case report of pyridoxine-dependent epilepsy in 1954.[2] Pyridoxine-responsive seizures have been described not only in association with inborn errors, leading to a vitamin dependency state, but also in deficiency states or with unknown etiology.[3] Vitamin B6 deficiency seizures, due to problems of intake or absorption, or the use of inhibitors such as isoniazid or penicillamine, will not respond to conventional antiseizure drugs but will remit with physiologic doses of vitamin B6.[4] Conversely, B6 dependency requires pharmacologic dosing, and the underlying defect in pyridoxine-dependent epilepsy was elucidated 50 years following its recognition (vide infra).

Pyridoxine (B6) is not itself an active cofactor. It is converted, together with the pyridoxal and pyridoxamine vitamers, to the biologically active PLP via phosphorylation through the action of a kinase followed by oxidation by PNPO. Autosomal recessively inherited PNPO deficiency causes PLP-dependent epilepsy, responsive to pharmacologic doses of PLP but otherwise associated with a severe early-onset epileptic encephalopathy with early mortality.[5,6]

Pyridoxine-dependent epilepsy occurs as a result of PLP inactivation caused by the accumulation of L-Δ'-piperidine-6-carboxylate in the pipecolic acid pathway of lysine degradation, associated with mutations in ALDH7A1/antiquitin.[7] Elevated pipecolic acid levels in the plasma and CSF of patients with vitamin B6 dependency led to the recognition of a defect in α-aminoadipic semialdehyde (αAASA) dehydrogenase (antiquitin) in the cerebral lysine degradation pathway and mutations in the antiquitin gene (ALDDH7A1) on chromosome 5q31. Pipecolic acid and αAASA have become useful diagnostic markers of vitamin B6–dependent seizures. Even though ALDH7A1 and PNPO deficiencies are rare inborn errors of vitamin B6 metabolism causing neonatal seizure disorders, the phenotypic variability is broad with an increasingly wide range of age of onset, seizure types, and systemic manifestations.[8] The classic syndrome is fetal- or neonatal-onset seizures unresponsive to traditional antiseizure medicines and associated encephalopathy, followed by partial response to pyridoxine and global developmental disorder, accompanied by elevations in AASA and pipecolic acid as well as pathogenic mutations in ALDH7A1. The variants include seizure onset later in infancy, mixed seizure types including the generalized forms as well as focal, infantile spasms, and status epilepticus, and systemic observations including poor feeding, strabismus, microcephaly, hepatomegaly, coagulopathy, and hypoglycemia. Neuroimaging has shown a variety of changes including dysplasia or hypoplasia of the corpus callosum, atrophy, and incomplete or delayed myelination.

In a study of 31 patients with pyridoxine-responsive seizures with normal biomarkers for antiquitin deficiency and normal sequencing of the ALDH7A1 gene, 11 patients were identified carrying three novel mutations of the PNPO gene: a homozygous missense mutation p.Arg225H in exon 7, compound heterozygosity for a novel missense mutation p.Arg141Cys in exon 5, and a deletion c.279_290del in exon 3.[9] Two unrelated patients experienced status epilepticus with homozygosity for the p.Arg225His mutation when switched to PLP. These findings challenged the paradigm of exclusive PLP responsiveness in patients with PNPO deficiency.

Pyridoxal, pyridoxamine, pyridoxine, PLP, pyridoxamine-5'-phosphate, and pyridoxine 5'-phosphate are different vitamers of vitamin B6 (Fig. 15.1). PLP is synthesized from dietary sources (pyridoxamine from meat and pyridoxine from vegetables) and via specific enzymes, e.g., PNPO, phosphatases, and kinases (Fig. 15.1). PNPO deficiency is treatable with PLP but generally not optimally with pyridoxine. A potential inhibitory effect of PLP on intrinsic PNPO activity has been postulated to explain why paradoxical worsening has been reported in some patients administered PLP with PNPO deficiency.

An initial clinical approach of utilizing PLP administration could theoretically cover the possibilities of both pyridoxine and PLP dependency, although sequential clinical trials of both may be needed because of overlap cases of PNPO deficiency responding partially to pyridoxine or even worsened by PLP.[10] PNPO mutations should be sought in patients with a positive pyridoxine response yet with normal PDE biomarkers and without any mutation in ALDH7A1. There have been a number of cases with confirmed antiquitin or PNPO, having a history compatible with a diagnosis of birth asphyxia. Such cases should be managed by trials of pyridoxine and PLP performed in neonates with drug-resistant seizures regardless of birth history.

Despite pyridoxine therapy in antiquitin deficiency, significant developmental delay and intellectual disability are reported. Hence, combinatorial therapy has utilized pyridoxine plus a lysine-restricted diet and L-arginine, the latter to compete for brain lysine influx and liver mitochondrial import.[11] This triple therapy reduces CSF, plasma, and urine biomarkers and appears to augment seizure control and neurodevelopmental outcome.

A related disorder, folinic acid–dependent epilepsy, was reported from a report of two siblings and two unrelated patients.[12] A representative phenotype was seizure onset within the first hours of life, showing partial amelioration to high-dose multiple anticonvulsant therapy, normal plasma amino acids or mild elevations in leucine and isoleucine, and an unidentified peak on CSF chromatography used for the detection of biogenic amines. Seizures ultimately showed responsiveness to folinic acid, which also led to a 50% decrease in the CSF peak. This syndrome was determined as allelic to pyridoxine-dependent epilepsy.[13]

A practical approach to the pyridoxine-related epilepsies is to administer a bolus of 100 mg of intravenous pyridoxine over 5–10 min with concomitant EEG and cardiorespiratory monitoring. If there is no response, a repeat dose of 100–500 mg may be administered.

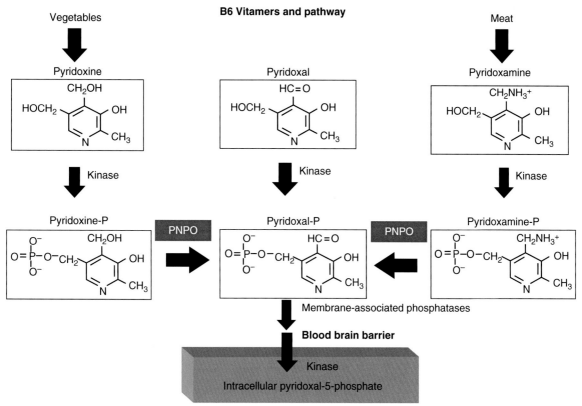

FIG. 15.1 B6 vitamers and their metabolic pathways.

In clinical and EEG responders, careful observation is important for a minimum of 48 h. If there is no response, alternative regimens have been recommended, including a trial of enteral pyridoxine 15–30 mg/kg/day divided twice daily, as well as P5P 30–50 mg/kg/day divided four to six times daily. The folinic acid dose typically recommended is 3–5 mg/kg/day divided twice daily over 3–5 days. Diagnostic studies, including plasma and urine AASA and pipecolic acid levels, and genotyping for ALDH7A1 and PNPO, can then be sent. A low threshold for diagnostic suspicion and therapeutic intervention is recommended for improved outcomes[14] (Fig. 15.2).

Biotinidase Deficiency

Biotinidase cleaves biotin from biocytin and, thus, provides the cofactor for the biotin-dependent carboxylases, which are involved in fatty acid synthesis, amino acid catabolism, and gluconeogenesis. Hence, its deficiency results in multiple carboxylase deficiency and secondary ketoacidosis, hyperammonemia, and organic aciduria. The neurologic manifestations of this autosomal recessive disorder include seizures, developmental impairment, hypotonia, spastic paraparesis, ataxia, sensorineural hearing loss, and optic atrophy. Seizures are typically tonic-clonic or myoclonic, or infantile spasms. Cutaneous abnormalities include alopecia and eczematous dermatitis. The diagnosis is based on demonstration of deficient enzymatic activity in serum or plasma. Biotinidase can recycle endogenous biotin so that most biotin can be preserved peripherally, but biotinidase activity is low in human brain and CSF, restricting the recycling of biotin in the CNS. Treatment is satisfying with low doses of biotin, 5–20 mg/day, but optic atrophy with vision loss and sensorineural hearing loss, once present, tend to persist.[15]

Cobalamin Deficiency

Case scenario: A 14-year-old boy presented at 6 weeks of age with failure-to-thrive, anemia, and recurrent status epilepticus. He developed profound cognitive impairment, visual impairment, spasticity, and a crouch gait. Laboratory evaluation showed megaloblastic anemia, thrombocytopenia, and elevated methylmalonic acid and homocysteine on urine organic and

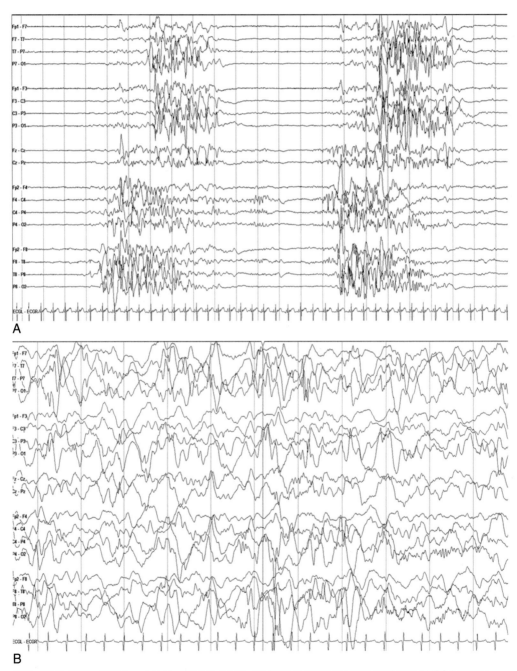

FIG. 15.2 EEG—P5P dependency. **(A)** A 3-month-old (former 33 week premature) with PNPO homozygous G686A, p.Arg229Gln mutations with burst-suppression EEG. Technical settings: HFF 70 Hz, LFF 1 Hz, sens 10 mcV/mm, time base 15 mm/s. **(B)** The same patient at 4.5 months of age on P5P therapy shows significant improvement with continuous background and intermittent multifocal spike discharges. Technical settings: LFF 1 Hz, HFF 70 Hz, sens 10 mcV/mm, time base 30 mm/s.

amino acids. He was diagnosed with cobalamin C deficiency. This was followed by two further pregnancies in this couple. A prenatal diagnosis was confirmed in the next pregnancy, leading to maternal cobalamin injections starting at 18 weeks of gestation, and treatment of the newborn with hydroxyl-cobalamin injections, folic acid, L-carnitine, and betaine. The second child had a far better outcome, affected only with mild learning disabilities and attention deficit hyperactivity disorder.

Cobalamin, a cobalt-containing vitamin, exists in multiple forms and is critical in the formation of vitamin B12 or cyanocobalamin. Cobalamin C deficiency is the most common of the cobalamin deficiencies and is integral in two chemical reactions, the conversion of homocysteine to methionine and of methylmalonyl-CoA to succinyl-CoA. The case exemplifies the value of an early diagnosis and the potential of even prenatal intervention in a condition that may present with status epilepticus in early childhood.

TRANSPORTOPATHIES
Glucose Transporter 1 Deficiency
This prototype transportopathy was recognized with the report of two probands with persistent hypoglycorrhachia and intractable epilepsy.[16] Glucose transporter 1 deficiency was initially described as what is now recognized as the classic phenotype of neonatal-onset or early infantile–onset seizures associated with acquired microcephaly and a severe associated epileptic encephalopathy. The clinical spectrum has widened to include later-onset phenotypes, including developmental delay, dysarthria, and dystonia and an extrapyramidal syndrome of choreoathetosis, dystonia, and paroxysmal exertional dyskinesias. CSF absolute glucose levels are less than 40–60 and a fasting CSF:serum glucose ratio should be <0.4. Neuroimaging may show T2-weighted hyperintensities involving subcortical white matter. The disorder is caused by haploinsufficiency of SLC2A1 and may be transmitted as autosomal dominant or recessive. In addition, SLC2A1 mutations are associated with as much as 10% of patients with onset of typical absence seizures before 3 years of age as well as cases of myoclonic-atonic epilepsy, i.e., Doose syndrome. The syndrome emerged as one of several specific indications for the ketogenic diet, offering increased fatty acids and thus an alternative fuel for the tricarboxylic acid cycle in the CNS.

It is notable that certain antiseizure medications may inhibit any residual glucose transporter 1 activity and should be avoided in this disorder, specifically phenobarbital, diazepam, and valproate. In addition, there are a variety of entities in the differential diagnosis of hypoglycorrhachia, including meningitis (especially bacterial and tuberculous), status epilepticus, mitochondrial disorders, systemic hypoglycemia, subarachnoid hemorrhage, and meningeal carcinomatosis. The lessons of glucose transport continue to evolve, with recent findings demonstrating a contribution of defective transporter activity in Alzheimer disease.[17]

Cerebral Folate Deficiency
Cerebral folate deficiency is characterized by a severe neurodevelopmental disorder usually presenting between 4 and 6 months of age with recurrent and ultimately intractable epilepsy, spastic paraplegia, choreoathetosis, and cerebellar ataxia.[18] Cases have been attributed to both folate receptor mutations and autoantibodies.[19,20] Active transport of folate across the blood-brain barrier influences brain development. The folate receptor-1 (FOLR1) protein is localized at the basolateral surface of the choroid plexus, which is characterized by a high binding affinity for circulating 5-methyltetrahydrofolate (5-MTHF).

Two folate transfer mechanisms have been identified in humans: the proton coupled folate transporter 1 (PCFT1) and the folate receptor proteins (FOLR1 and FOLR2). Both mechanisms are involved in the transport of folate from plasma to the cell interior, as well as the folate transport across the placental and blood-brain barriers. PCFT1 represents an integral membrane protein operating only at relatively high folate concentration, within the micromolar range and driven by anionic gradients. A genetic defect of the PCFT1 system is thought to be the most likely cause of a rare hereditary disease of intestinal malabsorption of folic acid. The membrane-attached folate receptors, FOLR1 and FOLR2, possess high affinity to folate in the nanomolar range. FOLR1 has higher affinity for 5-MTHF when compared with FOLR2. The most important site of folate transport to the nervous system is localized at the choroid plexus. The active transport of 5-MTHF from plasma to CSF depends mainly on membrane folate receptors, which primarily accumulate folate at the basolateral surface of choroid epithelium, mediate the transport against a concentration gradient into choroid epithelial cells, and subsequently deliver 5-MTHF to the CSF.

The cerebral folate level can be normalized by administration of folinic acid (leucovorin).[21] There are, however, conditions beyond proton-coupled folate transporter-1 deficiency and mutations or blocking/binding antibodies of the FOLR1 receptor with folate responsiveness. These include 5,10-MTHFR deficiency, the serine synthetic defect 3-phosphoglycerate dehydrogenase deficiency (vide infra), deficient dietary intake, and exogenous administration of valproic acid. In addition, cases of Rett, Aicardi-Goutieres, and Kearns-Sayre syndromes as well as channelopathies (e.g., KCNH1) have been associated with low concentrations of CSF folate measurements.

Biotin-Thiamine–Responsive Basal Ganglia Disease

A basal ganglia disorder resembling Leigh syndrome with biotin responsiveness was ultimately identified as deficiency of the thiamine transporter hTHTR2.[22] The clinical presentation is that of a subacute encephalopathy with confusion, seizures, dysarthria, and dystonia usually following a history of febrile illness. The disorder can progress to severe quadriparesis and even death. The disorder was mapped to chromosome 2q36.3 and was found to result from a mutation in the SLC19A3 gene. Thus, combined biotin and thiamine treatment is recommended in the setting of an acute or subacute presentation with symmetrical basal ganglia lesions and neurologic symptoms until this disorder is ruled out.

AMINO AND ORGANIC ACIDOPATHIES

There are a number of amino and organic acidopathies that can present with acute seizures, especially in the neonate presenting with a sepsislike picture. Rapid assessment of plasma glucose, ammonia, and lactic acid are important measures to screen for many of these conditions, including the classic organic acidopathies, e.g., isovaleric, propionic, and methylmalonic acidurias. Some examples of disorders having specific therapeutic strategies to address the associated metabolic defect are presented in the following sections.

Serine Biosynthesis Disorder

3-Phosphoglycerate dehydrogenase (3-PGDH) deficiency is a potentially treatable disorder of L-serine synthesis. The disease is characterized by congenital microcephaly, severe psychomotor retardation, and intractable epilepsy ranging from neonatal seizures to infantile spasms. Low concentrations of the amino acid serine in CSF and to a lesser extent in plasma are characteristic. Oral therapy with L-serine alone or in combination with glycine has beneficial effects. The presence of microcephaly indicates impairment of fetal brain growth, emphasizing that prenatal intervention is recommended when possible.[23] The pathophysiology of the disorder is unknown, although the X-linked cyclin dependent kinase-like 5 (CDKL5) gene has been

implicated. This gene encodes for a 1035-amino-acid-long protein with a highly conserved serine threonine kinase domain in the N-terminal region and is critical for brain development.[24]

Creatine Synthesis Disorder

Creatine deficiency syndromes comprise synthesis and transport of creatine, resulting in deficiency of creatine/phosphocreatine mainly in the brain. Guanidinoacetate methyltransferase (GAMT) deficiency has the most severe phenotype. Patients are clinically affected by severe intellectual deficiency, lack of speech, autistic behavior, extrapyramidal movement disorder, and epilepsy. Creatine deficiency and accumulation of guanidoacetoacetate (GAA), known for its neurotoxic and epileptogenic effects, contribute to the pathophysiology. Treatment in GAMT deficiency is directed toward replenishment of creatine and reduction of GAA.[25] GAA reduction is achieved by dietary arginine restriction combined with low-dose ornithine supplementation to avoid deficiency of the latter. Less commonly, patients may have deficiency of the enzyme upstream to GAMT, arginine-glycine aminotransferase (AGAT), treated with creatine supplementation. There are also defects of the X-linked creatine transporter CT1. In all three of the conditions of creatine synthesis or transport, epilepsy is a common feature and the phenotypic overlap mandates laboratory confirmation to distinguish between the entities.

Molybdenum Cofactor Deficiency

Molybdenum cofactor deficiency is a rare metabolic disorder characterized by severe and rapidly progressive neurologic damage caused by the functional loss of sulfite oxidase, one of four molybdenum-dependent enzymes. Until recently, no effective therapy was available, and early fatality was the usual outcome. Recent studies revealed that substitution therapy with the cofactor precursor cyclic pyranopterin monophosphate (cPMP) normalized all urinary markers of sulfite oxidase (sulfite, S-sulfocysteine, thiosulfate) and xanthine oxidase deficiency. This has been associated with improved neurodevelopmental outcomes including seizure resolution and responsiveness of EEG background with a reduction in epileptiform activity.[26,27] Imaging follow-up demonstrates preservation of parenchyma in sharp contrast to the natural history of the disorder.

An additional point is that α-AASA, previously discussed as the accumulating substrate in pyridoxine-dependent epilepsy, is also increased in molybdenum cofactor deficiency and sulfite oxidase deficiency. Sulfite appears to inhibit α-AASA dehydrogenase activity, as well as glutamate dehydrogenase. Patients with molybdenum cofactor deficiency or sulfite oxidase deficiency might benefit from pyridoxine supplementation. Increased urinary excretion of α-AASA should raise consideration of molybdenum cofactor or sulfite oxidase deficiency.[28]

Other broad groups of small-molecule disorders to consider in reversible metabolic epilepsies are mitochondrial and urea cycle disorders. Of the mitochondrial disorders, deficiency of pyruvate dehydrogenase (PDH) complex, a tetrameric protein, has the specific intervention of the ketogenic diet. This allows for increased free fatty acids to obviate the conversion of glucose to pyruvate and the subsequent PDH-mediated entry of pyruvate into the Krebs cycle. As for the urea cycle disorders, early recognition is important at the time of symptomatic presentation to cease protein intake and implement ammonia-lowering therapies. This is especially important to consider in the toxic neonate, particularly the breast-fed infant deteriorating after starting to feed and ingest protein. Of the various enzymes in the urea cycle, deficiencies of all can present in the neonatal period other than arginase, which tends to present somewhat later but still may become manifest in early infancy. EEG abnormalities in these disorders may show profound generalized disturbances including features reminiscent of Lennox-Gastaut syndrome (Fig. 15.3).

NEUROTRANSMITTER DEFECTS

Case scenario: A 7-year-old girl presented with recurrent weakness and rash. She had been diagnosed with "atypical PKU" from a newborn screen and treated with phenylalanine restriction until 4 years of age, at which point the family emigrated from El Salvador to the United States and became progressively less compliant with the diet. She developed gait difficulty, manifest as fluctuating weakness and stiffness, as well as knee pain and a rash over the thighs. Her neurologic evaluation included normal magnetic resonance imaging studies. A rheumatologic evaluation led to a diagnosis of seronegative juvenile rheumatoid arthritis and she was treated with prednisolone. This was ineffective and she was then given a trial of methotrexate.

She became bedridden and was unable to speak within days, although mentation was preserved. She was hospitalized and determined to have an elevated phenylalanine level (163 mg/dL). Subsequent workup showed very low urine biopterin (3.7%, with a normal range of

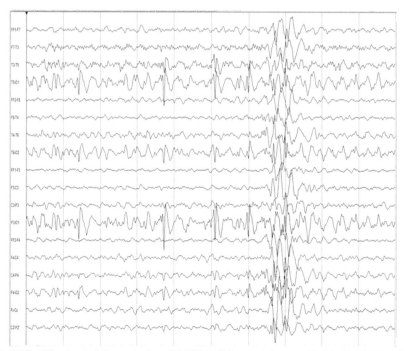

FIG. 15.3 EEG—Dihydropteridine reductase (DHPR) deficiency. A 7-year-old girl with DHPR deficiency; monoamine precursors and folinic acid were introduced at 3 years. EEG shows active occipital and generalized spike-wave discharges. HFF 70 Hz, LFF 1 Hz, sens 10 mcV/mm, time base 30 mm/s.

18%–70%). Enzymatic and genetic analysis confirmed the most common of the biopterin synthesis disorders, PTPS (pyruvoyl-tetrahydropterin synthase) deficiency.

Deficiencies of biopterin synthesis or recycling should be considered in any infant or child with an unexplained neurologic phenotype, including seizures as well as pyramidal and extrapyramidal manifestations. These disorders may be picked up on newborn screening and are sometimes called atypical PKU. Urine pterin quantification will be normal in classic PKU (usually 18%–70%), but low in the biopterin synthesis defects (0.7%–3%) and elevated in the defect of tetrahydrobiopterin (BH4) recycling, dihydropteridine reductase (DHPR) deficiency (81%–92%).

There is a salvage pathway from BH4 to BH2 using dihydrofolate reductase as an alternative to DHPR. In the example given, the patient's compensatory pathway to recycle and thus replenish BH4 became inhibited by the folate antagonist methotrexate, unmasking the underlying biopterin synthesis defect and leading to severe deficit in dopamine formation and thus the picture of profound motor arrest. In DHPR deficiency, quinonoid-dihydrobiopterin, formed during hydroxylation of aromatic amino acids, cannot reduce to BH4 and the unstable quinonoid-dihydrobiopterin is isomerized to dihydrobiopterin (7,8-dihydrobiopterin). These patients may also present with seizures, and more commonly developmental delay, hypotonia, and extrapyramidal manifestations. Basal ganglia calcifications may occur, but may resolve, along with clinical improvement, with therapy using monoamine precursors and folinic acid. Late treated patients have persistent extrapyramidal deficits and epilepsy (Fig. 15.4).

DISORDERS OF GLUCOSE HOMEOSTASIS

Disorders of glucose homeostasis that may present as severe early-onset epilepsy include both hypoglycemia due to congenital hyperinsulinism and neonatal diabetes. The discovery of the hyperinsulinism/hyperammonemia syndrome (HI/HA), a novel hypoglycemic disorder, has drawn attention to glutamate dehydrogenase (GDH) as a key regulator of amino acid and ammonia metabolism in pancreatic islet cells, the liver, and the brain.[29] The HI/HA syndrome is caused by missense mutations of GDH that reduce the sensitivity of the enzyme to allosteric inhibition by the high-energy phosphates, GTP and ATP. These mutations lead to a gain of enzyme function and are expressed in dominant fashion. The major clinical feature of children with the HI/HA syndrome is recurrent episodes of symptomatic hypoglycemia and these episodes can be provoked by protein feeding and present as postprandial hypoglycemia. The hypoglycemia is not usually as severe as that seen in infants with hyperinsulinism because of defects of the KATP channel (mutations of SUR1 or Kir6.2). Thus, children with HI/HA syndrome may not be macrosomic or recognized as hypoglycemic until several months of age. Plasma amino acid concentrations are normal in HI/HA patients. Specifically, they do not show the elevations of plasma glutamine that are typically seen in states of hyperammonemia. The HI/HA syndrome provides a rare example of an inborn error of intermediary metabolism in which the effect of the mutation on enzyme activity is a gain of function. The disorder is readily diagnosed by demonstrating mild hyperammonemia on a random blood sample in a patient with a history of hypoglycemia. The net biochemical effect of GDH gain-of-function is increased conversion of glutamate to α-ketoglutarate, which furthermore yields ammonia as a by-product, as well as stimulation of closure of the pancreatic β-islet cell KATP channel, which leads to cellular depolarization, entry of calcium through a voltage-gated channel, and subsequent exocytosis of insulin. The patients tend to have generalized spike-wave on EEG and require ongoing treatment with antiseizure medicines (Fig. 15.5). At least intermittent use of diazoxide becomes necessary, which allows for opening of the KATP channel and inhibition of insulin release during periods of acute, symptomatic hypoglycemia.

Conversely, neonatal diabetes mellitus, defined as peripheral hyperglycemia, requiring insulin therapy that presents within 6 months of birth may be associated with the syndrome acronymized as DEND, or Developmental delay with Epilepsy and Neonatal Diabetes. This syndrome may be caused by mutations in several different genes, including glucokinase1 and the ATP-sensitive potassium (KATP) channel subunits Kir6.2 and SUR1, as well as by abnormal imprinting at chromosome 6q24. Most cases result from heterozygous mutations in *KCNJ11*, the gene encoding Kir6.2, which constitutes the pore-forming subunit of the KATP channel. About 20% of patients also have neurologic features varying from mild psychomotor impairment to severe neurodevelopmental disability combined with medically intractable epilepsy. KATP channels couple cell metabolism to changes in cell excitability in numerous tissues including pancreatic β-islet cells, the brain, and the muscle. They consist of four pore-forming Kir6.2 subunits and four regulatory SUR subunits (SUR1 in β-cells and brain; SUR2 in muscle).

Insulin therapy can control the blood glucose level but does not ameliorate the consequences of the

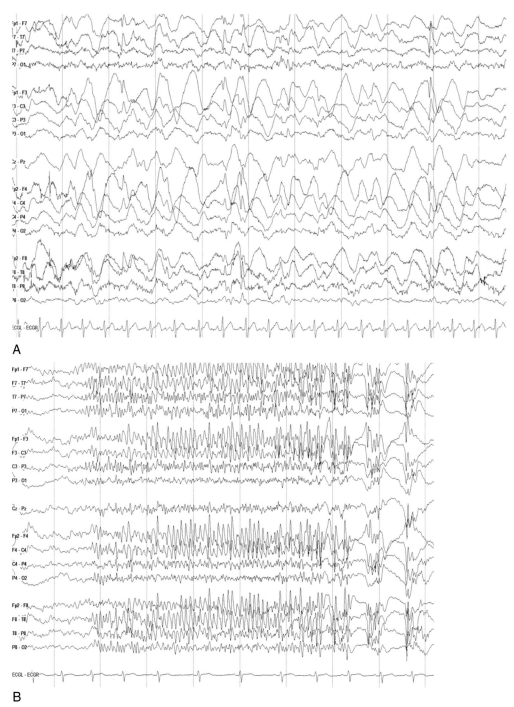

FIG. 15.4 EEG—Arginase deficiency. **(A)** An 18-year-old boy with arginase deficiency. EEG background shows generalized slow spike-and-wave activity. HFF 70 Hz, LFF 1 Hz, sens 10 mcV/mm, time base 30 mm/s. **(B)** The same patient with arginase deficiency, with recurrent paroxysmal fast activity during sleep, variably associated with tonic seizures. HFF 70 Hz, LFF 1 Hz, sens 10 mcV/mm, time base 30 mm/s.

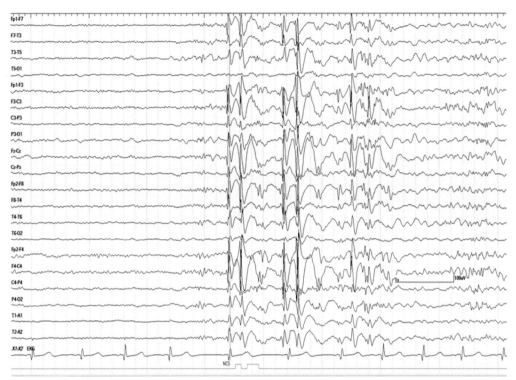

FIG. 15.5 EEG—HI/HA syndrome. An 8-year-old boy with HI/HA syndrome; EEG shows high voltage predominantly generalized spike-wave with some fragmentary discharges. HFF 70 Hz, LFF 1 Hz, sens 20 mcV/mm, 30 mm/s.

enhanced activity of extrapancreatic KATP channels, such as epilepsy, hypotonia, and developmental impairment. Alternatively, sulfonylureas block KATP channels in all tissues to which they have access, suggesting they may be able to reverse some of the extrapancreatic problems. Although the extent to which tolbutamide or glibenclamide cross the blood-brain barrier is unknown in man, it has been documented for other sulfonylureas in rodents. Improvement of neurologic symptoms has been noted with sulfonylurea treatment, suggesting central action although the pathophysiology of the encephalopathy associated with DEND is not well understood.[30]

CONCLUSION

There are a host of genetic-metabolic disorders that may present as acute, but reversible, severe epilepsy. These are presented herein as vitamin-responsive disorders (including pyridoxal vitamers and its variants, biotinidase, and cobalamin), transport disorders (including glucose, folate, and biotin-thiamine), amino and organic acid disorders (including synthetic pathways of serine and creatine, and molybdenum cofactor type A deficiency due to cPMP deficiency), neurotransmitter disorders (focusing on disorders of biopterin synthesis and recycling), and disorders of glucose homeostasis (including HI/HA and DEND). A high index of suspicion leading to efficient diagnosis and implementation of targeted therapy can have significant influences on outcome.

REFERENCES

1. Pearl PL, Hyland K, Chiles J, McGavin CL, Yu Y, Taylor D. Partial pyridoxine responsiveness in PNPO deficiency. In: *JIMD Reports-Case and Research Reports, 2012/6*. Springer; 2012:139–142.
2. Hunt AD, Stokes J, McCrory WW, Stroud H. Pyridoxine dependency: report of a case of intractable convulsions in an infant controlled by pyridoxine. *Pediatrics*. 1954;13(2):140–145.
3. Riikonen R, Mankinen K, Gaily E. Long-term outcome in pyridoxine-responsive infantile epilepsy. *Eur J Paediatr Neurol*. 2015;19(6):647–651.

4. Ohtahara S, Yamatogi Y, Ohtsuka Y. Vitamin B6 treatment of intractable seizures. *Brain Dev*. 2011;33(9):783–789.

5. Mills PB, Surtees RA, Champion MP, et al. Neonatal epileptic encephalopathy caused by mutations in the PNPO gene encoding pyridox(am)ine 5′-phosphate oxidase. *Hum Mol Genet*. 2005;14(8):1077–1086.

6. Mills PB, Camuzeaux SS, Footitt EJ, et al. Epilepsy due to PNPO mutations: genotype, environment and treatment affect presentation and outcome. *Brain*. 2014;137:1350–1360.

7. Mills PB, Struys E, Jakobs C, et al. Mutations in antiquitin in individuals with pyridoxine-dependent seizures. *Nat Med*. 2006;12:307–309.

8. van Karnebeek CD, Tiebout SA, Niermeijer J, et al. Pyridoxine-dependent epilepsy: an expanding clinical spectrum. *Pediatr Neurol*. 2016;59:6–12.

9. Plecko B, Paul K, Mills P, et al. Pyridoxine responsiveness in novel mutations of the PNPO gene. *Neurology*. 2014;82(16):1425–1433.

10. Pearl PL, Gospe SM. Pyridoxine or pyridoxal-5′-phosphate for neonatal epilepsy the distinction just got murkier. *Neurology*. 2014;82(16):1392–1394.

11. Coughlin CR, van Karnebeek CD, Al-Hertani W, et al. Triple therapy with pyridoxine, arginine supplementation and dietary lysine restriction in pyridoxine-dependent epilepsy: neurodevelopmental outcome. *Mol Genet Metab*. 2015;116(1):35–43.

12. Hyland K, Buist N, Powell B, et al. Folinic acid responsive seizures: a new syndrome? *J Inherit Metab Dis*. 1995;18(2):177–181.

13. Gallagher RC, Van Hove JL, Scharer G, et al. Folinic acid–responsive seizures are identical to pyridoxine-dependent epilepsy. *Ann Neurol*. 2009;65(5):550–556.

14. Hatch J, Coman D, Clayton P, et al. Normal neurodevelopmental outcomes in PNPO deficiency: a case series and literature review. *JIMD Rep*. 2016;26:91–97.

15. Wolf B. Clinical issues and frequent questions about biotinidase deficiency. *Mol Genet Metab*. 2010;100:6–13.

16. De Vivo DC, Trifiletti RR, Jacobson RI, et al. Defective glucose transport across the blood-brain barrier as a cause of persistent hypoglycorrhachia, seizures, and developmental delay. *N Engl J Med*. 1991;325(10):703–709.

17. Winkler EA, Nishida Y, Sagare AP, et al. GLUT1 reductions exacerbate Alzheimer's disease vasculo-neuronal dysfunction and degeneration. *Nat Neurosci*. 2015;18(4):521–530.

18. Ramaekers V, Häusler M, Opladen T, et al. Psychomotor retardation, spastic paraplegia, cerebellar ataxia and dyskinesia associated with low 5-methyltetrahydrofolate in cerebrospinal fluid: a novel neurometabolic condition responding to folinic acid substitution. *Neuropediatrics*. 2002;33(06):301–308.

19. Bonkowsky JL, Ramaekers VT, Quadros EV, Lloyd M. Progressive encephalopathy in a child with cerebral folate deficiency syndrome. *J Child Neurol*. 2008;23(12).

20. Steele SU, Cheah SM, Veerapandiyan A, et al. Electroencephalographic and seizure manifestations in two patients with folate receptor autoimmune antibody-mediated primary cerebral folate deficiency. *Epilepsy Behav*. 2012;24(4):507–512.

21. Al-Baradie RS, Chudary MW. Diagnosis and management of cerebral folate deficiency: a form of folinic acid-responsive seizures. *Neurosciences*. 2014;19(4):312.

22. Zeng W-Q, Al-Yamani E, Acierno JS, et al. Biotin-responsive basal ganglia disease maps to 2q36. 3 and is due to mutations in SLC19A3. *Am J Hum Genet*. 2005;77(1):16–26.

23. De Koning T, Klomp L, Van Oppen A, et al. Prenatal and early postnatal treatment in 3-phosphoglycerate-dehydrogenase deficiency. *Lancet*. 2004;364(9452):2221–2222.

24. Moseley BD, Dhamija R, Wirrell EC, Nickels KC. Historic, clinical, and prognostic features of epileptic encephalopathies caused by CDKL5 mutations. *Pediatr Neurol*. 2012;46(2):101–105.

25. Schulze A, Hoffmann G, Bachert P, et al. Presymptomatic treatment of neonatal guanidinoacetate methyltransferase deficiency. *Neurology*. 2006;67(4):719–721.

26. Veldman A, Santamaria-Araujo JA, Sollazzo S, et al. Successful treatment of molybdenum cofactor deficiency type A with cPMP. *Pediatrics*. 2010;125(5):e1249–e1254.

27. Schwahn BC, Van Spronsen FJ, Belaidi AA, et al. Efficacy and safety of cyclic pyranopterin monophosphate substitution in severe molybdenum cofactor deficiency type A: a prospective cohort study. *Lancet*. 2015;386(10007):1955–1963.

28. Struys EA, Nota B, Bakkali A, et al. Pyridoxine-dependent epilepsy with elevated urinary α-amino adipic semialdehyde in molybdenum cofactor deficiency. *Pediatrics*. 2012;130(6):e1716–e1719.

29. MacMullen C, Fang J, Hsu BY, et al. Hyperinsulinism/hyperammonemia syndrome in children with regulatory mutations in the inhibitory guanosine triphosphate-binding domain of glutamate dehydrogenase. *J Clin Endocrinol Metab*. 2001;86:1782–1787.

30. Shimomura K, Hörster F, De Wet H, et al. A novel mutation causing DEND syndrome A treatable channelopathy of pancreas and brain. *Neurology*. 2007;69(13):1342–1349.

CHAPTER 16

Acute Encephalopathy in Infants With Sulfite Oxidase Deficiency and Molybdenum Cofactor Deficiency

DR. HSIU-FEN LEE, MD • DR. CHING-SHIANG CHI, MD

INTRODUCTION

Human isolated sulfite oxidase deficiency (ISOD) and molybdenum cofactor deficiency (MoCoD) are very rare autosomal recessive neurometabolic diseases. ISOD and MoCoD share a common biochemical pathomechanism. Molybdenum cofactor–dependent enzymes include xanthine oxidase (XO), aldehyde oxidase (AO), and sulfite oxidase (SO). Once SO is deficient, either by ISOD or MoCoD, toxic sulfite accumulates in fluid and tissues and mainly affects the central nervous system.

ISOD and MoCoD have similar clinical manifestations characterized by neonatal-onset severe and progressive neurologic deterioration, seizures, and feeding difficulty. This is followed by facial dysmorphism, microcephaly, intractable seizures, and profound neurologic sequelae. The striking neuroimaging findings of ISOD and MoCoD are multicystic encephalomalacia and/or signal changes over bilateral globus pallidi and thalami, which resemble hypoxic-ischemic encephalopathy. A urine sulfite strip test, along with hypohomocysteinemia in plasma amino acids, could assist physicians in identifying patients with ISOD and MoCoD. Plasma uric acid level is a biochemical marker to differentiate ISOD and MoCoD.

In this section, we will provide an overview regarding the neuropathogenesis of the biochemical pathway, clinical manifestations, neuroimaging features, laboratory findings, and treatment in human ISOD and MoCoD.

NEUROPATHOGENESIS

Molybdenum cofactor synthesis is important for humans because essential metabolic functions are molybdenum dependent. As shown in Fig. 16.1, molybdenum cofactor is synthesized in a step by step process,

from guanosine triphosphate (GTP), cyclic pyranopterin monophosphate (cPMP), molybdopterin (MPT) via molybdenum cofactor synthetase 1A, 2A, 2B, and the synaptic organizing protein gephyrin. Molybdenum cofactor–dependent enzymes play central roles in many biologically important processes such as purine and sulfur catabolism in mammals, including xanthine oxidase (XO), aldehyde oxidase (AO), and sulfite oxidase (SO). XO and AO are the two key enzymes in purine degradation pathway. XO oxidizes hypoxanthine to xanthine, and xanthine to uric acid in the cytosol. AO, like XO, is a cytosolic molybdo-iron flavoenzyme that catalyzes the oxidation of a variety of aromatic and nonaromatic aldehydes to their corresponding carboxylic acid. The enzyme SO catalyzes the oxidation of sulfite to sulfate. As sulfite is a strong nucleophile that can react with a wide variety of cellular components, it is assumed that SO has a sulfite-detoxifying function and is therefore required for removing excess sulfite from the cell. Human SO uses cytochrome c as an electron acceptor, and coincident with this is that it has been shown to be localized in the mitochondrial intermembrane space. Human SO catalyzes the final step in the degradation of sulfur-containing amino acids.[1-4]

SO transforms sulfites into sulfates with the aid of a molybdenum cofactor. Normally, sulfur amino acids methionine and cysteine degrade through the metabolic pathway to transform sulfites into sulfates, which are subsequently excreted through the urine. Once SO is deficient, either by ISOD or MoCoD, sulfite accumulates in both physiologic fluids and tissues. If MoCoD occurs, the result is an accumulation of xanthine and hypoxanthine, and moreover, a uric acid deficiency. The biochemical consequence of sulfite accumulation is increased levels of S-sulphocysteine and thiosulfate, which would activate the NMDA receptor, and thus increase intracellular magnesium and calcium.[5] These

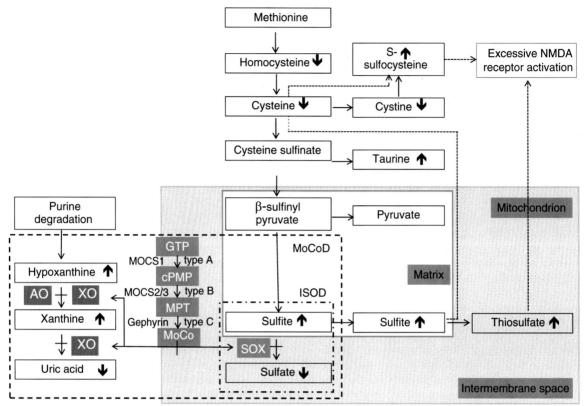

FIG. 16.1 Human sulfite oxidase and molybdenum cofactor deficiency. This biochemical pathway demonstrates the enzymes sulfite oxidase (SO) and molybdenum cofactor (MoCo) in their role of purine and sulfur amino acid degradation. Once SO is deficient, either by isolated sulfite oxidase deficiency (ISOD) or by molybdenum cofactor deficiency (MoCoD), sulfite accumulates in fluid and tissues. The biochemical consequence of sulfite accumulation is increased levels of both S-sulphocysteine and thiosulfate. These reactions are neurotoxic. *AO*, aldehyde oxidase; *cPMP*, cyclic pyranopterin monophosphate; *GPHN*, gephyrin; *GTP*, guanosine triphosphate; *MoCo*, molybdenum cofactor; *MPT*, molybdopterin; *SO*, sulfite oxidase; *XO*, xanthine oxidase. *Dotted lines* represent ISOD (·····) and MoCoD (- - -).

reactions are neurotoxic. Because SO resides within the mitochondrial intermembrane space, sulfite accumulation will damage mitochondrial function, with resultant energy failure.

A succession of biochemical effects will result in severe pathologic changes in the central nervous system, as proven in autopsy cases. The postmortem findings in patients with ISOD and MOCoD show gross generalized brain atrophy, cerebral cystic encephalomalacia, and rostral displacement of the pons and cerebellum, along with hypoplastic tentorium cerebellum.[5,6] Microscopic examination reveals extensive small cavities and spongiosis with essentially astrocytic gliosis and microgliocytic granular bodies in the cerebral gray and white matter. This is accompanied by extensive neuronal loss along with an accumulation of microgliocytic granular

bodies in all areas of the cortex and centrum semiovale; focal neuronal loss and astrogliosis in the basal ganglia, thalami, and brain stem; and bilateral early Wallerian degeneration of the corticospinal tracts in the spinal cord.[5,6]

CLINICAL MANIFESTATIONS

Patients with ISOD or MoCoD share common clinical features because of having the same biochemical and neuropathic consequences of sulfite accumulation. The major cause for the observed clinical symptoms is the deficiency of SO that protects the organisms from elevated levels of toxic sulfite, which is formed on the degradation of sulfur-containing amino acids and sulfur-lipids.[1] The initial clinical manifestations develop shortly after birth, when the baby's metabolism begins to operate and toxic metabolites accumulate within the body.

Newborns with either ISOD or MoCoD display severe neurologic abnormalities, including intractable seizures, irritability, and feeding difficulty. Lethality may occur during this acute stage, or survival may ensue with severe neurologic sequelae.[7,8] The later clinical manifestations are dysmorphic features, including microcephaly, coarse face with a narrow and very sloping forehead, broad nasal bridge, prominent philtrum nasi, and sagging skin, along with psychomotor retardation, spastic tetraplegia, and intractable seizures. Lens dislocation may be present months to years later.[9]

Milder phenotypes with later presentation and survival into the third decade of life are now being recognized. Clinical features of late-onset variants include episodic lethargy during viral infections, motor delay with fluctuating tone with or without seizures, isolated lens dislocation, and/or a mild speech problem during the infantile and early childhood stages. The later clinical manifestations are progressive, slow deterioration, choreoathetoid movements with a dystonic posture, and/or lens dislocation, without displaying dysmorphic features.[10–12]

NEUROIMAGING FEATURES

The characteristics of neuroimaging findings in patients with ISOD and MoCoD during neonatal and early infantile stages are distinctive. The most frequently reported neuroimaging features are diffuse cerebral edema rapidly evolving into multicystic encephalomalacia in the cerebral hemispheres within days to weeks.[13] Other features include signal changes over the basal ganglia[14] or extensive encephalomalacia in the bilateral cerebral hemispheres with prominent intracranial hemorrhage.[15] These findings resemble severe hypoxic-ischemic changes. During the period of follow-up, severe generalized cortical atrophy, ventriculomegaly, signal changes over bilateral basal ganglia, multicystic encephalomalacia in bilateral subcortical white matter (Fig. 16.2), and/or dilatation of the posterior fossa with vermian hypoplasia mimicking the Dandy-Walker malformation are observed.[14,16,17] A hypothesis on the maternal-placental clearance of sulfite had been postulated to explain this phenomenon regarding the rapid onset and rapid deterioration of clinical symptoms, along with the dramatic acceleration in the destruction of the subcortical white matter after clamping the cord. Maternal-placental clearance of sulfite is supposed to be quite effective until late pregnancy in the majority of cases. Once the cord is clamped, the enzyme of SO from

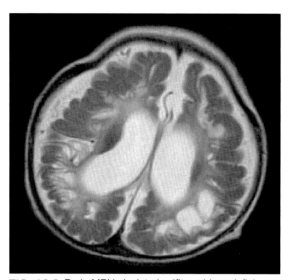

FIG. 16.2 Brain MRI in isolated sulfite oxidase deficiency at age of 13 months. Axial view (TE 94.8 ms/TR 4000 ms) shows generalized brain atrophy, ventriculomegaly, atrophic basal ganglia, and extensive multicystic encephalomalacia in the bilateral cerebral subcortical white matter.

the mother to the baby is much decreased, while sulfite accumulation in the brain and bodily fluids increases.[18]

Although the initial neuroimaging findings of ISOD and MoCoD are similar to that of severe neonatal hypoxic-ischemic encephalopathy, there are some differentiating clinical manifestations and radiologic findings. Patients with hypoxic-ischemic injury do not have facial dysmorphism or lens dislocation, and they exhibit static neurologic deficits. Neuroimaging findings of acute neonatal hypoxic-ischemic encephalopathy are predominantly located at the posterior and lateral putamina and ventral and lateral thalami.[19,20]

Regarding the milder phenotypes with late-onset variants, the neuroimaging manifestations are quite different from the neonatal-onset form. Brain MRI findings show signal changes over bilateral globus pallidi with various clinical manifestations of developmental delay, nysagmus followed by strokelike episodes, hypotonia and movement disorder, or initially isolated lens dislocation without any neurologic symptoms at early childhood but parkinsonism-dystonia syndrome during adulthood.[11,12,21]

LABORATORY FINDINGS

When cases are suspected to have ISOD or MoCoD with clinical and radiologic features, a urine sulfite strip test is useful to screen for sulfite accumulation. However, the sulfite strip test is not always reliable.

TABLE 16.1
Biochemical Findings in Cases With Early-Onset Neonatal Form and Late-Onset Variant of Isolated
Sulfite Oxidase Deficiency (ISOD) and Molybdenum Cofactor Deficiency (MoCoD)

Laboratory Tests	Biochemical Marker	Early Onset Neonatal Form	Late Onset Variant
Urine sulfite strip test	Sulfite	Increased in ISOD Increased in MoCoD	Increased in ISOD Increased in MoCoD
Urine amino acids	Sulfite	Increased in ISOD Increased in MoCoD	Increased in ISOD Increased in MoCoD
	S-sulfocysteine	Increased in ISOD Increased in MoCoD	Increased in ISOD Increased in MoCoD
	Taurine	Increased in ISOD Increased in MoCoD	Increased in ISOD Increased in MoCoD
	Thiosulfate	Increased in ISOD Increased in MoCoD	Increased in ISOD Increased in MoCoD
	Cysteine	Much decreased in ISOD Much decreased in MoCoD	Much decreased in ISOD Much decreased in MoCoD
	Sulfate	Much decreased in ISOD Much decreased in MoCoD	Mild decreased or normal in ISOD Mild decreased or normal in MoCoD
Urine purine analysis	Xanthine and hypoxanthine	Normal in ISOD Much increased in MoCoD	Normal in ISOD Increased in MoCoD
Urine uric acid	Uric acid	Normal in ISOD Much decreased in MoCoD	Normal in ISOD Normal but at low level in MoCoD
Blood uric acid	Uric acid	Normal in ISOD Much decreased in MoCoD	Normal in ISOD Normal but at low level in MoCoD

For the test, the urine should be fresh, kept on ice after being collected, and tested as soon as possible. False negative results may appear with stored urine because of autooxidation of sulfite to sulfate and when urine pH is less than 6. A false positive result occurs in the presence of drugs containing a free, reactive, aliphatic sulfhydryl group, such as N-acetylcysteine, mercaptamine, and dimercaprol; a mucolytic drug (2-mercapto-ethane-sulphonate; Mistabron), mesna therapy (a mixed disulfide of the drug and cysteine), and bacterial growth (reduction of sulfate to sulfite).

As shown in Table 16.1, detection of plasma uric acid levels is an important biochemical marker to assist physicians to both diagnose and differentiate ISOD and MoCoD. MoCoD can often, although not always, be diagnosed when pronounced hypouricemia is found, while ISOD is easily overlooked because of a normal level of plasma uric acid. In addition to MoCoD, the differential diagnoses of hypouricemia include the use of allopurinol, Dalmatian dog syndrome, Fanconi syndrome (cystinosis), purine nucleotide phosphorylase deficiency, renal absorption of urate, Wilson disease,

and XO deficiency.[22] In cases presenting with late-onset milder phenotypes, sulfate in urine amino acids could be normal or mildly decreased. Blood and urine uric acid in late-onset MoCoD may be normal, but at the lower end of the normal range, and the diagnosis may be overlooked.

ISOD and MoCoD both experience the accumulation of reactive sulfite, which may result in the degradation of thiol compounds such as homocysteine. A homocysteinemia or hypohomocysteinemia has previously been reported in ISOD and MoCoD.[23,24] Quantification of total homocysteine amounts in plasma is widely available and inexpensive. This measurement should be considered during selective screening for metabolic disorders, not only with regard to hyperhomocysteinemias, but also for the detection of ISOD and MoCoD by hypohomocysteinemia.

TREATMENT

No treatment had been found to be effective for the early-onset neonatal form of ISOD and MoCoD until recently, when studies showed the benefit of cPMP substitution in severe MoCoD type A patients,[25–27] which is a precursor of the cofactor lacking in two-thirds of patients with MoCoD. cPMP substitution has a favorable safety profile. When introduced sufficiently early, the restoration of molybdenum cofactor-dependent enzyme activity results in a greatly improved neurodevelopment outcome. For late-onset variant cases, diet therapy including methionine restriction and a special formula without cysteine and methionine seem to be effective in preventing neurologic and mental deterioration.[28]

CONCLUSION

The diagnoses of ISOD and MoCoD rely on clinical manifestations and neuroimaging findings, together with biochemical tests and genetic analysis. Clinical manifestations may include irritability, feeding difficulty, and abnormal tone, along with neonatal seizures. These are followed by prominent dysmorphic features, movement disorders, spastic tetraplegia, intractable seizures with or without lens dislocation, and profound psychomotor impairment during infancy. The neuroimaging findings show multicystic encephalomalacia and/or signal changes over the bilateral globus pallidi and/or thalami. In such cases without an obvious history of severe hypoxic-ischemic injury during the prenatal and postnatal periods, the detection of plasma uric acid and metabolic survey, including a urine sulfite strip test, and assay of tandem mass spectroscopy and plasma amino acids for detection of hypohomocysteinemia should be performed to obtain an early diagnosis of ISOD and MoCoD. This early diagnosis is important for genetic counseling and, furthermore, offers effective treatment of cPMP in patients with MoCoD type A to improve neurologic outcome.

DECLARATION OF CONFLICTING INTERESTS

The authors declared no conflicts of interest with respect to the research, authorship, and/or publication of this article.

REFERENCES

1. Mendel RR. Metabolism of molybdenum. *Met Ions Life Sci.* 2013;12:503–528.
2. Schwarz G, Mendel RR, Ribbe MW. Molybdenum cofactors, enzymes and pathways. *Nature.* 2009;460:839–847.
3. Reiss J, Hahnewald R. Molybdenum cofactor deficiency: mutations in GPHN, MOCS1, and MOCS2. *Hum Mutat.* 2011;32:10–18.
4. Ragg R, Natalio F, Tahir MN, et al. Molybdenum trioxide nanoparticles with intrinsic sulfite oxidase activity. *ACS Nano.* 2014;8:5182–5189.
5. Salman MS, Ackerley C, Senger C, Becker L. New insights into the neuropathogenesis of molybdenum cofactor deficiency. *Can J Neurol Sci.* 2002;29:91–96.
6. Roth A, Nogues C, Monnet JP, Ogier H, Saudubray JM. Anatomo-pathological findings in a case of combined deficiency of sulphite oxidase and xanthine oxidase with a defect of molybdenum cofactor. *Virchows Arch A Pathol Anat Histopathol.* 1985;405:379–386.
7. Hansen LK, Wulff K, Dorche C, Christensen E. Molybdenum cofactor deficiency in two siblings: diagnostic difficulties. *Eur J Pediatr.* 1993;152:662–664.
8. Bayram E, Topcu Y, Karakaya P, et al. Molybdenum cofactor deficiency: review of 12 cases (MoCD and review). *Eur J Paediatr Neurol.* 2013;17:1–6.
9. Parini R, Briscioli V, Caruso U, et al. Spherophakia associated with molybdenum cofactor deficiency. *Am J Med Genet.* 1997;73:272–275.
10. Hughes EF, Fairbanks L, Simmonds HA, Robinson RO. Molybdenum cofactor deficiency – phenotypic variability in a family with a late-onset variant. *Dev Med Child Neurol.* 1998;40:57–61.
11. Johnson JL, Coyne KE, Rajagopalan KV, et al. Molybdopterin synthetase mutations in a mild case of molybdenum cofactor deficiency. *Am J Med Genet.* 2001;104:169–173.
12. Alkufri F, Harrower T, Rahman Y, et al. Molybdenum cofactor deficiency presenting with a parkinsonism-dystonia syndrome. *Mov Disord.* 2013;28:399–400.
13. Serrano M, Lizarraga I, Reiss J, et al. Cranial ultrasound and chronological changes in molybdenum cofactor deficiency. *Pediatr Radiol.* 2007;37:1043–1046.
14. Schuierer G, Kurlemann G, Bick U, Stephani U. Molybdenum-cofactor deficiency: CT and MRI findings. *Neuropediatrics.* 1995;26:51–54.
15. Teksam O, Yurdakok M, Coskun T. Molybdenum cofactor deficiency presenting with severe metabolic acidosis and intracranial hemorrhage. *J Child Neurol.* 2004;19:155–157.
16. Slot HMJ, Overweg-Plandsoen WCG, Bakker HD, et al. *Neuropediatrics.* 1993;24:139–142.
17. Pintos-Morell G, Naranjo MA, Artigas M, et al. Molybdenum cofactor deficiency associated with Dandy-Walker malformation. *J Inherit Metab Dis.* 1995;18:86–87.
18. Veldman A, Hennermann JB, Schwarz G, et al. Timing of cerebral developmental disruption in molybdenum cofactor deficiency. *J Child Neurol.* 2011;26:1059–1060.
19. Bindu PS, Christopher R, Mahadevan A, Bharath RD. Clinical and imaging observations in isolated sulfite oxidase deficiency. *J Child Neurol.* 2011;26:1036–1040.
20. Nagappa M, Bindu PS, Taly AB, Sinha S, Bharath RD. Child neurology: molybdenum cofactor deficiency. *Neurology.* 2015;85:e175–e178.
21. Del Rizzo M, Burlina AP, Sass JO, et al. Metabolic stroke in a late-onset form of isolated sulfite oxidase deficiency. *Mol Genet Metab.* 2013;108:263–266.

22. Nyhan WL. Disorders of purine and pyrimidine metabolism. *Mol Genet Metab.* 2005;86:25–33.

23. Graf WD, Oleinik OE, Jack RM, Weiss AH, Johnson JL. Ahomocysteinemia in molybdenum cofactor deficiency. *Neurology.* 1998;51:860–862.

24. Sass JO, Nakanishi T, Sato T, Shimizu A. New approaches toward laboratory diagnosis of isolated sulphite oxidase deficiency. *Ann Clin Biochem.* 2004;41:157–159.

25. Veldman A, Santamaria-Araujo JA, Sollazzo S, et al. Successful treatment of molybdenum cofactor deficiency type A with cPMP. *Pediatrics.* 2010;125:e1249–e1254.

26. Hitzert MM, Bos AF, Bergman KA, et al. Favorable outcome in a newborn with molybdenum cofactor type A deficiency treated with cPMP. *Pediatrics.* 2012;130:e1005–e1010.

27. Schwahn BC, Van Spronsen FJ, Belaidi AA, et al. Efficacy and safety of cyclic pyranopterin monophosphate substitution in severe molybdenum cofactor deficiency type A: a prospective cohort study. *Lancet.* 2015;386:1955–1963.

28. Touati G, Rusthoven E, Depondt E, et al. Dietary therapy in two patients with a mild form of sulphite oxidase deficiency. Evidence for clinical and biological improvement. *J Inherit Metab Dis.* 2000;23:45–53.

CHAPTER 17

Autoimmune Encephalitis: Overview of Clinical Recognition, Autoantibody Diagnostic Markers, and Treatment of Autoimmune Encephalitis

RUSSELL C. DALE, PHD

BACKGROUND: BRAIN INFLAMMATION AND ENCEPHALITIS

Encephalitis is a pathologic description of inflammation of the brain. Technically to make a diagnosis of encephalitis a brain biopsy, which would classically show a lymphocytic inflammatory infiltrate of the brain parenchyma, is required. Because of the invasive nature of brain biopsies, a pragmatic diagnosis of encephalitis, instead, requires clinical features of encephalopathy, plus focal neurologic clinical features, as well as CSF, MRI, or EEG features compatible with encephalitis.[1] Until recently, the causes of encephalitis were obscure. The challenge is that there are over 100 different recognized causes of encephalitis including not only viral, bacterial, parasitic, and fungal infections but also immune and autoimmune causes.[1] These autoimmune encephalitis syndromes are the focus of this chapter. Recent cohort studies suggest autoimmune and immune-mediated encephalitis syndromes constitute about 30% of all encephalitis, with acute disseminated encephalomyelitis (ADEM) and anti-N-methyl-D-aspartate receptor (anti-NMDAR) encephalitis being most common.[2]

These autoimmune encephalitis syndromes are not new, but biomarkers to diagnose them have enabled the clinician to "see them." In the past, anti-NMDA receptor encephalitis was likely called dyskinetic encephalitis lethargica, immune chorea encephalopathy syndrome, or other clinical descriptive syndromes.[3] A major leap forward in the understanding of autoimmune encephalitis occurred after taking lessons from peripheral autoimmune diseases such as myasthenia gravis, which is associated with the presence of autoantibodies that bind to the acetylcholine receptor.[4]

The paradigm that has improved our understanding of autoimmune encephalitis is that patients with autoimmune encephalitis have autoantibodies that bind to cell surface proteins, such as receptors or synaptic proteins. The methodology to detect these autoantibodies is important, which must be a "cell-based assay" that presents the antigen of interest in its conformational state at the cell surface, so that immunoglobulins bind to extracellular epitopes of these proteins. These cell-based assays are now the major methodology employed to detect autoantibodies in autoimmune encephalitis.[4]

CLINICAL SYNDROMES

Although the autoantibodies have been very important in improving our understanding, there are many patients who do not have a diagnostic autoantibody biomarker. Therefore the clinical syndromes of the patients remain important diagnostic clues. For example, limbic encephalitis (LE) has been described, for many decades, mostly in adults with paraneoplastic association; however, LE is described in children as well. LE affects the limbic system, predominantly the medial temporal region and hippocampus, and presents with temporal lobe seizures, cognitive alteration, personality change, and psychiatric features.[5] Magnetic resonance imaging shows inflammatory features and swelling of the temporal lobe, particularly the medial temporal lobe and amygdala, typically bilaterally (Fig. 17.1), and CSF may demonstrate some inflammatory changes. Similarly, with the help of the anti-NMDA receptor antibody, it is now possible to make a clinical diagnosis of anti-NMDA receptor encephalitis while

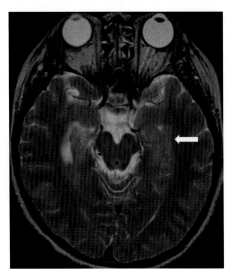

FIG. 17.1 Magnetic resonance imaging (MRI) T2 axial brain image of a 12-year-old girl with acute encephalitis, temporal lobe seizures, confusion, and behavioral change. Imaging shows bilateral limbic swelling more on arrowed side, compatible with limbic encephalitis. (Courtesy of Dr. Sekhar Pillai, Sydney, Australia.)

awaiting results from the antibody testing.[5] Because the clinical syndrome of anti-NMDAR encephalitis is quite recognizable (described below), the clinician can now start immune therapy based on a suspected diagnosis rather than waiting for the antibody results. Indeed a diagnosis of clinical autoimmune encephalitis is now encouraged, and a consensus recommendation paper was published in 2016, to allow a diagnosis of autoimmune encephalitis to be considered.[5]

CELL SURFACE AUTOANTIBODIES

The initial discoveries of autoimmune encephalitis syndromes associated with cell surface autoantibodies were made after it was recognized that these patients had CSF and serum immunoglobulin G (IgG), which bound to neuronal tissue, particularly the hippocampal region, using immunofluorescence or immunohistochemistry ("neuropil antibodies").[6] Subsequently, when using live neuronal cultures, it was further recognized that these patients had IgG that bound to the cell surface of these live neurons. This provided, in principle, evidence that these patients had a cell surface antibody, although the exact nature of the autoantigen involved in antibody binding using this technique is unknown; however, these are useful screening tests but are available in

only research laboratories. Using immunoprecipitation and mass spectrometry, it was subsequently possible to identify the targets of these cell surface autoantibodies, and they mostly transpired to be important neuronal receptors or synaptic proteins.[4] The most common autoantibody in autoimmune encephalitis is NMDA receptor antibody, and in children, autoantibodies against myelin oligodendrocyte glycoprotein (MOG) are also important in autoimmune demyelination such as ADEM, optic neuritis, and transverse myelitis.[7] Other autoantibodies are significantly rarer in children; however, the most common are described in detail below.

Subsequent study of these cell surface autoantibodies has determined the following:

- The autoantibody is typically IgG, and IgM and IgA have limited significance as a biomarker or mediator of disease.
- There is often a restricted epitope involved in antibody binding, such as the amino terminus of the NR1 subunit of the NMDA receptor in anti-NMDAR encephalitis.[8]
- In anti-NMDAR encephalitis, there is intrathecal production of antibody, whereas this is less true for anti-MOG-associated demyelination.[6,9]
- The cell surface antibodies have in vitro pathogenic effects by downregulating the receptor from the cell surface, altering neuronal circuits, and animal models have shown pathogenic effects (mostly for anti-NMDAR encephalitis).[10]
- Most of the cell surface autoantibody syndromes respond to immune therapy and have "reversibility," whereas this is less true for paraneoplastic antibodies that bind to intracellular antigens and anti–glutamic acid decarboxylase (anti-GAD) antibody–associated disease.[4,11]

By far the most common and important autoimmune encephalopathy syndromes in children are anti-NMDAR encephalitis and anti-MOG antibody–associated demyelination, which are reviewed in detail, followed by some other rarer syndromes.

ANTI–N-METHYL-D-ASPARTATE RECEPTOR ENCEPHALITIS

Initially described in young women with ovarian teratoma, anti-NMDAR encephalitis has transpired to be a very important encephalitis syndrome. This disease probably accounts for between 3% and 10% of all encephalitis in children (excluding neonates) and can affect children from 6 months until 18 years of age. Indeed, the most common age for this disorder is between 5 and 40 years of age.[11] Females are affected more in adulthood, but the age distribution is more equal under the age of 10 years. The disorder is associated with ovarian teratoma (paraneoplastic) in a very small minority of young children (<5%), but this association increases in females during adolescence so that by the age of 20 years over half of females will have an associated ovarian teratoma.[11] Apart from ovarian teratoma, the causes of anti-NMDA receptor encephalitis are usually unclear. Some children have a nonspecific infection; however, a very small proportion of children will have a preceding direct viral encephalitis. This is most commonly seen in children with herpes simplex encephalitis; ~20% of children with herpes simplex encephalitis will get a secondary autoimmune NMDAR encephalitis ~3 weeks after the herpes encephalitis. These patients show initial recovery from herpes encephalitis and then get a secondary deterioration usually with the evolution of movement disorders and agitation. This has become an excellent example of viral-induced autoimmunity, and it is hypothesized that the destructive nature of HSV encephalitis and release of neuronal antigens results in loss of immune tolerance and activation of autoimmunity.[12,13]

In children with anti-NMDAR encephalitis, the initial symptoms are often seizures, behavioral change, or a movement disorder. There are six main clusters of symptoms of anti-NMDA receptor encephalitis[11]:

- Encephalopathy in which the child is often awake but not interacting with his/her environment
- Seizures that are typically focal or secondary generalized
- Movement disorders that are typically generalized involving trunk, limbs, and orofacial region and have a stereotypical, hyperkinetic characteristic with perseverative qualities, plus chorea and dystonia[14]
- Psychosis and agitation
- Autonomic features including temperature and cardiorespiratory fluctuations
- Mutism/aphasia

In its complete form, anti-NMDAR encephalitis is a highly recognizable clinical syndrome, and a clinical diagnosis can be suspected.[5] Occasionally, patients can have incomplete forms and the diagnosis is more challenging. Unlike many other encephalitis syndromes, anti-NMDA receptor encephalitis evolves more slowly over weeks and even months and the improvements can take many months and even up to 2 years.[11] In this disease there is clear evidence of intrathecal production of antibodies with an evolved autoimmune brain process—it is probably for this reason that the

patients improve slowly. Investigation using conventional tests such as MRI brain is often normal although may show nonspecific changes or limbic features, CSF testing shows a pleocytosis in ~60%, and about half of patients will also have mirrored or intrathecal oligoclonal bands (likely dependent on timing of CSF sampling).[11] CSF neopterin when available can also be very useful, which is a sensitive biomarker, but is not specific of any particular inflammatory process.[15] If the diagnosis is suspected and there is no apparent contraindication, immune therapy can be started and testing for NMDA receptor antibody can be sent. CSF testing is more specific than serum testing, but both are recommended. Improvements often take many months, and prolonged inpatient stays are often required, with 3 months being a common duration of inpatient stay, sometimes with prolonged rehabilitation requirements. Immunotherapy should be encouraged and is described in more detail below. However, some patients can make a spontaneous recovery and there are historical descriptions of this disease who did not receive immune therapy and who completely recovered spontaneously. However, given the mortality of 5% and the morbidity of ~50% (predominantly cognitive and psychiatric),[11] immunotherapy is encouraged to reduce the inflammatory process and maximize the chance of recovery. There has been no randomized controlled trials in this disorder, but retrospective observational data, including from a very large cohort of 577 adult and child patients, strongly suggest that patients given immune therapy do better than patients not given therapy, and patients who fail first-line therapy do better if they receive second-line therapy.[11] Therapeutics will be discussed in more detail below. Symptomatic management of this extremely challenging condition is often required during prolonged inpatient stays.[16] There is typically major psychiatric features with agitation and psychosis, major sleep disruption with reduced sleep and sleep inversion, and there is often pronounced movement disorders, which are often violent or self-injurious. There are also frequent seizures, but only occasionally patients have very severe epilepsy with status epilepticus. For this reason many patients require symptomatic management of agitation/sleep/movement problems, which typically includes sedating agents such as benzodiazepines, clonidine, chloral hydrate, and melatonin.[16] Neuroleptics are frequently used for the psychotic and agitated behavior, but these patients appear to have a higher incidence of dystonic side effects and even rhabdomyolysis and neuroleptic malignant syndrome; therefore, these agents should be used with caution.[16]

Anti-NMDAR encephalitis is a very severe disorder and a large proportion of patients are rendered bedbound and highly dependent, sometimes including intensive care and even ventilatory support for prolonged periods of time, and secondary complications may occur. Ongoing nursing, physiotherapy, psychologic support, and occupational therapy support are essential, and support for the family and medical staff is essential as this is typically extremely stressful disorder for all involved. As NMDA receptor is required for memory, typically patients with anti-NMDAR encephalitis do not remember the acute phase of the illness, although many parents are left with posttraumatic stress disorder (personal observations).

ANTI–MYELIN OLIGODENDROCYTE GLYCOPROTEIN ANTIBODY–ASSOCIATED DEMYELINATION

Myelin oligodendrocyte glycoprotein (MOG) is a minor component of myelin expressed on the outer surface of the myelin sheath, which wraps around neurons and axons to enable efficient action potential electrical conduction. Before using cell-based assays, anti-MOG antibodies had unknown significance in demyelination syndromes. However, since the first use of cell-based assays to measure anti-MOG antibodies in children, there have been highly consistent confirmatory studies demonstrating their anti-MOG antibodies strongly associate with an autoimmune demyelination spectrum of disease.[7] Patients with multiple sclerosis do not have these antibodies, instead anti-MOG antibodies are associated with pediatric ADEM, and adults and children with bilateral optic neuritis and myelitis, which can be relapsing.[17] Anti-MOG antibodies (ab) are found in ~50% of young children with ADEM.[18] The clinical syndrome of anti-MOG ab positive ADEM is similar to anti-MOG ab negative ADEM; however, the radiology shows that MOG positive patients have larger and more globular white matter lesions, which are less well demarcated, and also anti-MOG ab positive ADEM is more likely to have coexistent longitudinally extensive myelitis and sometimes bilateral optic neuritis radiologically (and clinically) (Fig. 17.2).[18] About 30% of patients will relapse, although the majority will be monophasic.[9] When relapse occurs it tends to again be ADEM, optic neuritis, or myelitis, although occasionally there can be posterior fossa relapses. Typically oligoclonal bands are negative although there can be peripheral evidence of inflammation such as raised erythrocyte sedimentation rate.[9] Patients typically respond to high-dose

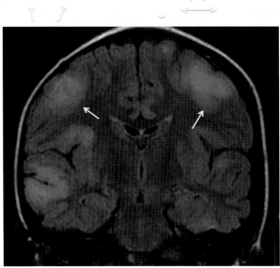

FIG. 17.2 Magnetic resonance imaging (MRI) T2 coronal brain image of a 2-year-old boy with acute disseminated encephalomyelitis (ADEM) and positive anti-MOG (anti–myelin oligodendrocyte glycoprotein) antibodies showing large globular lesions with poorly demarcated lesions. (Courtesy of Dr. Sekhar Pillai, Sydney, Australia.)

corticosteroids, patients who do not respond to corticosteroids may benefit from intravenous immunoglobulin or even plasma exchange, and it would be very unusual to require further immune suppression. Most patients do well, although residual attention problems and occasional focal seizures can remain, which may suggest persistent low-grade inflammation, and in some patients a trial of steroids for residual symptoms many months after the illness can determine if there is some persistent low-grade inflammation. Most patients with ADEM will typically show complete or partial resolution of lesions on repeat MRI 6–12 months after episode, and it would be very unusual to see new asymptomatic lesions, which would be more suggestive of multiple sclerosis.[18] Although 30% of patients may have a relapsing course, some of these patients will relapse in months after the first event but then to go into complete clinical and radiologic remission. However, occasionally patients can have a relapse many years or even a decade after the first event. In between events, the MRI brain can be normal, which again would be inconsistent with multiple sclerosis. Generally, anti-MOG antibody–associated autoimmune demyelination has a better prognosis than aquaporin-4 antibody–associated neuromyelitis optica, which is a more destructive pathologic process.[7]

ANTIGLYCINE RECEPTOR ANTIBODY–ASSOCIATED ENCEPHALITIS

Glycine (like γ-aminobutyric acid [GABA]) is a classic inhibitory neurotransmitter, and genetic mutations of glycine receptors and related proteins result in hyperekplexia resulting in rigidity and stimulus sensitive myoclonus. An acquired form of autoimmune hyperekplexia was first described associated with glycine receptor antibodies in adults, but children including very young children can present with acquired hyperekplexia.[19] The classic syndrome associated with glycine receptor antibodies is called progressive encephalomyelitis rigidity and myoclonus (PERM), although glycine receptor antibodies are also associated with LE, brainstem syndromes, and even demyelination syndromes such as optic neuritis. These disorders are immune responsive and can result in good outcomes.[19]

ANTI–γ-AMINOBUTYRIC ACID-A RECEPTOR ANTIBODY–ASSOCIATED ENCEPHALITIS

Anti-GABA-A receptor antibodies are associated with an encephalitis characterized by refractory seizures and status epilepticus, sometimes epilepsia partialis continua.[20] There can also be movement disorders and be "anti-NMDAR encephalitis-like." MRI is unusual, showing globular lesions affecting cerebral cortex and the associated white matter. Despite being very sick, the patients can do well with immune therapy.

BASAL GANGLIA ENCEPHALITIS

Basal ganglia inflammation is seen in ADEM; however, there is a restricted encephalitic syndrome that is referred to as "basal ganglia encephalitis (BGE)," which is considered to be autoimmune. Unlike patients with ADEM, patients with BGE have a restricted extrapyramidal clinical syndrome with akinesia, dystonia, or chorea plus emotional or attentional behavioral change.[21] Seizures are uncommon and if present are often isolated. CSF may show some inflammatory changes such as mild pleocytosis or mirrored/intrathecal oligoclonal bands, and MRI (which is abnormal in 50%) shows restricted basal ganglia inflammation with symmetrical involvement of the striatum (caudate and putamen) particularly, and to a lesser extent the substantia nigra (Fig. 17.3).[21] A diagnosis can be made clinically based on the clinicoradiological syndrome. A majority of these patients have serum antibodies that bind to dopamine 2 receptor in a cell-based assay (negative to other dopamine receptors), and these patients respond to immune therapy such as high-dose corticosteroids and

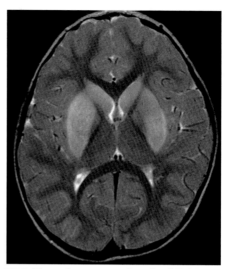

FIG. 17.3 Magnetic resonance imaging (MRI) T2 axial brain image of a 10-year-old boy with postinfectious acute-onset akinesia with behavioral change, and imaging showing restricted inflammation to caudate and putamen bilaterally. The clinicoradiological syndrome is basal ganglia encephalitis.

intravenous immunoglobulin or plasma exchange.[21] Early therapy may be important because a significant proportion of patients can have residual attention issues and executive dysfunction, sometimes in association with striatal atrophy or gliosis.[22] There is likely to be a cellular component of disease (B or T cell), in addition to the autoantibody.

ANTI–GLUTAMIC ACID DECARBOXYLASE ANTIBODY–ASSOCIATED ENCEPHALITIS

GAD antibodies are technically not a cell surface antibody, because GAD is an intracellular antigen, and the detection method does not use a cell-based assay but instead uses a radioimmunoassay (RIA) or ELISA. GAD65 is the main antigen, and low titers, as found in diabetes, have no relevance to neurologic disease. By contrast, titers 100-fold higher than the "diabetic titers" have been strongly associated with neurologic phenotypes such as LE, cerebellar ataxia, and stiff person syndrome.[23] Although patients with high-titer GAD antibody–associated CNS phenotypes should receive an immune therapy trial, these patients are often more refractory to immune therapy, and there is often persistent disability in the LE patients, which may relate to the fact that GAD antibodies are not cell surface antibodies, and there may be a T cell–driven process.

OTHER RARE SYNDROMES

DPPX is a regulatory subunit of neuronal potassium channel Kv4.2, and DPPX antibodies are found in a spectrum of autoimmune encephalitis with PERM (myoclonus and rigidity) or encephalopathy with psychiatric features. One of the most important diagnostic features of the disorder is the association with gut symptoms of diarrhea and weight loss (presumably as DPPX is expressed in gut) plus other dysautonomic features.[24] Anti-DPPX antibody–associated encephalitis has been described in children.

Syndromes associated with GABA-B-receptor, CASPR2, LGI-1, AMPAR, IgLON5, and neurexin 3a antibody are described in adults but either described or not described in children or only in single case reports.

The issue of voltage-gated potassium channel (VGKC) antibodies requires specific consideration. VGKC antibodies are typically detected using radioimmunoassay (RIA), which precipitates VGKC as well as other associated proteins (called the VGKC complex). Although the VGKC assay defined a LE and resulted in the discovery of LGI1 and CASPR2 antigens (which are the dominant antibody targets in the VGKC complex), many observers now recommend testing for only LGI1 and CASPR2 using cell-based assays, and not using VGKC RIA, because both adult and child patients who are VGKC antibody positive but LGI1 and CASPR2 negative lack syndrome specificity and do not clearly have immune responsive conditions.[25]

RELAPSING COURSE

Although many patients have monophasic disease, a relapsing course occurs in ~12% of anti-NMDAR encephalitis patients[11] and ~30% of anti-MOG-associated demyelination.[9] Likewise, relapsing disease is reported in the other rarer syndromes. Relapses tend to be milder, more subtle, and monosymptomatic in anti-NMDAR encephalitis, which can present a diagnostic challenge. The patient with severe anti-NMDAR encephalitis who is improving, but after 6 months, starts having seizures again or becomes more agitated should be assessed for a possible relapse. Worsening symptoms associated with B cell repopulation after use of rituximab should be considered to represent a possible relapse. Monitoring the clinical course is not straightforward, because antibodies often remain positive, and although antibody titers decline, the titers are not adequately reliable for monitoring disease course. If a relapse is considered possible, escalation of immune therapy can be considered, such as a retrial of pulsed steroids/IVIG/plasma exchange or redosing rituximab.

CLINICAL CRITERIA

Anti-NMDAR encephalitis is a highly recognizable syndrome in its complete form, indeed a previously healthy child with acquired encephalopathy, psychotic features, a movement disorder, and mutism probably has a high pretest probability of being anti-NMDAR antibody positive. For this reason, and to encourage clinicians to start first-line immune therapy early (see below), a clinical criterion of "suspected anti-NMDAR encephalitis" has been proposed by Graus et al.,[5] and it has good sensitivity and specificity in the context of children with encephalitis (unpublished observations). Fig. 17.4 presents the criteria outlined by Graus et al. If a patient fulfills these criteria and anti-NMDAR encephalitis is suspected, and other causes have been reasonably excluded, first-line immune therapy can be commenced while awaiting antibody testing. This clinical criterion has potentially highest utility in countries of limited resources, where antibody testing is not possible.

SERONEGATIVE SUSPECTED AUTOIMMUNE ENCEPHALITIS

A patient who is suspected to have autoimmune encephalitis but is negative on autoantibody testing is a challenge to the clinician. The reasons for "seronegativity," meaning negative CSF and serum autoantibody testing, can be due to any of the following:

- The assay lacks sensitivity.
- The patient has an unknown or untested autoantibody.
- The patient does not have a cell surface autoantibody syndrome, instead has an alternative immune disorder due to an aberrant B cell, T cell, or innate immune process.
- The patient has an alternate disease etiology, such as genetic autoinflammation, or genetic/metabolic disease. Common scenarios include the following:
  - An infant with preceding normal development who starts regressing, loses skills and develops a syndrome of four-limbed hypertonia (rigidity or spasticity or dystonia). The patient has evidence of CSF inflammation such as raised neopterin, but normal or nonspecific imaging, and is not or only partially responsive to first-line immune therapy. In this scenario, a genetic autoinflammatory condition such as ADAR1 or IFIH1 genetic interferonopathy (also called Aicardi

Probable anti-NMDA receptor encephalitis

Diagnosis can be made when all three of the following criteria have been met:
1. Rapid onset (less than 3 months) of at least four* of the six following major groups of symptoms:
   - Abnormal (psychiatric) behavior or cognitive dysfunction
   - Speech dysfunction (pressured speech, verbal reduction, mutism)
   - Seizures
   - Movement disorder, dyskinesias, or rigidity/abnormal postures
   - Decreased level of consciousness
   - Autonomic dysfunction or central hypoventilation

2. At least one of the following laboratory study results:
   - Abnormal EEG (focal or diff use slow or disorganized activity, epileptic activity, or extreme delta brush)
   - CSF with pleocytosis or oligoclonal bands

3. Reasonable exclusion of other disorders

*Diagnosis can also be made in the presence of three of the above groups of symptoms accompanied by a systemic teratoma

Definite anti-NMDA receptor encephalitis

Diagnosis can be made in the presence of one or more of the six major groups of symptoms, and IgG anti-GluN1 (NR1 subunit of NMDAR) antibodies, after reasonable exclusion of other disorders.

FIG. 17.4 Proposed clinical criteria for a diagnosis of anti-NMDAR (anti–*N*-methyl-D-aspartate receptor) encephalitis. (From Graus F, Titulaer MJ, Balu R, et al. A clinical approach to diagnosis of autoimmune encephalitis. *Lancet Neurol*. 2016;15(4):391–404.)

Goittieres syndrome types 6 and 7) should be considered.[26,27]

- A previously neurodevelopmentally normal child or a child with autistic spectrum disorder appears to regress or change in function with development of worsening cognitive problems, obsessive compulsive disorder, tics, or epilepsy. This is a specific diagnostic challenge, and biomarkers are lacking for this scenario. Possible diagnostic terms include pediatric acute neuropsychiatric syndrome[28] although the exact immunopathogenesis of this is unclear and may not be autoimmune, but some other immunologic mechanism.

THERAPEUTICS

Fig. 17.5 outlines the generally agreed therapeutic pathway in the treatment of autoimmune encephalitis. For anti-NMDAR encephalitis and other severe autoimmune encephalitis syndromes, high-dose corticosteroids with intravenous immunoglobulin are recommended.[29] Plasma exchange is an alternative or can be used before IVIG.[30] After commencing this first-line therapy, the clinician should try to wait and observe for effect, generally for 10–14 days if possible.

Some patients will respond to this first-line therapy, and second-line therapy is not required. If the disease is severe and life-threatening, or if there is no apparent response to this first-line therapy, second-line therapy with rituximab can be considered, given according to local protocols.[31] Cyclophosphamide can be used as an alternative, or in addition for severe disease, and is usually given intravenously monthly for 3–6 months.

In anti-NMDAR encephalitis, the disease course is often prolonged, and ongoing pulsed steroids and IVIg are required for 6–12 months. Many clinicians now prefer pulsed steroids (oral or IV) rather than regular daily prednisolone, although there is little evidence to say which is better.

In some patients who are poorly responsive to therapy, or patients who have relapsing disease, a "chronic therapeutic plan" will be required, which may include redosing rituximab regularly,[32] or the use of chronic immune suppression such as mycophenolate mofetil.

If patients fail to respond to these therapies and active disease is suspected, there are some reports of the use of intrathecal methotrexate,[33] tocilizumab (interleukin-6 blocker),[34] or bortezomib (a protease inhibitor that inhibits proinflammatory signalling cascades and reduces plasma cells and antibody production).[35]

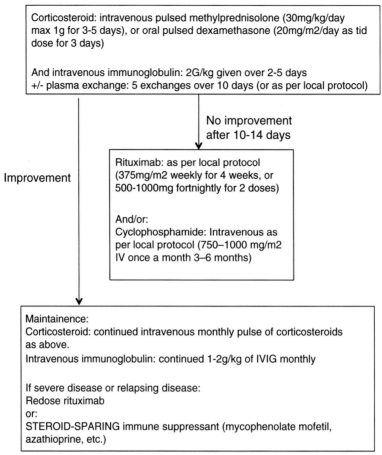

Corticosteroid: intravenous pulsed methylprednisolone (30mg/kg/day max 1g for 3-5 days), or oral pulsed dexamethasone (20mg/m2/day as tid dose for 3 days)

And intravenous immunoglobulin: 2G/kg given over 2-5 days +/- plasma exchange: 5 exchanges over 10 days (or as per local protocol)

No improvement after 10-14 days

Improvement

Rituximab: as per local protocol (375mg/m2 weekly for 4 weeks, or 500-1000mg fortnightly for 2 doses)

And/or:
Cyclophosphamide: Intravenous as per local protocol (750–1000 mg/m2 IV once a month 3–6 months)

Maintainence:
Corticosteroid: continued intravenous monthly pulse of corticosteroids as above.
Intravenous immunoglobulin: continued 1-2g/kg of IVIG monthly

If severe disease or relapsing disease:
Redose rituximab
or:
STEROID-SPARING immune suppressant (mycophenolate mofetil, azathioprine, etc.)

FIG. 17.5 Therapeutic decision-making of anti-NMDAR (anti–N-methyl-D-aspartate receptor) encephalitis and other severe autoimmune encephalitis syndromes.

As discussed above, in a patient who was improving who appears to deteriorate, it is important to consider a possible relapse, and a retrial or escalation of immune therapy can be considered.

As is true for all therapeutic interventions, it is important to weigh up the "risk versus benefit" of the treatments and involve clinicians with experience in the use of immune suppressive agents, to counsel families appropriately.

Although the recommendations in Fig. 17.5 are applicable to severe autoimmune encephalitis syndromes such as anti-NMDAR encephalitis, anti-MOG antibody–associated demyelination usually does not require the same pathway. Generally, patients with autoimmune demyelination with anti-MOG antibodies will respond to high-dose corticosteroids. If they do not respond to corticosteroids, intravenous immunoglobulin or plasma exchange can be used. In the relapsing form of MOG antibody–associated demyelination, the following options are reasonable: low-dose corticosteroid (10 mg alternate days of prednisolone), or monthly intravenous immunoglobulin, or mycophenolate mofetil, or if severe rituximab. More data on relapsing MOG antibody–associated disorders are required to determine the best approach.

FUTURE PRIORITIES

There are many unanswered issues in autoimmune encephalitis, including the role of infection, an improved definition of seronegative autoimmune encephalitis, consideration of the role of neuroprotection, and better understanding of ethnic or genetic vulnerability factors.[36] In addition, there are still no randomized controlled trials to guide clinicians in the treatment of these conditions.

FUNDING

RCD has an NHMRC Practitioner Fellowship, funding from the Petre Foundation and support from the University of Sydney.

REFERENCES

1. Granerod J, Cunningham R, Zuckerman M, et al. Causality in acute encephalitis: defining aetiologies. *Epidemiol Infect.* 2010;138(6):783–800.
2. Pillai SC, Hacohen Y, Tantsis E, et al. Infectious and autoantibody-associated encephalitis: clinical features and long-term outcome. *Pediatrics.* 2015;135(4):e974–e984.
3. Dale RC, Irani SR, Brilot F, et al. N-methyl-D-aspartate receptor antibodies in pediatric dyskinetic encephalitis lethargica. *Ann Neurol.* 2009;66(5):704–709.
4. Leypoldt F, Armangue T, Dalmau J. Autoimmune encephalopathies. *Ann N Y Acad Sci.* 2015;1338:94–114.
5. Graus F, Titulaer MJ, Balu R, et al. A clinical approach to diagnosis of autoimmune encephalitis. *Lancet Neurol.* 2016;15(4):391–404.
6. Dalmau J, Gleichman AJ, Hughes EG, et al. Anti-NMDA-receptor encephalitis: case series and analysis of the effects of antibodies. *Lancet Neurol.* 2008;7(12):1091–1098.
7. Ramanathan S, Dale RC, Brilot F. Anti-MOG antibody: the history, clinical phenotype, and pathogenicity of a serum biomarker for demyelination. *Autoimmun Rev.* 2016;15(4):307–324.
8. Gleichman AJ, Spruce LA, Dalmau J, Seeholzer SH, Lynch DR. Anti-NMDA receptor encephalitis antibody binding is dependent on amino acid identity of a small region within the GluN1 amino terminal domain. *J Neurosci.* 2012;32(32):11082–11094.
9. Dale RC, Tantsis EM, Merheb V, et al. Antibodies to MOG have a demyelination phenotype and affect oligodendrocyte cytoskeleton. *Neurol Neuroimmunol Neuroinflamm.* 2014;1(1):e12.
10. Hughes EG, Peng X, Gleichman AJ, et al. Cellular and synaptic mechanisms of anti-NMDA receptor encephalitis. *J Neurosci.* 2010;30(17):5866–5875.
11. Titulaer MJ, McCracken L, Gabilondo I, et al. Treatment and prognostic factors for long-term outcome in patients with anti-NMDA receptor encephalitis: an observational cohort study. *Lancet Neurol.* 2013;12(2):157–165.
12. Armangue T, Moris G, Cantarin-Extremera V, et al. Autoimmune post-herpes simplex encephalitis of adults and teenagers. *Neurology.* 2015;85(20):1736–1743.
13. Mohammad SS, Sinclair K, Pillai S, et al. Herpes simplex encephalitis relapse with chorea is associated with autoantibodies to N-Methyl-D-aspartate receptor or dopamine-2 receptor. *Mov Disord.* 2014;29(1):117–122.
14. Mohammad SS, Fung VS, Grattan-Smith P, et al. Movement disorders in children with anti-NMDAR encephalitis and other autoimmune encephalopathies. *Mov Disord.* 2014;29(12):1539–1542.
15. Dale RC, Brilot F, Fagan E, Earl J. Cerebrospinal fluid neopterin in paediatric neurology: a marker of active central nervous system inflammation. *Dev Med Child Neurol.* 2009;51(4):317–323.
16. Mohammad SS, Jones H, Hong M, et al. Symptomatic treatment of children with anti-NMDAR encephalitis. *Dev Med Child Neurol.* 2016;58(4):376–384.
17. Hacohen Y, Absoud M, Deiva K, et al. Myelin oligodendrocyte glycoprotein antibodies are associated with a non-MS course in children. *Neurol Neuroimmunol Neuroinflamm.* 2015;2(2):e81.
18. Baumann M, Sahin K, Lechner C, et al. Clinical and neuroradiological differences of paediatric acute disseminating encephalomyelitis with and without antibodies to the myelin oligodendrocyte glycoprotein. *J Neurol Neurosurg Psychiatry.* 2015;86(3):265–272.
19. Carvajal-Gonzalez A, Leite MI, Waters P, et al. Glycine receptor antibodies in PERM and related syndromes: characteristics, clinical features and outcomes. *Brain.* 2014;137(Pt 8):2178–2192.
20. Petit-Pedrol M, Armangue T, Peng X, et al. Encephalitis with refractory seizures, status epilepticus, and antibodies to the GABAA receptor: a case series, characterisation of the antigen, and analysis of the effects of antibodies. *Lancet Neurol.* 2014;13(3):276–286.
21. Dale RC, Merheb V, Pillai S, et al. Antibodies to surface dopamine-2 receptor in autoimmune movement and psychiatric disorders. *Brain.* 2012;135(Pt 11):3453–3468.
22. Pawela C, Brunsdon RK, Williams TA, Porter M, Dale RC, Mohammad SS. The neuropsychological profile of children with basal ganglia encephalitis: a case series. *Dev Med Child Neurol.* 2017;59(4):445–448.
23. Saiz A, Blanco Y, Sabater L, et al. Spectrum of neurological syndromes associated with glutamic acid decarboxylase antibodies: diagnostic clues for this association. *Brain.* 2008;131(Pt 10):2553–2563.
24. Tobin WO, Lennon VA, Komorowski L, et al. DPPX potassium channel antibody: frequency, clinical accompaniments, and outcomes in 20 patients. *Neurology.* 2014;83(20):1797–1803.
25. Hacohen Y, Singh R, Rossi M, et al. Clinical relevance of voltage-gated potassium channel-complex antibodies in children. *Neurology.* 2015;85(11):967–975.
26. Crow YJ, Zaki MS, Abdel-Hamid MS, et al. Mutations in ADAR1, IFIH1, and RNASEH2B presenting as spastic paraplegia. *Neuropediatrics.* 2014;45(6):386–393.
27. Rice GI, del Toro Duany Y, Jenkinson EM, et al. Gain-of-function mutations in IFIH1 cause a spectrum of human disease phenotypes associated with upregulated type I interferon signaling. *Nat Genet.* 2014;46(5):503–509.
28. Chang K, Frankovich J, Cooperstock M, et al. Clinical evaluation of youth with pediatric acute-onset neuropsychiatric syndrome (PANS): recommendations from the 2013 PANS Consensus Conference. *J Child Adolesc Psychopharmacol.* 2015;25(1):3–13.
29. Nosadini M, Mohammad SS, Ramanathan S, Brilot F, Dale RC. Immune therapy in autoimmune encephalitis: a systematic review. *Expert Rev Neurother.* 2015;15(12):1391–1419.

30. Suppiej A, Nosadini M, Zuliani L, et al. Plasma exchange in pediatric anti-NMDAR encephalitis: a systematic review. *Brain Dev.* 2016;38(7):613–622.

31. Dale RC, Brilot F, Duffy LV, et al. Utility and safety of rituximab in pediatric autoimmune and inflammatory CNS disease. *Neurology.* 2014;83(2):142–150.

32. Nosadini M, Alper G, Riney CJ, et al. Rituximab monitoring and redosing in pediatric neuromyelitis optica spectrum disorder. *Neurol Neuroimmunol Neuroinflamm.* 2016;3(1):e188.

33. Tatencloux S, Chretien P, Rogemond V, Honnorat J, Tardieu M, Deiva K. Intrathecal treatment of anti-N-Methyl-D-aspartate receptor encephalitis in children. *Dev Med Child Neurol.* 2015;57(1):95–99.

34. Lee WJ, Lee ST, Moon J, et al. Tocilizumab in autoimmune encephalitis refractory to rituximab: an institutional cohort study. *Neurotherapeutics.* 2016;13(4):824–832.

35. Behrendt V, Krogias C, Reinacher-Schick A, Gold R, Kleiter I. Bortezomib treatment for patients with anti-N-methyl-D-aspartate receptor encephalitis. *JAMA Neurol.* 2016;73(10):1251–1253.

36. Dale RC, Gorman MP, Lim M. Autoimmune encephalitis in children: clinical phenomenology, therapeutics, and emerging challenges. *Curr Opin Neurol.* 2017;30(3):334–344.

CHAPTER 18

Acute Disseminated Encephalomyelitis

SUVASINI SHARMA, MD, DM • RUSSELL C. DALE, MBCHB, MSC, MRCPHCH, PHD

INTRODUCTION

Acute disseminated encephalomyelitis (ADEM) is an acute immune-mediated inflammatory demyelinating condition involving the brain and spinal cord, which presents clinically with new-onset polyfocal neurologic features, which by definition include encephalopathy.[1] The MRI shows characteristic multifocal demyelinating abnormalities. There is often a history of infection or immunization, and ADEM is considered a postinfectious/parainfectious condition. This condition is a common cause of encephalitis in children and must be considered in the differential diagnosis of a child presenting with acute febrile encephalopathy and altered sensorium with or without fever. Children with ADEM respond well to immunosuppressive treatment (steroids) with the majority having a single event, i.e., a monophasic course. A small proportion of children with ADEM may have relapses, and in this subset, multiple sclerosis (MS) is a diagnostic consideration. In this chapter we discuss the epidemiology, pathophysiology, clinical features, investigations, treatment, and outcome of ADEM in children.

DEFINITIONS

ADEM is a clinicoradiological diagnosis because there are currently no diagnostic blood or CSF abnormalities or biomarkers (apart from anti–myelin oligodendrocyte protein [anti-MOG] antibodies, discussed later). Therefore in earlier studies there was a marked heterogeneity regarding the criteria for diagnosis. In 2007, the International Pediatric Multiple Sclerosis Study Group (IPMSSG) proposed consensus definitions for pediatric acquired demyelinating disorders of the central nervous system (CNS) to improve consistency in terminology.[2] These criteria were revised in 2013.[3]

For the diagnosis of ADEM, all of the following criteria are required[3]:

1. A first polyfocal, clinical CNS event with presumed inflammatory demyelinating cause.

2. Encephalopathy that cannot be explained by fever. Encephalopathy refers to an alteration in consciousness (e.g., stupor, lethargy) or behavioral change unexplained by fever, systemic illness, or postictal symptoms.

3. No new clinical and MRI findings emerge 3 months or more after the onset. This implies that the confirmation of the monophasic course requires follow-up and can only be done retrospectively.

4. Brain MRI is abnormal during the acute (3 months) phase.

5. Typically on brain MRI, there are diffuse poorly demarcated, large (>1–2 cm) lesions involving predominantly the cerebral white matter. T1 hypointense lesions in the white matter are rare. Deep gray matter lesions (e.g., thalamus or basal ganglia lesions) can be present.

If a child has a first monofocal or polyfocal clinical CNS event with presumed inflammatory demyelinating cause in the *absence* of encephalopathy and the MRI criteria for MS are not met, this is known as clinically isolated syndrome (CIS).[3] Examples of CIS include optic neuritis, transverse myelitis, hemiparesis, monoparesis, and brainstem syndromes. CIS has a higher likelihood of progression to MS as compared with ADEM.[4]

The clinical symptoms and radiologic findings of ADEM can fluctuate in severity and evolve in the first 3 months after onset. Accordingly, a second event is defined as the development of new symptoms more than 3 months after the start of the incident illness. There is no strong biological rationale of the use of 3 months as a cutoff, although it is hypothesized that monophasic immune dysregulation is usually resolved within a 3-month period.

A small proportion of children with ADEM (10%) will have a relapse of an inflammatory demyelinating event with encephalopathy.[2] In the 2007 criteria, two terms were used for relapses of ADEM: recurrent and multiphasic ADEM. Recurrent ADEM was defined as a new event of ADEM with a recurrence of the same symptoms and signs, 3 or more months after the first ADEM event.[2] Multiphasic ADEM was defined as a new event of ADEM involving new anatomic areas of the CNS and occurring at least 3 months after the onset of the initial ADEM event and at least 1 month after completing steroid therapy. In the 2013 revision, the term recurrent ADEM has been dropped.[3] Multiphasic ADEM now encompasses both new as well as reemergence of previous clinical and MRI findings. Also, the timing criterion in relation to steroids for recurrent/multiphasic ADEM has been removed.

A third ADEM-like event is not consistent with a diagnosis of multiphasic ADEM but indicates a chronic relapsing demyelinating disorder, such as relapsing optic neuritis, neuromyelitis optica spectrum disorder associated with antiaquaporin-4 antibodies, relapsing anti-MOG antibody–associated demyelination, or MS depending the clinical phenotype, biomarker, and neuroimaging findings.[1]

EPIDEMIOLOGY

Population-based studies have shown varying incidence rates of ADEM: 0.07 per 100,000 children per year (Germany),[5] 0.3 per 100,000 children per year (China),[6] 0.4 per 100,000 children per year (San Diego),[7] and 0.64 per 100,000 person years (Japan).[8] The varying incidence may be influenced by factors such as genetic predisposition, latitude, environmental and socioeconomic factors, and study methodology.[9,10] The median age at presentation of ADEM is 5–8 years, with male predominance.[1] A recent study from a single center showed that ADEM was the most common cause of encephalitis (21% of all encephalitis).[11]

ADEM is preceded by infection or vaccination in 50%–85% of cases.[9] Common antecedent infections include flu-like illnesses (56%–61%), followed by nonspecific upper respiratory tract infections (12%–17%) and gastroenteritis (7%).[9,12,13] In children, exanthematous diseases are also reported as an infectious antecedent. ADEM has been reported more commonly in winter and spring. This seasonal distribution is likely due to seasonal viral illnesses and epidemics. Viruses (coronavirus, Coxsackie B, dengue, hepatitis A virus, hepatitis C virus, herpes simplex virus, varicella zoster virus, Epstein-Barr virus, human herpesvirus-6, human immunodeficiency virus, measles, mumps, rubella, and parainfluenza) are the infectious agents most frequently associated with

ADEM.[9] Bacteria (*Streptococcus*, *Mycoplasma*, *Legionella*, *Chlamydia*, *Borrelia*, *Rickettsia*, *Campylobacter*) and parasites (*Plasmodium vivax*, *Toxoplasma gondii*) may be rarely involved.[14] The mean latency between the infectious prodrome and the onset of neurologic symptoms varies, often being between 4 and 12 days (range: 1–42 days).[9]

Postimmunization ADEM accounts for only 5% of cases of ADEM.[14] Postvaccination ADEM has been associated with several vaccines such as rabies, diphtheria-tetanus-polio, smallpox, measles, mumps, rubella, Japanese B encephalitis, pertussis, influenza, hepatitis B vaccine, and human papillomavirus vaccine. In a recent retrospective review of Vaccine Adverse Event Reporting System (VAERS) database and the EudraVigilance Postauthorisation Module (EVPM) from 2005 to 2012, a total of 404 cases of postvaccination ADEM were reported,[15] and half of the patients were less than 18 years of age and with a slight male predominance. The time interval from vaccination to ADEM onset was 2–30 days in 61% of the cases. Vaccine against seasonal flu and human papillomavirus vaccine were those most frequently associated with ADEM, accounting for almost 30% of the total cases.

The risk of developing ADEM following vaccination is relatively low, compared with the risk of ADEM following infections against which the vaccines are aimed to protect.[1] The benefits of vaccinations are considered to far surpass the potential risk of postvaccine ADEM.

PATHOPHYSIOLOGY

The exact pathogenesis of ADEM is unclear. Postinfectious immune-mediated mechanisms are implicated. Molecular mimicry with T cell–mediated cross-activation and response against myelin proteins, such as myelin basic protein, proteolipid protein, and MOG plus B cell activation and autoantibody production, may play a role.[14] This hypothesis is supported by studies showing the presence of anti-MOG antibodies in the serum and cerebrospinal fluid (CSF) during the acute phase and their progressive decline along with disease resolution.[16] In a single study comparing the profile of myelin peptide autoantibodies in children with ADEM versus MS, ADEM was characterized by IgG autoantibodies targeting epitopes derived from myelin basic protein, proteolipid protein, myelin-associated oligodendrocyte basic glycoprotein, and α-B-crystallin.[17] In contrast, MS was characterized by IgM autoantibodies targeting myelin basic protein, proteolipid protein, myelin-associated oligodendrocyte basic glycoprotein, and oligodendrocyte specific protein.

There may also be a nonspecific self-sensitization of reactive T cells (bystander activation) against myelin proteins secondary to infections.[18] In a recent study comparing the CSF cytokine profiles in children with ADEM, enterovirus encephalitis, and anti-NMDA receptor encephalitis, patients with ADEM showed predominant elevation of Th1 (IFN-γ, TNF-α, CXCL9, CXCL10), Th2 (IL-4, eotaxin, CCL17, IL-13), Th17 (IL-23, G-CSF, IL-6, IL-8, and IL-17A), B cell (CXCL13, BAFF, CCL19), and other cytokine (CXCL1, IFN-α 2, IL-1ra) molecules, which supports the hypothesis that both cell-mediated and humoral effector mechanisms may play a role.[19]

In a recent study comparing the cytokine profile of anti-MOG positive versus anti-MOG negative demyelinating disorders it was found that the CSF in anti-MOG antibody positive patients showed predominant elevation of B cell–related cytokines/chemokines (CXCL13, APRIL, BAFF, and CCL19) as well as some of Th17-related cytokines (IL-6 AND G-CSF) compared with anti-MOG antibody seronegative patients.[20] These findings suggest that patients with anti-MOG antibodies have a more pronounced CNS inflammatory response with elevation of predominant humoral-associated cytokines/chemokines, as well as some Th 17- and neutrophil-related cytokines/chemokines, suggesting a differential inflammatory pathogenesis associated with MOG antibody seropositivity.[20] These findings also suggest that there is a considerable pathophysiologic heterogeneity in patients with ADEM, suggesting a spectrum of inflammatory demyelination rather than a single disease entity.

Histopathologically, the hallmarks of ADEM include perivenular sleeves of demyelination, perivenous inflammation with infiltrates of myelin-laden macrophages, T and B lymphocytes, plasma cells and granulocytes, axonal injury, and edema.[1,14] The axonal damage is demonstrated by the increased level of a phosphorylated microtubule-associated protein, primarily located in neuronal axons, known as Tau protein, in the CSF, indicative of the clinical severity of ADEM.[21] Moreover, the CSF tau protein concentration in patients with partial lesion resolution in follow-up brain MRI has been shown to be significantly higher than in patients with complete lesion resolution.[21] In addition, there are diffuse cortical microglial alterations (multifocal microglial aggregates), which may be partly responsible for the encephalopathy seen in children with ADEM.[22]

CLINICAL FEATURES

ADEM clinically presents as an acute onset encephalopathy along with polyfocal neurologic deficits. The neurologic symptoms are preceded by prodromal symptoms such a fever, malaise, irritability, somnolence, headache, nausea, and vomiting.[1] Encephalopathy presents as a change in behavior and/or consciousness, varying in severity from lethargy to coma. Commonly headache/vomiting (58%–32%), seizures (13%–47%), and meningismus (5%–43%) may be associated.[9] The patient may also have focal or multifocal neurologic deficits such as hemiparesis, ataxia, aphasia, diplopia, and rarely dystonia and choreiform movements.[14] Multiple cranial nerve involvement may occur. Spinal cord involvement may be present in up to 24% of cases, with clinical features of flaccid paralysis, constipation, or urinary retention.[23,24] Myelitis is significantly more common in anti-MOG antibody–associated ADEM and is associated with longitudinally extensive lesions on the MRI.[25]

The clinical course of ADEM is rapidly progressive, with the development of maximal deficits within 2–5 days.[23] Rarely, respiratory failure occurs because of brainstem involvement. Fever and seizures are described more frequently in ADEM compared with other acute demyelinating syndromes.[1] Combined central and peripheral demyelination has been reported but is very rare in children. Clinical manifestations of peripheral neuropathy may occur simultaneously along with the CNS manifestations or after them.[9]

NEUROIMAGING

The diagnosis of ADEM is clinicoradiological. The characteristic MRI lesions are T2-weighted and fluid-attenuated inversion recovery hyperintense multifocal, irregular, poorly marginated areas with diameters between 5 mm and 5 cm.[14] ADEM lesions typically involve the subcortical and central white matter and cortical gray-white matter junction, thalami, basal ganglia, cerebellum, and brainstem (Figs. 18.1–18.4).[1] The reported frequency of gadolinium-enhancing lesions is highly variable between studies (10%–95%), perhaps depending on the timing of obtaining MRI in the course of the illness.[9] Spinal cord involvement is seen in 10%–28% of patients.[9]

Five radiologic patterns have been described in ADEM[26]: (1) ADEM with small lesions (<5 mm), (2) ADEM with large confluent white matter asymmetric lesions, (3) ADEM with symmetric bithalamic involvement, (4) ADEM with a leukodystrophic pattern with diffuse bilateral and usually nonenhanced white

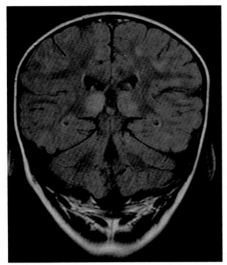

FIG. 18.1 T2 FLAIR Coronal image showing hyperintense signal abnormalities in bilateral subcortical white matter and bilateral thalami in a patient with acute disseminated encephalomyelitis.

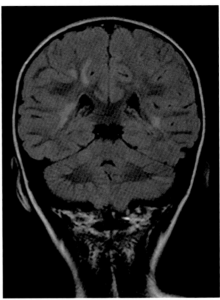

FIG. 18.3 T2 FLAIR Coronal image showing subcortical white matter, and cerebellar white matter abnormalities in a patient with acute disseminated encephalomyelitis.

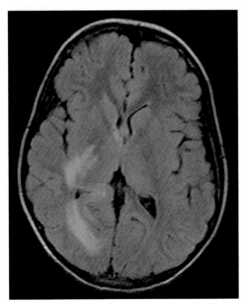

FIG. 18.2 T2 FLAIR Axial image showing large fluffy hyperintense signal abnormalities in right-sided parietooccipital white matter in a patient with acute disseminated encephalomyelitis. Abnormalities also noted in the internal and external capsule on the right side.

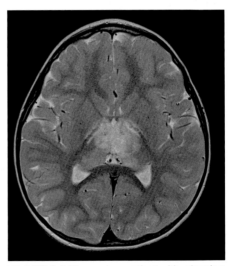

FIG. 18.4 T2 Axial image in a patient with relapsing anti-MOG seropositive patient showing bilateral symmetric thalamic hyperintensities.

matter–sited lesions, and (5) ADEM with acute hemorrhagic encephalomyelitis. The latter two phenotypes are uncommon.

MRI abnormalities may appear later than the clinical symptoms, and progression of MRI lesions has been reported during the course of illness despite clinical improvement.[9] MRI at presentation can even be normal,[27] and delays of between 5 days and 8 weeks between symptom onset and the appearance of MRI alterations have been reported.[28] In a recent

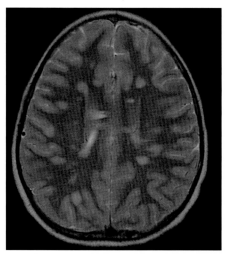

FIG. 18.5 T2 Axial image in a patient with multiple sclerosis showing multiple discrete ovoid hyperintensities involving both the subcortical and periventricular white matter. Note the periventricular Dawson fingers.

study on the evolution of MRI during ADEM episodes, it was noted that new lesions and enlargement of existing MRI lesions occurred in the first 3 months in about 50% of the performed MRIs, despite clinical recovery.[29] However, this was not noted 3 months after first onset of ADEM. Therefore it should be recommended that convalescent MRI scans performed during the first 3 months after ADEM that show new lesions should not necessarily infer the patient has MS.

To differentiate from MS, lesions of MS tend be smaller, discrete and ovoid, and periventricular, especially perpendicular to corpus callosum (Dawson fingers), in contrast to the fluffy poorly marginated subcortical lesions in ADEM.[1] The main differentiating features of ADEM compared with MS are periventricular sparing and the absence of periventricular Dawson finger lesions and black holes on T1 sequences, which are typical of MS (Fig. 18.5).

Follow-up imaging is important to demonstrate resolution of lesions and confirming that no new lesions have developed. In asymptomatic children, repeat imaging is recommended 9–12 months after the episode of ADEM.[1] An earlier repeat imaging at 3 months would be optimal.[1] In children with new symptoms, imaging should be considered earlier.

Advanced neuroimaging techniques such as diffusion-weighted imaging (DWI) and magnetic resonance spectroscopy appear useful to exclude other diseases, such as strokes and neoplasms, to discriminate between acute and chronic lesions, and to add

information about the extent of the affected areas.[14] In a recent study of DWI in 16 children with ADEM, vasogenic edema was demonstrated on DWI and corresponding apparent diffusion coefficient (ADC) maps in 12 of 16 patients; cytotoxic edema was identified in 2 patients while the other 2 patients displayed no changes on DWI/ADC.[30]

CEREBROSPINAL FLUID ABNORMALITIES

Because the presentation of ADEM frequently mimics acute encephalitis, CSF studies are often done, and although they may confirm an inflammatory process, they are nondiagnostic in ADEM. CSF examination is, however, important, especially to exclude an infectious pathology, which is a common differential diagnosis. CSF examination in ADEM reveals inflammatory findings in most patients, consisting of elevated protein levels, up to 1.1 g/L (seen in 15%–60% of patients) and lymphocytic pleocytosis, which is typically mild (seen in 25%–65% of patients).[1,9] The CSF may be normal in 25%–33% of patients.[9,13,31] Intrathecal oligoclonal bands are rare, and if present should raise consideration of MS.[1] In three recent series, of 53 patients, oligoclonal bands were reported in only 1 patient (1.9%).[32-34]

ANTI–MYELIN OLIGODENDROCYTE PROTEIN ANTIBODIES

Recently, it has been shown that serum IgG antibodies to MOG are present in up to 40% of children with ADEM. High-titer anti-MOG antibodies have also been found in children with bilateral often relapsing optic neuritis and aquaporin-4 seronegative neuromyelitis optica.[35] Although some relapsing patients with positive anti-MOG antibodies can fulfill 2013 consensus criteria for MS, anti-MOG antibodies generally do not associate with MS and, instead, suggest anti-MOG–associated autoimmune demyelination.[36,37] These antibodies are seen almost exclusively in demyelinating illnesses and may help to differentiate from viral encephalitis.[38]

In patients with ADEM, the majority of children with anti-MOG antibodies have a monophasic course with a rapid decline of anti-MOG antibodies.[16] The presence of anti-MOG antibodies is likely to be a negative predictor for a future diagnosis of MS.[36] In a study comparing children with ADEM with and without positivity for anti-MOG antibodies, children with ADEM who were seropositive for anti-MOG antibodies had MRI characterized by large, bilateral, and widespread lesions with an increased frequency of longitudinal extensive transverse myelitis and a favorable clinical outcome in contrast to children lacking MOG antibodies.[25] Corpus callosal lesions have been found to be uncommon in children with anti-MOG antibodies.[39] CSF pleocytosis is more common in children with anti-MOG antibodies, suggesting more inflammatory burden in the acute phase as compared with seronegative patients. Some children with ADEM and seropositivity for anti-MOG antibodies may have a relapsing course with future development of optic neuritis or myelitis,[40] or multiphasic ADEM,[41] but development of MS is rare.[42]

DIFFERENTIAL DIAGNOSIS

The diagnosis of ADEM is based on the clinical features and suggestive MRI findings. The clinical picture mimics acute meningoencephalitis, and excluding infectious causes is the first priority. This is done by CSF examination for Gram stain, bacterial culture, and viral studies. Peripheral smear should be obtained for malarial parasites in endemic areas. The MRI obtained should be a gadolinium-enhanced image to look for any leptomeningeal enhancement or any other feature of infection (e.g., basal exudates, brain abscess).

In a child with unexplained altered sensorium and neurologic deficits, other possibilities include autoimmune encephalitis (especially anti-NMDA receptor encephalitis), viral-associated encephalopathies such as acute necrotizing encephalopathy, Hashimoto encephalopathy, CNS vasculitis, primary and secondary (systemic lupus erythematosus, anti-phospholipid antibody syndrome), metabolic (both inherited and acquired) disorders, and rarely toxins and nutritional deficiencies. Anti-NMDA receptor encephalitis must be suspected if the patient has behavior problems, psychosis, sleep disturbances, and movement disorders (especially orofacial dyskinesias) along with encephalopathy.

Other inflammatory demyelinating conditions must also be considered in the differential diagnosis. If the patient has monofocal or polyfocal symptoms in the absence of encephalopathy, then clinically isolated syndrome is diagnosed. If the predominant presentation is optic neuritis and myelitis, then neuromyelitis optica must be considered, and testing for aquaporin antibodies must be done if possible. Neuromyelitis optica with anti-aquaporin-4 antibodies is an uncommon form of CNS demyelination in children; therefore autoantibody testing for aquaporin 4 antibodies should probably be done only with optic neuritis,

myelitis, and brainstem symptoms with typical AQP4 antibody–associated features.[43] The diagnosis of MS is not made during the first event but may be considered if the MRI findings are suggestive, such as the presence of old and new lesions, and fulfillment of McDonald or other criteria.[44,45]

TREATMENT

The treatment of ADEM is based on observational studies and expert guidelines, because there are no randomized controlled trials. High-dose intravenous corticosteroids are generally considered the first-line treatment. The treatment regimen consists of IV methylprednisolone at a dose of 30 mg/kg/day (maximally 1000 mg/d) for 3–5 days, sometimes followed by an oral taper over 4–6 weeks with a starting dose of prednisone of 1–2 mg/kg/day.[1] The risk of relapse is increased if the steroid tapering period is less than 3 weeks, although not all experts use tapered prednisolone.[24] The aim of steroid treatment is primarily to reduce the CNS inflammatory reaction and accelerate clinical recovery. Recovery rates with steroid treatment are generally good, with full recovery reported in 60%–85% of the patients.[23,24] A repeat pulse of intravenous steroids may be considered in the case of unsatisfactory clinical improvement or early relapse.[46]

IV immunoglobulin (IVIg) treatment has been described in case reports and small case series, mostly in combination with corticosteroids or as a second-line treatment in steroid unresponsive ADEM.[47] The usual total dose is 2 g/kg, administered over 2–5 days. Treatment with IVIg has proven effective in about 40%–50% of steroid-resistant patients.[12,48] IVIg presumably acts by binding and neutralizing autoantibodies, inhibiting cytokine release, and modulating lymphocyte activation.[14]

Plasmapheresis may be considered in therapy-refractory patients with fulminant disease, with an estimated efficacy of 40%.[49] The usual regimen is five to seven exchanges but there are not infrequent complications in the form of anemia, hypotension, hypocalcemia, thrombosis, and line infections.[14] Moreover, plasmapheresis is technically difficult to perform in young children. Rarely, patients with fulminant ADEM and cerebral edema have been treated with hypothermia in which the body temperature is reduced to 34°C and intracranial pressure and cerebral perfusion pressure levels are maintained low using mannitol and dopamine.[50,51] Decompressive craniectomy may be considered in cases of refractory intracranial hypertension.[52]

OUTCOME

In pediatric series, ADEM has a favorable prognosis, with a good functional recovery reported in 60%–85% of patients. Neurologic improvement is usually seen within days following initiation of treatment, and recovery to baseline usually occurs within weeks.[1] Mortality has been reported in 1%–3% of affected patients in recent series.[53,54] Residual severe disability is rare, reported in 7% of children in recent studies.[55]

About 10%–40% of children are reported to experience residual cognitive impairment or changes in mood and behavior, and the neurocognitive burden of ADEM is probably underappreciated.[24,31,33] Few studies have analyzed the neuropsychological profile of monophasic ADEM patients. Although, overall, these patients showed a satisfactory global performance, a number of children demonstrated isolated deficits in one or more cognitive domains, most frequently the attentive and executive domains.[9] Greater vulnerability to cognitive dysfunction and behavioral problems has been noted in ADEM patients diagnosed before the age of 5 years.[56] Optic nerve involvement at presentation[23] and antecedent viral infection[24] have also been suggested as indicative of a poor outcome. In a recent study of the long-term neurocognitive outcome of children with ADEM, the most common residual symptoms were concentration difficulties (30%), behavior problems (28%), and learning difficulties (26%).[55] On the Kaufman intelligence test, a full-scale IQ of more than 85 was found in only 60% of patients, and 44% of patients fulfilled the criteria for ADHD. Male gender was a predictor for a worse neurocognitive outcome in this study.[55] The attention and behavioral impairment in ADEM may be attributed to the cerebral white matter damage that may interfere with information processing and attention skills, which are critical for emotional functioning and behavioral regulation.[56] When persisting symptoms continue after ADEM, persisting chronic immune activation should be considered, and a retrial of immune therapy can be used to determine if there is a reversible cause for ongoing symptoms.

RELAPSES

Although in most cases ADEM has a monophasic course, a variable number of patients (10%–30% in previous studies) experience relapses.[9] Because of the high interstudy variability and inconsistency of definitions in the past studies, it is difficult to have conclusive findings on relapsing patients from the current literature. Latency from first episode to relapse is variable, ranging from 2 months to 8 years,[23] and even after 33 years

in one case.[41] Relapses have been reported to be more common in the first 6 months after the first episode, mostly occurring in children who underwent oral steroid tapering for 3 weeks or less.[57] Most children experience a single relapse, but as many as three relapses are reported in some studies.[23,57] An increased risk of relapse after ADEM has been associated with coexistent optic neuritis, familial history of CNS inflammatory demyelination, the presence of MS findings criteria on MRI, and the absence of sequelae after the first attack in one study.[58]

Multiphasic ADEM is uncommon. In literature, multiphasic ADEM was diagnosed in only 2 of 117 (1.7%) children in one series,[59] and in 5 of 132 (3.8%) children in another series.[58]

After the initial episode of ADEM, a subsequent diagnosis of MS is not common. A long-term follow-up study using the 2007 International Pediatrics Multiple Sclerosis Study Group criteria evaluated the parameters at initial diagnosis and eventual conversion to MS in a cohort of 123 children with a first episode of acute CNS demyelination.[4] Of the 47 patients initially diagnosed with ADEM, only 4 (8.5%) were eventually diagnosed with MS at follow-up versus 38.8% of those initially diagnosed with clinically isolated syndrome had MS. On multivariate analysis, the following predictors for developing MS were identified: female gender, clinical presentation with monofocal brainstem or hemispheric dysfunction, and fulfillment of the MRI criteria for MS. In a patient with first episode of ADEM, criteria for MS are met, if after the initial ADEM, a second clinical event (1) is non-encephalopathic, (2) occurs 3 or more months after the incident neurologic illness, and (3) is associated with new MRI findings consistent with revised radiologic criteria for dissemination in space.[3]

Patients with anti-MOG antibodies who relapse typically have further episodes of ADEM[60] or optic neuritis,[61] and typically do not have new lesions on MRI during asymptomatic periods.

CONCLUSION

ADEM is a polyfocal immune-mediated inflammatory demyelinating disease of the CNS that involves multiple areas of the white matter, which mostly affects children under 10 years of age. Common antecedents include a recent viral or bacterial infection or more rarely immunization. The diagnosis is made in the clinical setting of acute onset of encephalopathy with other neurologic deficits and MRI findings of multifocal demyelination after excluding CNS infections. Commonly, ADEM has a monophasic course in

70%–80% of cases, with most children having a good recovery with high-dose intravenous steroid pulse treatment. IVIg and plasmapheresis may be considered as second- and third-line therapies. ADEM overall has a good prognosis, but 10%–40% of children may have neurocognitive dysfunction on follow-up. Relapses may occur in 10%–30% of patients in the form of multiphasic ADEM, optic neuritis, myelitis, or MS. There is need for further evaluation of biomarkers such as anti-MOG antibodies for prediction of relapses and prognosis.

REFERENCES

1. Pohl D, Alper G, Van Haren K, et al. Acute disseminated encephalomyelitis: updates on an inflammatory CNS syndrome. *Neurology.* 2016;87(9 suppl 2):S38–S45.
2. Krupp LB, Banwell B, Tenembaum S. Consensus definitions proposed for pediatric multiple sclerosis and related disorders. *Neurology.* 2007;68(16 suppl 2):S7–S12.
3. Krupp LB, Tardieu M, Amato MP, et al. International Pediatric Multiple Sclerosis Study Group criteria for pediatric multiple sclerosis and immune-mediated central nervous system demyelinating disorders: revisions to the 2007 definitions. *Mult Scler.* 2013;19(10):1261–1267.
4. Peche SS, Alshekhlee A, Kelly J, Lenox J, Mar S. A long-term follow-up study using IPMSSG criteria in children with CNS demyelination. *Pediatr Neurol.* 2013;49(5):329–334.
5. Pohl D, Hennemuth I, von Kries R, Hanefeld F. Paediatric multiple sclerosis and acute disseminated encephalomyelitis in Germany: results of a nationwide survey. *Eur J Pediatr.* 2007;166(5):405–412.
6. Xiong CH, Yan Y, Liao Z, et al. Epidemiological characteristics of acute disseminated encephalomyelitis in Nanchang, China: a retrospective study. *BMC Public Health.* 2014;14:111.
7. Leake JA, Albani S, Kao AS, et al. Acute disseminated encephalomyelitis in childhood: epidemiologic, clinical and laboratory features. *Pediatr Infect Dis J.* 2004;23(8):756–764.
8. Torisu H, Kira R, Ishizaki Y, et al. Clinical study of childhood acute disseminated encephalomyelitis, multiple sclerosis, and acute transverse myelitis in Fukuoka Prefecture. *Jpn Brain Dev.* 2010;32(6):454–462.
9. Berzero G, Cortese A, Ravaglia S, Marchioni E. Diagnosis and therapy of acute disseminated encephalomyelitis and its variants. *Expert Rev Neurother.* 2016;16(1):83–101.
10. Pellegrino P, Radice S, Clementi E. Geoepidemiology of acute disseminated encephalomyelitis. *Epidemiology.* 2014;25(6):928–929.
11. Pillai SC, Hacohen Y, Tantsis E, et al. Infectious and autoantibody-associated encephalitis: clinical features and long-term outcome. *Pediatrics.* 2015;135(4):e974–e984.
12. Marchioni E, Ravaglia S, Montomoli C, et al. Postinfectious neurologic syndromes: a prospective cohort study. *Neurology.* 2013;80(10):882–889.
13. Panicker JN, Nagaraja D, Kovoor JM, Subbakrishna DK. Descriptive study of acute disseminated encephalomyelitis and evaluation of functional outcome predictors. *J Postgrad Med.* 2010;56(1):12–16.
14. Esposito S, Di Pietro GM, Madini B, Mastrolia MV, Rigante D. A spectrum of inflammation and demyelination in acute disseminated encephalomyelitis (ADEM) of children. *Autoimmun Rev.* 2015;14(10):923–929.
15. Pellegrino P, Carnovale C, Perrone V, et al. Acute disseminated encephalomyelitis onset: evaluation based on vaccine adverse events reporting systems. *PLoS One.* 2013;8(10):e77766.
16. Probstel AK, Dornmair K, Bittner R, et al. Antibodies to MOG are transient in childhood acute disseminated encephalomyelitis. *Neurology.* 2011;77(6):580–588.
17. Van Haren K, Tomooka BH, Kidd BA, et al. Serum autoantibodies to myelin peptides distinguish acute disseminated encephalomyelitis from relapsing-remitting multiple sclerosis. *Mult Scler.* 2013;19(13):1726–1733.
18. Ishizu T, Minohara M, Ichiyama T, et al. CSF cytokine and chemokine profiles in acute disseminated encephalomyelitis. *J Neuroimmunol.* 2006;175(1–2):52–58.
19. Kothur K, Wienholt L, Mohammad SS, et al. Utility of CSF cytokine/chemokines as markers of active intrathecal inflammation: comparison of demyelinating, anti-NMDAR and enteroviral encephalitis. *PLoS One.* 2016;11(8):e0161656.
20. Kothur K, Wienholt L, Tantsis EM, et al. B cell, Th17, and neutrophil related cerebrospinal fluid cytokine/chemokines are elevated in MOG antibody associated demyelination. *PLoS One.* 2016;11(2):e0149411.
21. Oka M, Hasegawa S, Matsushige T, et al. Tau protein concentrations in the cerebrospinal fluid of children with acute disseminated encephalomyelitis. *Brain Dev.* 2014;36(1):16–20.
22. Young NP, Weinshenker BG, Parisi JE, et al. Perivenous demyelination: association with clinically defined acute disseminated encephalomyelitis and comparison with pathologically confirmed multiple sclerosis. *Brain.* 2010;133(Pt 2):333–348.
23. Tenembaum S, Chamoles N, Fejerman N. Acute disseminated encephalomyelitis: a long-term follow-up study of 84 pediatric patients. *Neurology.* 2002;59(8):1224–1231.
24. Dale RC, de Sousa C, Chong WK, Cox TC, Harding B, Neville BG. Acute disseminated encephalomyelitis, multiphasic disseminated encephalomyelitis and multiple sclerosis in children. *Brain.* 2000;123(Pt 12):2407–2422.
25. Baumann M, Sahin K, Lechner C, et al. Clinical and neuroradiological differences of paediatric acute disseminating encephalomyelitis with and without antibodies to the myelin oligodendrocyte glycoprotein. *J Neurol Neurosurg Psychiatry.* 2015;86(3):265–272.
26. Tenembaum SN. Disseminated encephalomyelitis in children. *Clin Neurol Neurosurg.* 2008;110(9):928–938.
27. Murray BJ, Apetauerova D, Scammell TE. Severe acute disseminated encephalomyelitis with normal MRI at presentation. *Neurology.* 2000;55(8):1237–1238.

28. Lakhan SE. Teaching neuroimages: MRI time lag with acute disseminated encephalomyelitis. *Neurology.* 2012; 78(22):e138–e139.

29. Wong YY, van Pelt ED, Ketelslegers IA, Catsman-Berrevoets CE, Hintzen RQ, Neuteboom RF. Evolution of MRI abnormalities in paediatric acute disseminated encephalomyelitis. *Eur J Paediatr Neurol.* 2017;21(2):300–304.

30. Zuccoli G, Panigrahy A, Sreedher G, et al. Vasogenic edema characterizes pediatric acute disseminated encephalomyelitis. *Neuroradiology.* 2014;56(8):679–684.

31. Hynson JL, Kornberg AJ, Coleman LT, Shield L, Harvey AS, Kean MJ. Clinical and neuroradiologic features of acute disseminated encephalomyelitis in children. *Neurology.* 2001;56(10):1308–1312.

32. Pavone P, Pettoello-Mantovano M, Le Pira A, et al. Acute disseminated encephalomyelitis: a long-term prospective study and meta-analysis. *Neuropediatrics.* 2010;41(6):246–255.

33. Erol I, Ozkale Y, Alkan O, Alehan F. Acute disseminated encephalomyelitis in children and adolescents: a single center experience. *Pediatr Neurol.* 2013;49(4):266–273.

34. Alper G, Heyman R, Wang L. Multiple sclerosis and acute disseminated encephalomyelitis diagnosed in children after long-term follow-up: comparison of presenting features. *Dev Med Child Neurol.* 2009;51(6):480–486.

35. Ramanathan S, Dale RC, Brilot F. Anti-MOG antibody: the history, clinical phenotype, and pathogenicity of a serum biomarker for demyelination. *Autoimmun Rev.* 2016;15(4):307–324.

36. Ketelslegers IA, Van Pelt DE, Bryde S, et al. Anti-MOG antibodies plead against MS diagnosis in an acquired demyelinating syndromes cohort. *Mult Scler.* 2015;21(12):1513–1520.

37. Hacohen Y, Absoud M, Deiva K, et al. Myelin oligodendrocyte glycoprotein antibodies are associated with a non-MS course in children. *Neurol Neuroimmunol Neuroinflamm.* 2015;2(2):e81.

38. Lalive PH, Hausler MG, Maurey H, et al. Highly reactive anti-myelin oligodendrocyte glycoprotein antibodies differentiate demyelinating diseases from viral encephalitis in children. *Mult Scler.* 2011;17(3):297–302.

39. Fernandez-Carbonell C, Vargas-Lowy D, Musallam A, et al. Clinical and MRI phenotype of children with MOG antibodies. *Mult Scler.* 2016;22(2):174–184.

40. Miyauchi A, Monden Y, Watanabe M, et al. Persistent presence of the anti-myelin oligodendrocyte glycoprotein autoantibody in a pediatric case of acute disseminated encephalomyelitis followed by optic neuritis. *Neuropediatrics.* 2014;45(3):196–199.

41. Numa S, Kasai T, Kondo T, et al. An adult case of anti-myelin oligodendrocyte glycoprotein (MOG) antibody-associated multiphasic acute disseminated encephalomyelitis at 33-year intervals. *Intern Med.* 2016;55(6):699–702.

42. Dale RC, Tantsis EM, Merheb V, et al. Antibodies to MOG have a demyelination phenotype and affect oligodendrocyte cytoskeleton. *Neurol Neuroimmunol Neuroinflamm.* 2014;1(1):e12.

43. Marignier R, Cobo Calvo A, Vukusic S. Neuromyelitis optica and neuromyelitis optica spectrum disorders. *Curr Opin Neurol.* 2017;30(3):208–215.

44. Sadaka Y, Verhey LH, Shroff MM, et al. 2010 McDonald criteria for diagnosing pediatric multiple sclerosis. *Ann Neurol.* 2012;72(2):211–223.

45. Tantsis EM, Prelog K, Brilot F, Dale RC. Risk of multiple sclerosis after a first demyelinating syndrome in an Australian Paediatric cohort: clinical, radiological features and application of the McDonald 2010 MRI criteria. *Mult Scler.* 2013;19(13):1749–1759.

46. Apak RA, Anlar B, Saatci I. A case of relapsing acute disseminated encephalomyelitis with high dose corticosteroid treatment. *Brain Dev.* 1999;21(4):279–282.

47. Sahlas DJ, Miller SP, Guerin M, Veilleux M, Francis G. Treatment of acute disseminated encephalomyelitis with intravenous immunoglobulin. *Neurology.* 2000;54(6): 1370–1372.

48. Ravaglia S, Piccolo G, Ceroni M, et al. Severe steroid-resistant post-infectious encephalomyelitis: general features and effects of IVIg. *J Neurol.* 2007;254(11):1518–1523.

49. Keegan M, Pineda AA, McClelland RL, Darby CH, Rodriguez M, Weinshenker BG. Plasma exchange for severe attacks of CNS demyelination: predictors of response. *Neurology.* 2002;58(1):143–146.

50. Ichikawa K, Motoi H, Oyama Y, Watanabe Y, Takeshita S. Fulminant form of acute disseminated encephalomyelitis in a child treated with mild hypothermia. *Pediatr Int.* 2013;55(6):e149–e151.

51. Miyamoto K, Kozu S, Arakawa A, et al. Therapeutic hypothermia with the use of intracranial pressure monitoring for acute disseminated encephalomyelitis with brainstem lesion: a case report. *J Child Neurol.* 2014;29(9). NP69-73.

52. Granget E, Milh M, Pech-Gourg G, et al. Life-saving decompressive craniectomy for acute disseminated encephalomyelitis in a child: a case report. *Childs Nerv Syst.* 2012;28(7):1121–1124.

53. Absoud M, Parslow RC, Wassmer E, et al. Severe acute disseminated encephalomyelitis: a paediatric intensive care population-based study. *Mult Scler.* 2011;17(10):1258–1261.

54. Ketelslegers IA, Visser IE, Neuteboom RF, Boon M, Catsman-Berrevoets CE, Hintzen RQ. Disease course and outcome of acute disseminated encephalomyelitis is more severe in adults than in children. *Mult Scler.* 2011;17(4):441–448.

55. Shilo S, Michaeli O, Shahar E, Ravid S. Long-term motor, cognitive and behavioral outcome of acute disseminated encephalomyelitis. *Eur J Paediatr Neurol.* 2016;20(3):361–367.

56. Jacobs RK, Anderson VA, Neale JL, Shield LK, Kornberg AJ. Neuropsychological outcome after acute disseminated encephalomyelitis: impact of age at illness onset. *Pediatr Neurol.* 2004;31(3):191–197.

57. Anlar B, Basaran C, Kose G, et al. Acute disseminated encephalomyelitis in children: outcome and prognosis. *Neuropediatrics*. 2003;34(4):194–199.

58. Mikaeloff Y, Caridade G, Husson B, Suissa S, Tardieu M. Acute disseminated encephalomyelitis cohort study: prognostic factors for relapse. *Eur J Paediatr Neurol*. 2007;11(2):90–95.

59. Neuteboom RF, Boon M, Catsman Berrevoets CE, et al. Prognostic factors after a first attack of inflammatory CNS demyelination in children. *Neurology*. 2008;71(13):967–973.

60. Baumann M, Hennes EM, Schanda K, et al. Children with multiphasic disseminated encephalomyelitis and antibodies to the myelin oligodendrocyte glycoprotein (MOG): extending the spectrum of MOG antibody positive diseases. *Mult Scler*. 2016;22(14):1821–1829.

61. Huppke P, Rostasy K, Karenfort M, et al. Acute disseminated encephalomyelitis followed by recurrent or monophasic optic neuritis in pediatric patients. *Mult Scler*. 2013;19(7):941–946.

CHAPTER 19

Epidemiology of Acute Disseminated Encephalomyelitis

HIROYUKI TORISU, MD, PHD

INTRODUCTION

Acute disseminated encephalomyelitis (ADEM) is a monophasic demyelinating encephalomyelitis presumably caused by autoreactive immune responses in the central nervous system (CNS). ADEM generally demonstrates multiple lesions with perivenous demyelination in the CNS. Hence, ADEM is pathologically a CNS demyelinating disease. The other diseases in this category include multiple sclerosis (MS) and neuromyelitis optica (NMO). The manifestations of these demyelinating diseases often resemble each other, and therefore, it is difficult for clinicians to distinguish ADEM clinically from other demyelinating diseases, especially at the first demyelinating event.

ADEM could be considered as an autoimmune disease related to infections, and hence, it has been referred to as postinfectious encephalomyelitis.

In this chapter, the epidemiologic characters of ADEM will be discussed on the basis of findings of previous studies on ADEM.

DEFINITION OF ACUTE DISSEMINATED ENCEPHALOMYELITIS

ADEM is defined mainly by pathologic characteristics as multiple inflammatory demyelination in the CNS and by clinical characteristics as a monophasic disease. Brain biopsy is rarely performed because ADEM is usually not fatal. Therefore, most ADEM cases have been clinically diagnosed mainly based on neurologic findings, neuroimaging findings, and the clinical course. After the widespread use of MRI in the early 2000s, which enabled clinicians to easily identify white matter lesions in the CNS, ADEM could be diagnosed at a number of medical facilities, and the clinical features were investigated eagerly. As a result, common clinical diagnostic criteria were needed to promote international research about demyelinating diseases in the late 2000s.

International Pediatric Multiple Sclerosis Study Group Definition

In 2007, the International Pediatric Multiple Sclerosis Study Group (IPMSSG) proposed a definition of pediatric ADEM for the purpose of the early diagnosis of MS at the first demyelinating event. Pediatric ADEM was defined as the first acute or subacute clinical event with multifocal lesions in the CNS presumably caused by inflammation or demyelination. Additionally, children with ADEM should be polysymptomatic and should present with encephalopathy, alternation of behavior and/or consciousness. A clinical change within 3 months after onset should be considered as a single episode.[1]

The IPMSSG revised the definition in 2013 and included the criteria that children with ADEM should show abnormalities on MRI in the acute phase and new symptoms or MRI abnormalities should not appear 3 months after onset.[2]

Brighton Collaboration Case Definition

Regarding ADEM preceded by vaccination, the Brighton Collaboration Encephalitis Working Group proposed a definition according to the certainty from level 1 to level 3.[3] ADEM of level 1 was defined as confirmation of pathologic diagnosis or fulfillment of the following three conditions: presentation with focal or multifocal signs and symptoms related to CNS lesions, characteristic MRI abnormalities, and monophasic course. ADEM of level 2 was defined as fulfillment of only the following two conditions: presentation with focal or multifocal signs and symptoms related to CNS lesions and characteristic MRI abnormalities; therefore, this level of ADEM is not observed after an extended period following the event. ADEM of level 3 was defined as fulfillment of only the following condition: presentation with focal or multifocal signs and symptoms related to CNS lesions. A case should not be considered as ADEM if it fulfills any of the following conditions: presence of apparent infection, unsuitable MRI or pathologic findings, and relapse within 3 months.

After the definition was proposed, many cases were analyzed by using the definition, and it was found that the proposed definition was useful for defining ADEM.[4]

Subtypes of Acute Disseminated Encephalomyelitis by Antecedent Events

ADEM is generally classified into the following three subtypes according to antecedent events: infection-associated ADEM, vaccination-associated ADEM, and idiopathic ADEM. Most previous studies on ADEM generally investigated previous events within 1 month of the onset of ADEM. However, there is no consensus on the period of time that enables the determination of whether a preceding event is related to ADEM. The World Health Organization considers an association between ADEM and vaccination within 3 months of the disease onset.

EPIDEMIOLOGY OF ACUTE DISSEMINATED ENCEPHALOMYELITIS

Although ADEM has been carefully defined as mentioned above, it remains difficult to exclude some acute encephalitis conditions or other demyelinating diseases from ADEM at the clinical level. IPMSSG proposed that

ADEM should not be considered as a single disease but as a syndrome in the revised definition.[2] The epidemiology of ADEM should be considered as that of ADEM syndrome, which has a heterogeneous etiology.

Incidence of Pediatric Acute Disseminated Encephalomyelitis

The annual incidence of pediatric ADEM has been reported to be 0.07–0.64/100,000 children (Table 19.1).[5-14]

Population-based studies of patients with ADEM performed in Asian countries showed a relatively high incidence of pediatric ADEM. A nationwide survey in Japan revealed that the annual incidence of pediatric ADEM was 0.40/100,000,[5] and multicenter studies in Fukuoka, Japan,[6] and Nanchang, China,[10] demonstrated that the incidences were 0.64/100,000 and 0.47/100,000, respectively.

Population-based studies performed in the United States and the United Kingdom showed a slightly lower or almost same incidence of pediatric ADEM compared with that in Asian countries (0.40/100,000 in San Diego[9] and 0.30/100,000 in Southern California[11]). A nationwide survey in the United Kingdom revealed that the annual incidence of pediatric ADEM was 0.30.[12]

Some studies reported a lower annual incidence of pediatric ADEM than that in the above mentioned

TABLE 19.1
Overview of the Epidemiologic Features of Acute Disseminated Encephalomyelitis (ADEM) From Population-Based Studies

| Studies on ADEM | Country | SURVEILLANCE STYLE | | | | Estimated Annual Incidence of ADEM, (/100,000 Children) |
		Region	Period	Diagnostic Criteria	Age Group	
Yamaguchi et al.[5]	Japan	Nationwide	2005–07	2007 IPMSSG	Under 16	0.40
Torisu et al.[6]	Japan	Fukuoka	1998–2003	Others	Under 17	0.64
Pohl et al.[7]	Germany	Nationwide	1997–99	Others	Under 18	0.07
Banwell et al.[8]	Canada	Nationwide	2004–07	2007 IPMSSG	Under 18	0.20
Leake et al.[9]	United States	San Diego	1991–2000	Others	Under 20	0.40
Xiong et al.[10]	China	Nanchang	2008–10	2007 IPMSSG	Under 15	0.47
Langer-Gould et al.[11]	United States	Southern California	2004–09	Others	Under 19	0.30
Absoud et al.[12]	United Kingdom	Nationwide	2009–10	2007 IPMSSG	Under 16	0.31
Ketelslegers et al.[13]	Netherlands	Nationwide	2007–10	Others	Under 18	0.16[a]
Gudbjornsson et al.[14]	Iceland	Nationwide	1990–2009	2007 IPMSSG	Under 18	0.13

[a]Polysymptomatic acquired demyelinating syndrome with encephalopathy.

countries (0.20/100,000 in Canada,[8] 0.16/100,000 in Netherlands,[13] 0.16/100,000 in Iceland,[14] and 0.07/100,000 in Germany[7]).

The variety of incidences suggests that pediatric ADEM might be influenced by geographic, ethnic, or genetic factors.

Incidence of Adult Acute Disseminated Encephalomyelitis

The incidence of adult ADEM has been reported in few studies. A retrospective study in Nanchang, China, presented the age-based incidence of ADEM. The annual incidence of ADEM in adults was variable from 0.55/100,000 in individuals aged over 60 years to 0.08/100,000 in those aged 30–39 years, and the mean annual incidence of ADEM was 0.27/100,000 in those aged over 15 years.[10] The incidence of ADEM in adults tended to be lower than that in children (0.47/100,000 in individuals aged under 15 years).

Ethnicity

There have been few studies on the relation between pediatric ADEM and ethnicity. The study in San Diego revealed that the proportional ethnicity of cases was nearly identical to the ethnicity of the assessed area.[9] On the other hand, a study performed to examine pediatric acquired demyelinating syndrome (ADS), including ADEM, MS, and NMO, in Southern California revealed a relation between pediatric ADS

and ethnicity. The study showed that the annual incidence of ADS (except MS), which included ADEM and other demyelinating diseases, such as optic neuritis and myelitis, was higher in black and Asian children than in Hispanic and white non-Hispanic children.[11] The findings suggest that environmental or genetic risk factor for ADS, except MS, might be more common in black and Asian children.

Sex

Most previous studies on pediatric ADEM showed slight or no male dominance (Table 19.2); however, studies in Japan demonstrated high male dominance at almost 70%.[5,6]

A study in China demonstrated that the incidence of ADEM among males was nearly equal to that among females.[10] These findings differ from those of other demyelinating diseases, such as MS.

Age

The mean onset age was the lowest for ADEM among all demyelinating diseases.

The onset age of pediatric ADEM extends throughout childhood from infancy to adolescence, and the most frequent onset age is around 5–7 years in most countries (Table 19.2),[5–9, 11, 12] indicating that ADEM tends to develop in children who are acquiring sufficient immunity against common infections. Additionally, the findings suggest that vaccination programs, which

TABLE 19.2
Demographic Features of Children With Acute Disseminated Encephalomyelitis (ADEM)

Studies on ADEM	Country	Number	Male Sex, %	Mean Age at Onset, Years	Antecedent Infection, %	Antecedent Vaccination, %
Yamaguchi et al.[5]	Japan	66	67	5.5	62	18
Torisu et al.[6]	Japan	26	69	5.7	73	15
Pohl et al.[7]	Germany	28	57	6.6	ND	ND
Banwell et al.[8]	Canada	49	56	7.7	ND	4 in all ADS
Leake et al.[9]	United States	42	57	6.5	93 within 21 days	5
Xiong et al.[10]	China	16	ND	ND	38 within 2 months	0
Langer-Gould et al.[11]	United States	15	47	5.6	ND	ND
Absoud et al.[12]	United Kingdom	40	60	5.3	ND	ND
Ketelslegers et al.[13]	Netherlands	21	48	3.9	48	5
Gudbjornsson et al.[14]	Iceland	2	50	3–5 and 15–17 years	ND	ND

ADS, acquired demyelinating syndrome; ND, not described.

are mainly performed for infants or younger children, do not strongly affect the occurrence of ADEM.

There is limited information on the onset age of adult ADEM. A study performed in Nanchang demonstrated that ADEM developed at a higher rate in children than in adults of all age groups, except those aged over 60 years.[10] The incidence of ADEM in individuals aged over 60 years was comparable to that in children.

Infection

It is well known that ADEM develops after various types of infections, including bacterial infection. The susceptibility to ADEM and the severity of ADEM depend on the pathogen causing the infection. ADEM develops at a high frequency after measles, rubella, varicella zoster, and other such diseases. It has been reported that about 1 in 1000 patients with measles will develop ADEM and about 25% of patients with ADEM will die. Therefore, the incidence of ADEM might depend on the types of prevalent pathogens and the status of vaccination in the target area.

However, a large number of ADEM children having the same specific infection (measles or other exanthemas) has never been reported in previous studies since the late 1990s, and an outbreak of ADEM has never occurred. Moreover, previous studies reported that the pathogens causing the infection associated with ADEM were mostly unknown. These findings might indicate that vaccination prevented infections that were strongly related to ADEM.

Vaccination

Vaccination-associated ADEM is generally rare. Previous studies demonstrated that 0%–5% of children with ADEM had received vaccination within 1 month from ADEM onset (Table 19.2).[8–10,13] This finding suggests that most cases of pediatric ADEM might not be associated with vaccination. On the other hand, Japanese studies revealed that a relatively high percentage (18% and 15%) of children with ADEM had received vaccination within 1 month from ADEM onset.[5,6] The reported vaccines were not specific, and there was no definite difference in the reported vaccines between Japan and other countries. The Japanese studies reported on the influenza vaccine; combination vaccine for measles and rubella; combination vaccine for diphtheria, pertussis, and tetanus; poliovirus vaccine; rubella vaccine; Japanese encephalitis vaccine; and hepatitis B vaccine. Meanwhile, the Canadian nationwide study of ADS children reported on hepatitis B vaccine; influenza vaccine; measles, mumps, and rubella vaccine; human papillomavirus vaccine; pertussis vaccine; and combination vaccine for diphtheria, pertussis, and tetanus (Tdap).[8]

The incidence of vaccine-associated ADEM has fluctuated since 1920s. This can be related to the methods of vaccine production, the amount of myelin antigen included, and the type of adjuvant.[15] At present, vaccines are generally assumed to cause ADEM at a rate of almost 1–2 cases in 1 million vaccinations.

The incidence of vaccine-associated ADEM is different among the various kinds of vaccines. The common vaccines related to ADEM include measles, varicella zoster, rubella, small pox, and influenza.[16] Postmarketing study on vaccine adverse events from 1994 to 2004 in Japan revealed that ADEM developed at a rate of 7 cases in 67.2 million vaccinations, and the rates were 0 case in 3.64 million measles vaccinations, 1 case in 4.0 million rubella vaccinations, 1 case in 1.53 million mumps vaccinations, 2 cases in 9.45 million Japanese encephalitis virus vaccinations, 3 cases in 38.02 million influenza vaccinations, and 0 case in 10.56 million diphtheria, pertussis, and tetanus vaccinations.[17]

The study on ADEM based on vaccine adverse events reporting systems in the United States and the European Union analyzed 404 ADEM cases reported between 2005 and 2012.[18] This study revealed that vaccine against seasonal flu and human papillomavirus vaccine were most frequently associated with ADEM, and that mean number of reports per year in VEARS database was 40 ± 21.7, decreasing after 2010 mainly because of a reduction of reports associated with human papillomavirus and diphtheria, pertussis, tetanus, polio, and *Hemophillus* influenza type B vaccines.

Therefore, the kind of vaccine and the immunization program might have a strong influence on the occurrence of vaccination-associated ADEM. The annual incidence of vaccination-associated ADEM in Fukuoka, Japan, was estimated to be about 1/1,000,000 children in 2000[6]; however, the incidence of vaccination-associated ADEM might change in the future.

Geography

The geographic factors influencing the incidence of ADEM remain unclear, although the prevalence of adult MS was known to be associated with the latitude of the area investigated.[19] A study performed in San Diego revealed that the geographic distribution of cases in households was proportionate to the population.[9] However, previous studies indicated that the incidence of pediatric ADEM tends to be low in Europe. A Japanese study demonstrated that the incidence of pediatric ADEM tended to be lower in the north of Japan than in other areas.[5] In addition, a Canadian study revealed the regional differences in the incidence of pediatric ADS, and reported that the incidence in the northern region of Canada appeared to be lower than that in other regions.[8] However, a study on ADEM, which was performed on the basis of medical records in the United Kingdom and the United States, demonstrated contradictory results.[20]

Assuming that there is some geographic factor associated with ADEM, the influence of this factor on the occurrence of ADEM would remain unknown. The influence of vitamin D or the sun exposure time in children with ADEM has not been appropriately investigated; however, this has been investigated in MS patients.

Genetics

There are few studies on genetic susceptibility to ADEM. One study demonstrated that ADEM was associated with the *HLA-DR* gene.[21] This result suggests that susceptibility to ADEM is associated with genetic immune characteristics. However, genetic susceptibility to ADEM might be different from genetic susceptibility to MS. A Canadian study revealed that 51% of MS patients had one or more *HLA-DRB1*15* alleles, whereas 30% of monophasic ADS patients had those alleles.[22] We had investigated the association between some MS susceptibility genes and ADEM; however, we did not find any association (unpublished data).

A single specific gene might not have a strong influence on susceptibility to ADEM. There has not yet been a report of large familial cases of ADEM. However, patients with incontinentia pigmenti are known to be relatively susceptible to acute demyelinating events, such as ADEM.[23] We experienced infants with incontinentia pigmenti who developed ADEM after oral polio vaccination. The *IKBKG* gene, which is related to NF-kB activation, is responsible for incontinentia pigmenti. This finding suggests that genetic factors associated with immune responsiveness might be related to acute demyelinating events, although we do not understand the precise pathophysiology.

Other Factors

Previous studies on ADEM did not mention the specific illnesses frequently observed among pediatric ADEM patients. Susceptibility to demyelination in ADEM patients remains unknown; however, some patients with congenital adrenal hyperplasia or acquired adrenal insufficiency have been reported to have a tendency to experience encephalopathy with white matter lesions.[24,25]

VACCINATION AND ACUTE DISSEMINATED ENCEPHALOMYELITIS

In the early stage of vaccination, vaccination for small pox or rabies caused "neuroparalytic accidents," which are currently considered to be vaccination-associated ADEM.[26] Since then, ADEM has been reported to be associated with a large variety of vaccines.[16]

Vaccination-associated ADEM aids in the assessment of the pathophysiology of ADEM. As the rabies vaccine was produced by using the spinal cord of rabbits, vaccine-associated ADEM was believed to be caused by an allergic reaction to neuronal components that might have contaminated the vaccine. In 1933, this hypothesis was supported by the induction of encephalomyelitis by injecting neural component and some adjuvants in an animal model. Moreover, in 1987, the sera and cerebrospinal fluid of patients with rabies vaccination–associated ADEM contained elevated antibodies against myelin.[27] Thereafter, the idea that the neural components of animals in vaccine products could cause ADEM spread widely.

However, this idea is no longer true for present vaccines. In the past, ADEM after receiving the Japanese encephalitis vaccine became a social problem in Japan, and the cause was assumed to be neural components of mouse present in the vaccine. This vaccine was changed to a vaccine that is produced using a cell-based assay. However, the incidence of ADEM did not change greatly after the introduction of this new vaccine. This fact implies that present vaccines do not cause ADEM by cross-reaction between animal's neural components and the CNS. Recent cases of vaccine-associated ADEM might have developed by other mechanisms, including molecular mimicry (e.g., similarities between a vaccine viral epitope and host myelin antigen) or nonspecific activation of preexisting myelin-reactive T cells.

Immunization programs could decrease the incidence of ADEM. The use of the measles vaccine was associated with the development of ADEM at a rate of 1/1,000,000, while patients with measles generally develop ADEM at a rate of 1/1000. Therefore, the probability of developing ADEM is much higher after the occurrence of measles than after measles vaccination. A study in China demonstrated that the number of patients with ADEM decreased with the increase in the number of vaccinations.[10]

LIMITATIONS IN ACUTE DISSEMINATED ENCEPHALOMYELITIS EPIDEMIOLOGIC STUDIES

It remains difficult to diagnose ADEM and elucidate the etiology of events precisely based on clinical information. ADEM is presently considered to be a syndrome with heterogeneous etiologies. Thus, research on ADEM revealed common characteristics among the different types of ADEM conditions having specific etiologies.

To elucidate the pathophysiology of ADEM, it is necessary to analyze the features of ADEM conditions having specific etiologies, such as ADEM related to a specific infectious agent or a specific vaccine. In addition, assessment of other clinically unique types of ADEM conditions, e.g., acute hemorrhage leukoencephalitis and ADEM with myelin oligodendrocyte glycoprotein antibody, might aid in the understanding of the pathophysiology of ADEM.

Epidemiologic Survey of Pediatric Diseases in Japan

The medical system for children in Japan has unique characteristics, and therefore, it is relatively easy to perform an epidemiologic study about specific rare diseases. In Japan, children easily receive medical care because infants and younger children have free medical services and all individuals are covered under health insurance. In addition, people can directly visit any hospital; therefore, there is little difference in medical services among places in Japan. Children experiencing an acute neurologic event are admitted to the department of pediatrics at a hospital where MRI is available and pediatricians can treat them.

REFERENCES

1. Krupp LB, Banwell B, Tenembaum S, et al. Consensus definitions proposed for pediatric multiple sclerosis and related disorders. *Neurology.* 2007;68(16 suppl 2): S7–S12.
2. Krupp LB, Tardieu M, Amato MP, et al. International Pediatric Multiple Sclerosis Study Group criteria for pediatric multiple sclerosis and immune-mediated central nervous system demyelinating disorders: revisions to the 2007 definitions. *Mult Scler.* 2013;19(10): 1261–1267.
3. Sejvar JJ, Kohl KS, Bilynsky R, et al. Encephalitis, myelitis, and acute disseminated encephalomyelitis (ADEM): case definitions and guidelines for collection, analysis, and presentation of immunization safety data. *Vaccine.* 2007;25(31):5771–5792.
4. Rath B, Magnus M, Heininger U. Evaluating the Brighton Collaboration case definitions, aseptic meningitis, encephalitis, myelitis, and acute disseminated encephalomyelitis, by systematic analysis of 255 clinical cases. *Vaccine.* 2010; 28(19):3488–3495.
5. Yamaguchi Y, Torisu H, Kira R, et al. A nationwide survey of pediatric acquired demyelinating syndromes in Japan. Neurology. 2016;87(19):2006–2015.
6. Torisu H, Kira R, Ishizaki Y, et al. Clinical study of childhood acute disseminated encephalomyelitis, multiple sclerosis, and acute transverse myelitis in Fukuoka Prefecture, Japan. *Brain Dev.* 2010;32(6):454–462.

7. Pohl D, Hennemuth I, von Kries R, Hanefeld F. Paediatric multiple sclerosis and acute disseminated encephalomyelitis in Germany: results of a nationwide survey. *Eur J Pediatr.* 2007;166(5):405–412.
8. Banwell B, Kennedy J, Sadovnick D, et al. Incidence of acquired demyelination of the CNS in Canadian children. *Neurology.* 2009;72(3):232–239.
9. Leake JA, Albani S, Kao AS, et al. Acute disseminated encephalomyelitis in childhood: epidemiologic, clinical and laboratory features. *Pediatr Infect Dis J.* 2004;23(8): 756–764.
10. Xiong CH, Yan Y, Liao Z, et al. Epidemiological characteristics of acute disseminated encephalomyelitis in Nanchang, China: a retrospective study. *BMC Public Health.* 2014;14:111.
11. Langer-Gould A, Zhang JL, Chung J, Yeung Y, Waubant E, Yao J. Incidence of acquired CNS demyelinating syndromes in a multiethnic cohort of children. *Neurology.* 2011;77(12):1143–1148.
12. Absoud M, Lim MJ, Chong WK, et al. Paediatric acquired demyelinating syndromes: incidence, clinical and magnetic resonance imaging features. *Mult Scler.* 2013;19(1): 76–86.
13. Ketelslegers IA, Catsman-Berrevoets CE, Neuteboom RF, et al. Incidence of acquired demyelinating syndromes of the CNS in Dutch children: a nationwide study. *J Neurol.* 2012;259(9):1929–1935.
14. Gudbjornsson BT, Haraldsson A, Einarsdottir H, Thorarensen O. Nationwide incidence of acquired central nervous system demyelination in icelandic children. *Pediatr Neurol.* 2015;53(6):503–507.
15. Karussis D, Petrou P. The spectrum of post-vaccination inflammatory CNS demyelinating syndromes. *Autoimmun Rev.* 2014;13(3):215–224.
16. Huynh W, Cordato DJ, Kehdi E, Masters LT, Dedousis C. Post-vaccination encephalomyelitis: literature review and illustrative case. *J Clin Neurosci.* 2008;15(12):1315–1322.
17. Nakayama T, Onoda K. Vaccine adverse events reported in post-marketing study of the Kitasato Institute from 1994 to 2004. *Vaccine.* 2007;25(3):570–576.
18. Pellegrino P, Carnovale C, Perrone V, et al. Acute disseminated encephalomyelitis onset: evaluation based on vaccine adverse events reporting systems. *PLoS One.* 2013;8(10):e77766.
19. Compston A, Coles A. Multiple sclerosis. *Lancet.* 2008; 372(9648):1502–1517.
20. Pellegrino P, Radice S, Clementi E. Geoepidemiology of acute disseminated encephalomyelitis. *Epidemiology.* 2014;25(6):928–929.
21. Idrissova Zh R, Boldyreva MN, Dekonenko EP, et al. Acute disseminated encephalomyelitis in children: clinical features and HLA-DR linkage. *Eur J Neurol.* 2003;10(5):537–546.
22. Banwell B, Bar-Or A, Arnold DL, et al. Clinical, environmental, and genetic determinants of multiple sclerosis in children with acute demyelination: a prospective national cohort study. *Lancet Neurol.* 2011;10(5):436–445.

23. Meuwissen ME, Mancini GM. Neurological findings in incontinentia pigmenti; a review. *Eur J Med Genet.* 2012; 55(5):323–331.

24. Lee S, Sanefuji M, Watanabe K, et al. Clinical and MRI characteristics of acute encephalopathy in congenital adrenal hyperplasia. *J Neurol Sci.* 2011;306(1–2):91–93.

25. Abe Y, Sakai T, Okumura A, et al. Manifestations and characteristics of congenital adrenal hyperplasia-associated encephalopathy. *Brain Dev.* 2016;38(7):638–647.

26. Baxter AG. The origin and application of experimental autoimmune encephalomyelitis. *Nat Rev Immunol.* 2007; 7(11):904–912.

27. Hemachudha T, Griffin DE, Giffels JJ, Johnson RT, Moser AB, Phanuphak P. Myelin basic protein as an encephalitogen in encephalomyelitis and polyneuritis following rabies vaccination. *N Engl J Med.* 1987;316(7):369–374.

28. Pohl D, Alper G, Van Haren K, et al. Acute disseminated encephalomyelitis: updates on an inflammatory CNS syndrome. *Neurology.* 2016;87(9 suppl 2):S38–S45.

CHAPTER 20

Autoimmune-Mediated Encephalitis With Antibodies to NMDA-Type GluRs: Early Clinical Diagnosis

YUKITOSHI TAKAHASHI, MD, PHD • TAKUJI NISHIDA, MD, PHD •
TOMOKAZU KIMIZU, MD • TAIKAN OBOSHI, MD • ASAKO HORINO, MD •
TAKAYOSHI KOIKE, MD • SHINSAKU YOSHITOMI, MD • TOKITO YAMAGUCHI, MD •
HIROWO OMATSU, MD

INTRODUCTION

Nonherpetic acute limbic encephalitis (NHALE) is diagnosed with the characteristic onset symptoms of limbic systems and the absence of herpes simplex virus in cerebrospinal fluid (CSF) and usually is not associated with tumors.[1,2] The initial neurologic symptoms originated from limbic systems in patients with NHALE are psychiatric symptoms, memory disturbances, disorientation, emotional disturbances, etc. (Fig. 20.1). Psychiatric symptoms include abnormal behavior, confusion, excitement, auditory hallucination, hallucination of smell, schizophrenic symptom, delirium, increased libido, etc. In patients with severe NHALE, these limbic symptoms are followed by seizures, clustering of seizures, profound impairment of consciousness, oral automatism, etc. Patients with NHALE have antibodies to GluN2B (GluR epsilon2), one of the N-methyl-D-aspartate receptor (NMDA)-type GluR subunits, which play pivotal roles in NHALE.[3,4] According to our data in 100 patients with NHALE, 71.4% and 82.4% of the patients had antibodies to n-terminal peptide of GluN2B (GluN2B-NT2) and n-terminal peptide of GluN1 (GluN1-NT) (ELISA) (not published).

Anti-NMDAR encephalitis is diagnosed with the presence of antibodies to the complex of NMDA-type GluR subunits by the cell-based assay in patients with encephalitis.[5,6] Most patients with anti-NMDAR encephalitis develop a multistage illness that progresses from psychosis, memory deficits, seizures, and language disintegration into a state of unresponsiveness with catatonic features often associated with abnormal movements, and autonomic and breathing instability.[6]

NHALE and anti-NMDAR encephalitis are causally related with antibodies to NMDA-type GluR, which internalize complex of NMDA-type GluR subunits on neural cell surface.[7,8] Internalization may lead to the antagonistic effects to NMDA-type GluR, resulting in limbic symptoms. On the other hand, antagonistic effects of the antibodies may bring protection from apoptosis by excitotoxicity of NMDA-type GluRs caused by increased levels of glutamate and cytokines in CSF in the severe stage NHALE and NMDAR encephalitis.

We examined the relationship between treatment at the onset stage and outcome in NHALE patients with antibodies to GluN2B-NT2 more than mean + 2SD of disease controls in CSF.[9] In 100 patients with confirmed outcome, death rate was 5%, and disability of ADL was observed in 27.4%, epileptic seizures in 21.1%, psychiatric disorder in 30.4%, cognitive disorder in 42.9%, memory disorder in 48.9%, and motor dysfunction in 18.9%. Outcome was significantly better in patients with earlier introduction of methylprednisolone pulse therapy, but intravenous immunoglobulin (IVIg) therapy and apheresis had insignificant relationship with outcome.[9] These data suggest that early clinical diagnosis of encephalitis mediated by antibodies to NMDA-type GluR is important for better outcome. Because confirmation of the antibodies needs at least several days in general hospitals, and the antibodies by cell-based assay and ELISA are found in CSF of many heterogeneous neurologic diseases[2] and sera of healthy individuals,[10,11] we need to establish clinical diagnosis of NHALE and probable evolution to NHALE, without confirmation of antibodies to NMDA-type GluRs, to start immunomodulatory treatment early.

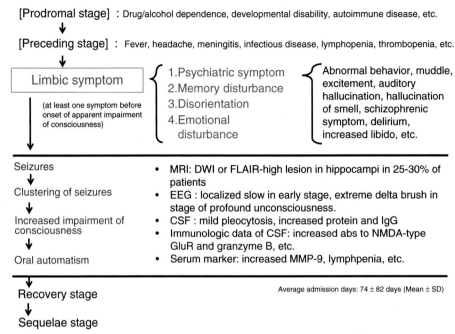

[Prodromal stage] : Drug/alcohol dependence, developmental disability, autoimmune disease, etc.

↓

[Preceding stage] : Fever, headache, meningitis, infectious disease, lymphopenia, thrombopenia, etc.

↓

Limbic symptom

(at least one symptom before onset of apparent impairment of consciousness)

1.Psychiatric symptom
2.Memory disturbance
3.Disorientation
4.Emotional disturbance

Abnormal behavior, muddle, excitement, auditory hallucination, hallucination of smell, schizophrenic symptom, delirium, increased libido, etc.

Seizures
↓
Clustering of seizures
↓
Increased impairment of consciousness
↓
Oral automatism

- MRI: DWI or FLAIR-high lesion in hippocampi in 25-30% of patients
- EEG : localized slow in early stage, extreme delta brush in stage of profound unconsciousness.
- CSF : mild pleocytosis, increased protein and IgG
- Immunologic data of CSF: increased abs to NMDA-type GluR and granzyme B, etc.
- Serum marker: increased MMP-9, lymphpenia, etc.

↓
Recovery stage

Average admission days: 74 ± 82 days (Mean ± SD)

↓
Sequelae stage

FIG. 20.1 Evolution of nonherpetic acute limbic encephalitis.

PATIENTS AND METHODS
Definition of Clinical Stages
We divide clinical stages of NHALE into five stages: prodromal stage, preceding stage, onset stage, recovery stage, and sequelae stage (Figs. 20.1 and 20.2). The prodromal stage is defined as the stage before the appearance of any symptoms preceding the onset of NHALE, and the symptoms in the prodromal stage are considered as history. The preceding stage is defined as the stage manifesting acute symptoms just before the appearance of encephalitis symptoms, for example, fever, diarrhea, and headache. The onset stage is defined as the stage from the appearance to disappearance of acute symptom of encephalitis, impairment of consciousness, etc. The recovery stage is defined as the stage from the disappearance of acute symptom of encephalitis to the end of acute hospitalization. The sequela stage is defined as the stage after the end of acute hospitalization.

Inclusion and Exclusion Criteria of Nonherpetic Acute Limbic Encephalitis Patients
Among patients with written agreement to contribute to the study of autoimmune-mediated encephalitis, we selected NHALE patients with the following criteria: (1) characteristic onset with limbic symptom (at least one limbic symptom from psychiatric symptoms, memory disturbances, disorientation, and emotional disturbances), (2) no HSV infection, (3) no association of tumor, and (4) subsequent acute impairment of consciousness after the limbic symptom. We excluded patients with the findings of direct infection of central nervous system diagnosed by polymerase chain reaction or significant increase in antibodies to microbes in CSF.

Healthy Controls and Disease Controls of Infection for Evaluation of Blood Data in the Preceding Stage
Among individuals with written agreement to contribute to the study of autoimmune-mediated encephalitis, we selected epilepsy patients without infection and healthy volunteers as healthy controls, with age- and sex-matched manner. Among individuals with written agreement to contribute to the study of autoimmune-mediated encephalitis, we selected epilepsy patients with infection as disease controls of infection with age- and sex-matched manner.

Disease Controls and Disease Controls of Aseptic Meningitis for Evaluation of Cerebrospinal Fluid Data in the Preceding Stage
Among individuals with written agreement to contribute to the study of autoimmune-mediated encephalitis,

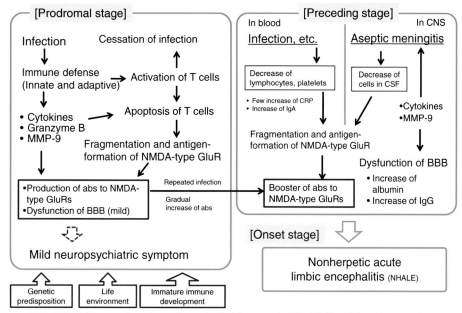

FIG. 20.2 Stages of nonherpetic acute limbic encephalitis. *GluRs*, glutamate receptors.

we selected epilepsy patients without infection as disease controls with age- and sex-matched manner. Among individuals with written agreement to contribute to the study of autoimmune-mediated encephalitis, we selected aseptic meningitis patients without evolution to encephalitis as disease controls of aseptic meningitis with age- and sex-matched manner.

Study for the Prodromal Stage

We examined history of NHALE patients, using clinical records provided by referring doctors, and compared the history of diseases in NHALE patients with that in Japanese population.[12]

Study for the Preceding Stage

We examined blood data and CSF data of NHALE patients at the preceding stage from records provided by referring doctors and compared blood data of NHALE patients with healthy controls and disease controls of infection, and compared CSF data of NHALE patients with disease controls and disease controls of aseptic meningitis.

Statistics

Nonparametric Mann-Whitney U test was used to compare data between two groups. A P value less than .05 was considered to indicate a statistically significant difference. The changes in CSF marker levels over time

were examined by linear regression analysis. Statistical analyses were performed using GraphPad Prism 6 (GraphPad Software, Inc. La Jolla, USA).

RESULTS

History of Nonherpetic Acute Limbic Encephalitis Patients

In 217 patients with NHALE, psychiatric diseases including related diseases were found in 21 patients (9.7%), and the frequency was significantly higher than the prevalence in Japanese population (~2.2%, 281 million)[12] (Fisher's exact test, $P<.05$). Mood disorder was found in eight patients (3.7%) and in 3.1% of Japanese population.[11] Addiction to alcohol, stimulant drugs, etc., was found in eight patients (3.7%), and alcohol abuse was in 1.4% of Japanese population.[12] Developmental disorder was found in five patients (2.3%) and in ~10% of Japanese population.[12]

A preceding history of encephalitis, meningitis, or epilepsy was not found in NHALE patients. Autoimmune and related diseases were found in nine patients (4.1%), and the frequency was higher than that in 107 patients with paraneoplastic acute encephalitis associated with ovarian teratoma (0%) (Fisher's exact test, $P<.05$). Prevalence of rheumatoid arthritis and type 1 diabetes mellitus was 1.0% and 0.4%, respectively, of Japanese population.[12]

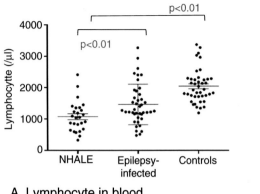

A. Lymphocyte in blood

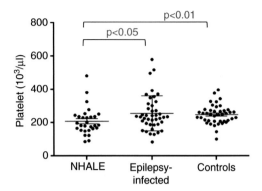

B. Platelet in blood

Cell counts in CSF

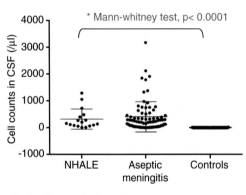

C. Cell counts in CSF

Evolution of cell counts

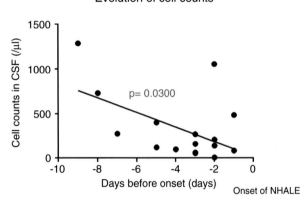

D. Evolution of cell counts

FIG. 20.3 Blood and cerebrospinal fluid (CSF) data of nonherpetic acute limbic encephalitis. *Controls*, healthy controls and epilepsy patients without infection; *Epilepsy infected*, epilepsy patients with infection; *NHALE*, nonherpetic acute limbic encephalitis; (Data from Takahashi Y, Mori T, Oboshi T, et al. Presence of autoantibodies to GluRε2 in intractable epilepsy by CNS infection in childhood, *Nihonshounikagakkaishi*. 2002;106:1402–1411.)

Preceding Symptoms of Nonherpetic Acute Limbic Encephalitis Patients

In 207 NHALE patients with enough clinical data (onset age [mean ± SD], 30.0 ± 19.6 years), 162 (78.3%) patients had preceding symptoms, and 23 of 162 (14.2%) patients had confirmed infectious etiologies (influenza virus, *Staphylococcus pyogenes*, *Mycoplasma*, etc.). Infectious etiologies were confirmed frequently in patients <20 years of age. Fever as a preceding symptom was observed in 135 patients and was frequent in younger onset patients. Headache was in 78 patients and frequent in patients with onset age of 30–49 years. Aseptic meningitis was in 18 of 18 patients with CSF examination (100%) in the preceding stage and was frequent in patients with onset age of 30–39 years (29%).

Blood Data in the Preceding Stage of Nonherpetic Acute Limbic Encephalitis Patients

In 207 NHALE patients with enough clinical data (onset age [mean ± SD], 30.0 ± 19.6 years), 42 patients had blood data in preceding stages (NHALE group), which were compared with data of healthy control group (n = 42) and disease control of infection group (n = 42). In NHALE group, mean WBC count was higher than that in healthy controls ($P < .04$).[13] Mean lymphocytes count in NHALE group was lower than that in healthy control group ($P < .01$) and disease control of infection group ($P < .01$) (Fig. 20.3). Mean platelets count in NHALE group was lower than that in healthy control group ($P < .01$) and disease control of infection group ($P < .05$). Mean level of CRP in NHALE group was lower than that in disease control of infection group ($P < .05$). Mean level of IgG in NHALE group was higher than that in healthy control group ($P < .02$). Mean level of IgA in NHALE group was higher than that in healthy control group ($P < .01$) and disease control of infection group ($P < .03$). Levels of IgA in NHALE group were not related with the days before onset of NHALE.

Cerebrospinal Fluid Data in the Preceding Stage of Nonherpetic Acute Limbic Encephalitis Patients

In 207 NHALE patients with enough clinical data (onset age [mean $\pm$ SD], 30.0 ± 19.6 years), 17 patients had CSF data in preceding stages (NHALE group), which were compared with data of disease control group (n = 86) and disease control of aseptic meningitis group (n = 78). In NHALE group, mean cell count was higher than that in disease controls ($P < .01$), and the cell counts decreased until the onset of encephalitis ($P = .03$) (Fig. 20.3).[13] Mean level of protein in NHALE group was higher than that in disease control group ($P < .01$) and disease control of aseptic meningitis group ($P < .01$). Mean level of glucose in NHALE group was lower than that in disease control group ($P < .01$) and disease control of aseptic meningitis group ($P < .03$). Mean level of IgG in NHALE group was higher than that in disease control group ($P < .01$). Mean level of albumin in NHALE group was higher than that in disease control group ($P < .01$).

DISCUSSION

We studied characteristics of history in the prodromal stage and blood and CSF data in the preceding stage of patients with NHALE, for the establishment of early clinical diagnosis of NHALE, with the aim of achieving better outcomes by starting immunomodulatory treatment early.

In the history of patients with NHALE, frequency of psychiatric diseases (9.7%) was high, compared with the Japanese population data. Schizophrenia, one of psychiatric diseases, is a common, heterogeneous, and complex disorder with unknown etiologies, and there is established evidence for NMDA-type GluR hypofunction as a central component of the functional dysconnectivity.[14] In a previous study, 3 of 46 patients with the first episode of schizophrenia, antibodies to NMDA-type GluR were detected by cell-based assay, and 2 patients recovered well at the last observation.[14] Furthermore, in a patient with neuromyelitis optica, aquaporin-4 antibody existed in sera more than 10 years before onset.[15] These data may suggest that individuals with the ability to produce antibodies to NMDA-type GluRs have chance to manifest tentative psychiatric symptoms before the onset of NHALE and to suffer from NHALE in the future.

Addiction including abuse of alcohol was also frequent in the history of NHALE patients. Ethanol exposure activates signaling pathways featuring high-mobility group box 1 and Toll-like receptor 4 (TLR4), resulting in the induction of the transcription factor nuclear factor kappa-light-chain-enhancer of activated B cells, which regulates expression of several cytokine genes involved in innate immunity, and its target genes.[16] Neuroimmune receptor stimulation leads to activation of NMDA-type GluR, resulting in increases in Ca^{2+} flux, triggering further induction of neuroimmune genes and promotion of glutamate hyperexcitability and excitotoxicity. Therefore, these proinflammatory and excitotoxic condition of CNS induced by alcohol may theoretically contribute to the onset of NHALE.

The frequency of autoimmune diseases was higher in the history of NHALE patients. This may suggest that genetic predisposition to autoimmune diseases contributes to the onset of NHALE. We need to study genetic predisposition markers in the future.

In the preceding periods of NHALE, lymphocyte and platelet counts in blood were decreased, compared with disease control of infection group. The cell counts in CSF decreased toward the onset of encephalitis. These data suggest possible apoptosis of lymphocytes and platelets in NHALE by immune mechanisms (Fig. 20.2). Because lymphocytes and platelets express NMDA-type GluRs,[17,18] it is hypothesized that their apoptosis provide fragmented NMDA-type GluRs, resulting in the production of autoantibodies to NMDA-type GluRs.

The level of CRP in NHALE group was lower than that in disease control of infection group. This may suggest that infection of microbes is not clearly evident at the onset of NHALE. The level of IgA in NHALE group was higher than that of disease control of infection group, and levels of IgA seem to be constitutionally high in patients who developed NHALE. Higher levels of IgA may suggest the predisposition to the onset of NHALE, because higher levels of IgA are known in collagen diseases including rheumatoid arthritis, systemic lupus erythematosus, etc.

The level of protein in CSF of NHALE group was higher than that in healthy control group and disease control of aseptic meningitis group, and levels of albumin in NHALE group were higher than those in disease control group. These may suggest dysfunction of blood-brain barrier (Fig. 20.2). The levels of IgG in

NHALE group were higher than those in disease control group. This may be attributed to the production of antibodies to NMDA-type GluR in CNS.[19]

CONCLUSIONS

In the history of patients with suspected NHALE, the presence of psychiatric diseases, addiction including abuse of alcohol, and autoimmune diseases suggest the diagnosis of possible evolution to NHALE from the preceding stage. In blood markers at the preceding stage before the appearance of encephalitis symptoms, decreased counts of lymphocytes and platelets in blood, relatively lower levels of CRP in sera, and relatively higher levels of IgA suggest possible contributors to the onset of NHALE. CSF markers at the preceding stage show relatively higher levels of protein, albumin, and IgG, which may suggest possible evolution to the onset of NHALE. These findings may improve our ability to identify patients at risk of developing NHALE and may provide an opportunity to intervene early with immune therapy.

ACKNOWLEDGMENTS

This study was funded in part by grants-in-aid for Scientific Research Nos. 23591238, 2451537, and 15K09634, Health and Labour Sciences Research Grants for Comprehensive Research on Disability Health and Welfare; Research on rare and intractable disease; and grants from Japan Epilepsy Research Foundation.

REFERENCES

1. Kushara T, Shoji H, Kaij M, Ayabe M, Hino H. Non-herpetic acute limbic encephalitis. *Clin Neurol.* 1994;34:1083–1088.
2. Takahashi Y, Kimizu Y, Koike T, Horino A. Autoimmune mediated encephalitis/encephalopathy. *Shinkeichiryougaku.* 2016;33:19–26.
3. Takahashi Y, Mori H, Mishina M, et al. Autoantibodies to NMDA receptor in patients with chronic forms of epilepsia partialis continua. *Neurology.* 2003;61:891–896. PMID: 14557555.
4. Mochizuki Y, Mizutani T, Isozaki E, Otake T, Takahashi Y. Acute limbic encephalitis: a new entity?. *Neurosci Lett.* 2006;394:5–8. PMID: 16364542.
5. Dalmau J, Tüzün E, Wu HY, et al. Paraneoplastic anti–N-methyl-D-aspartate receptor encephalitis associated with ovarian teratoma. *Ann Neurol.* 2007;61:25–36. PMID: 17262855.
6. Dalmau J, Lancaster E, Martinez-Hernandez E, Rosenfeld MR, Balice-Gordon R. Clinical experience and laboratory investigations in patients with anti-NMDAR encephalitis. *Lancet Neurol.* 2011;10(1):63–74. PMID: 21163445.
7. Hughes EG, Peng X, Gleichman AJ, et al. Cellular and synaptic mechanisms of anti-NMDA receptor encephalitis. *J Neurosci.* 2010;30(17):5866–5875. PMID: 20427647.
8. Takano S, Takahashi Y, Kishi H, et al. Detection of autoantibody against extracellular epitopes of N-methyl-D-aspartate receptor by cell-based assay. *Neurosci Res.* 2011;71(3):294–302. PMID: 21839784.
9. Takahashi Y, Nishimura S, Takao E, Kasai R, Enokida K, Kubota M. Study in 157 patients with non-herpetic acute limbic encephalitis: treatment in acute stage & outcome. *Neuroinfection.* 2016;21:121–127.
10. Dahm L, Ott C, Steiner J, et al. Seroprevalence of autoantibodies against brain antigens in health and disease. *Ann Neurol.* 2014;76(1):82–94. PMID: 24853231.
11. Takahashi Y, Nishimura S, Takao E, Kasai R, Hiramatsu H, Inoue Y. Study for pathophysiology of NHALE: antibodies to GluR and age in normal controls. *Neuroinfection.* 2014;19(2):170 (in Japanese abstract).
12. Governmental Survey of Patients in 2008. http://www.e-stat.go.jp/SG1/estat/NewList.do?tid=000001031167.
13. Takahashi Y, Mori T, Oboshi T, et al. Presence of autoantibodies to GluRε2 in intractable epilepsy by CNS infection in childhood. *Nihonshounikagakkaishi.* 2002;106:1402–1411.
14. Zandi MS, Irani SR, Lang B, et al. Disease-relevant autoantibodies in first episode schizophrenia. *J Neurol.* 2011;258:686–688. PMID: 20972895.
15. Nishiyama S, Ito T, Misu T, et al. A case of NMO seropositive for aquaporin-4 antibody more than10 years before onset. *Neurology.* 2009;72:1960–1961.
16. Crews FT, Sarkar DK, Qin L, Zou J, Boyadjieva N, Vetreno RP. Neuroimmune function and the consequences of alcohol exposure. *Alcohol Res.* 2015;37(2):331–341. 344-51.
17. Miglio G, Varsaldi F, Lombardi G. Human T lymphocytes express N-methyl-D-aspartate Receptors functionally active in controlling T cell activation. *Biochem Biophys Res Commun.* 2005;338:1875–1883. PMID: 16289038.
18. Mahaut-Smith MP. The unique contribution of ion channels to platelet and megakaryocyte function. *J Thromb Haemost.* 2012;10:1722–1732.
19. Irani SR, Bera K, Waters P, et al. N-methyl-D-aspartate antibody encephalitis: temporal progression of clinical and paraclinical observations in a predominantly non-paraneoplastic disorder of both sexes. *Brain.* 2010;133: 1655–1667. PMID: 20511282.

CHAPTER 21

Clinical Features of HHV-6B Encephalitis: Difference Between Primary Infection and Reactivation

TETSUSHI YOSHIKAWA, MD, PHD

VIROLOGIC INFORMATION OF HUMAN HERPESVIRUS 6B

Human herpesvirus 6 (HHV-6) belongs to β-herpes virinae subfamily similar to human cytomegalovirus and HHV-7. These viruses have lymphotropism and have similar genetic construction and sequence similarities. Additionally, HHV-6 is now divided into two different species: HHV-6A and HHV-6B; thus, there are four different human β-herpesviruses right now. Receptor of HHV-6A has been demonstrated to be CD46 that is expressed on all of the eukaryotic cells.[1] Meanwhile, CD134 that is expressed on activated T cells has been recently shown to be a receptor of HHV-6B.[2] Although CD46 might be a cellar receptor for invasion of HHV-6A into glial cell,[3] no remarkable cell receptor that is associated with neurotropism of HHV-6B has been identified to date.

Although clinical features of HHV-6A infection remains unclear, it has been clearly demonstrated that primary HHV-6B infection causes exanthem subitum (ES), which is a benign febrile illness in young children.[4] According to the seroepidemiologic analysis, because most of infants and young children receive primary HHV-6B infection,[5] older children and adults are considered to be seropositive for the virus. In contrast to Japan, the United States, and Europe, HHV-6A infection has been dominant in Ugandan children.[6] Although most of the ES patients demonstrate benign and self-limiting clinical course, several severe complications such as fulminant hepatitis, myocarditis, hemophagocytic syndrome, and encephalitis have been reported. Among the complications, central nervous system (CNS) complications, such as febrile seizure and encephalitis,[7–13] are the most common in ES patients.

After primary infection, HHV-6B can establish lifelong latency in peripheral blood mononuclear cells,[14,15] salivary glands,[16,17] and the CNS.[18,19] Similar to other human herpesviruses, HHV-6B can reactivate in immunocompromised patients such as hematopoietic stem cell transplant (HSCT) recipient and solid organ transplant recipients.[20,21] Additionally, the viral reactivation also occurs in patients with severe drug allergy (drug-induced hypersensitivity syndrome).[22,23] Although various types of clinical manifestations including bone marrow suppression, pneumonitis, acute graft-versus-host disease, and graft rejection have been suggested to be associated with HHV-6B reactivation, the strongest correlation has been demonstrated between HHV-6B reactivation and posttransplant acute limbic encephalitis.[24–26]

The unique characteristic of HHV-6 is integration of the entire viral genome into host chromosome, referred to as "chromosomally integrated HHV-6" (ciHHV-6).[27–30] Viral genome is integrated in germ line and is vertically transmitted in a Mendelian manner. It has been demonstrated that incidence of ciHHV-6 was lower in Japan (0.6%)[31] than in the United States and Europe (0.8%–1.0%).[32] Homologous recombination between the viral and host telomere repeats has been proposed for the mechanisms of viral genome integration in both ciHHV-6A[33] and ciHHV-6B.[34] Therefore, the entire viral genome can be integrated in the telomere region of host chromosome. Although several clinical impacts of ciHHV-6 have been suggested, the precise role of ciHHV-6 is still under investigation. As high copy of viral DNA is detected in peripheral blood or serum samples, misdiagnosis of active viral infection may occur, which results in unnecessary antiviral treatment.[35,36] Detection of viral DNA in cerebrospinal fluid (CSF) is a reliable marker for viral encephalitis including HHV-6 encephalitis. As extremely high copies of HHV-6 DNA can be detected in CSF obtained from ciHHV-6 patients,[36,37] physicians have to remember this unique phenomenon.

NEUROVIRULENCE OF HUMAN HERPESVIRUS 6B

Several investigators demonstrated viral latency and reactivation in the CNS based on the detection of HHV-6 DNA and antigens in brain tissues. HHV-6 infection was primarily restricted to oligodendrocytes and astrocytes, but rarely to neurons.[38,39] In addition, it is well established that HHV-6B reactivation is involved in posttransplant acute limbic encephalitis.[25,40,41] Several previous in vitro studies sought to elucidate the neurovirulence of HHV-6. It is well established that HHV-6 infects multiple types of cell lines, including hematopoietic cell lines,[42] epidermal and endothelial cell lines,[43] and glioma cell lines.[44] In fact, both glioma cell lines and primary human astrocytes are susceptible to HHV-6 infection.[45] HHV-6 latency and reactivation in an astrocytoma cell line resulted in an upregulation of cytokine synthesis.[44] These in vitro studies allowed us important information to better understand the pathogenesis of HHV-6B-associated neurologic complications. Furthermore, similar to herpes simplex virus, it has been suggested that the olfactory pathway may be implicated in the transmission of HHV-6 into the CNS.[46]

Although the main theme of this chapter is HHV-6B encephalitis, it has been suggested that HHV-6B may be associated with other intractable neurologic diseases such as multiple sclerosis (MS)[47–49] and mesial temporal lobe epilepsy (MTLE).[50] Either a high-frequency or a high viral DNA load has been demonstrated in the brain tissues obtained from MS[47,51] and MTLE[52] patients compared with control subjects. Additionally, it has been demonstrated that the immune response against HHV-6 was stronger in MS patients than in controls.[48,53,54] However, the finding of high levels of HHV-6 antibody titers and high frequency of viral detection in MS patients compared with control subjects has been controversial to date,[55,56] and the precise role of HHV-6 infection in the pathogenesis of MS remains unclear. HHV-6B DNA has been detected in hippocampal tissues resected from MTLE patients. The localization of HHV-6 to astrocytes was confirmed by the colocalization of viral antigens to glial fibrillary acidic protein (GFAP)-positive cells in vivo.[52] Additionally, HHV-6B may contribute to the pathogenesis of MTLE by altering the expression of glutamate transporters.[50] Recently our study demonstrated that HHV-6, primarily HHV-6B, was the most prevalent human herpesvirus that established latent infections in the hippocampus or amygdala of MTS patients.[57] The analyses of host gene expression levels suggested that latent HHV-6 infection may play an important role in

the pathogenesis of MTS via the upregulation of GFAP and MCP-1 expression. Thus, many pieces of in vivo and in vitro evidence have suggested neurovirulence of HHV-6 and an association between HHV-6 and several severe neurologic diseases.

HUMAN HERPESVIRUS 6B ENCEPHALITIS AT THE TIME OF PRIMARY INFECTION

Bulging fontanelle is a well-known characteristic manifestation in patients with primary HHV-6B infection, and intracranial pressure may occur, suggesting direct invasion of etiologic agent into the CNS. Before discovery of HHV-6, it has been suggested that ES might be caused by some viral agents, because of transmission of the disease in human experimental studies that would be impossible to perform today. Additionally, several ES cases with CNS complications such as hemiplegia and encephalitis have been reported in the late 1960s.[58–60] As virologic examinations have become available after discovery of HHV-6B as an etiologic agent for ES, direct invasion of the virus into the CNS has been demonstrated in ES patients with complex type of febrile seizures[8,10,19,61] and encephalitis based on the PCR analysis.[9,13] According to our survey, the annual incidence of ES-associated encephalitis was estimated to be ~60 cases per year in Japan, and almost half of the patients had severe neurologic sequelae including quadriplegia and mental retardation and two fatal cases.[11] Additionally, it has been demonstrated that HHV-6B was the second highest incidence of childhood encephalitis in Japan following influenza encephalitis. Thus, disease burden of HHV-6B encephalitis at the time of primary viral infection is considered to be high in Japanese children. It has been demonstrated that HHV-6B encephalitis showed various types of clinical courses, including acute necrotizing encephalopathy,[62] hemorrhagic shock and encephalopathy syndrome, and acute encephalopathy with biphasic seizures and late reduced diffusion (AESD).[63–66] In particular, although the reason is unclear, the number of HHV-6B-associated AESD cases has been increasing recently. As prognosis and kinetics of serum and CSF cytokines levels were different among these different types of HHV-6B encephalitis, an appropriate treatment protocol should be developed in each type of encephalitis in the future.

Although direct invasion of HHV-6B has been suggested by the initial studies for HHV-6B encephalitis using highly sensitive nested PCR assay, subsequently, not only frequency but also amounts of viral DNA have been limited in comparison with HHV-6B encephalitis in adult transplant recipients on the basis the real-time PCR analysis.[67] Additionally, it has been demonstrated that CSF cell counts and protein levels were normal in most of the patients. Meanwhile, levels of proinflammatory cytokines and chemokines have been elevated in the patients' serum or CSF.[67–71] These findings suggest that host immune response rather than direct viral invasion into the CNS may play an important role in the pathogenesis of HHV-6B encephalitis at the time of primary viral infection.

Although no reliable treatment protocol for HHV-6B encephalitis at the time of primary infection has been developed, in addition to the anti-hypercytokinemia treatments such as intravenous high dose of immunoglobulin and steroid pulse treatment, antiviral drug administration has been attempted in some of the patients. It is important to determine whether antiviral drug administration is effective or not and to establish reliable treatment protocol for these patients in the future. Furthermore, another important research question is why HHV-6B encephalitis frequently occurs in eastern Asian population including Japanese. As genetic background might be associated with susceptibility of encephalitis caused by HHV-6B infection, linkage analysis would be required for identification of the candidate genes in future study.

POSTTRANSPLANT HUMAN HERPESVIRUS 6B ENCEPHALITIS

It is well established that HHV-6B reactivation is involved in posttransplant acute limbic encephalitis.[25,40,41] As HHV-6B can reactivate in 2–4 weeks after transplant in almost half of the HSCT recipients, it has been demonstrated that posttransplant HHV-6B encephalitis also occurs in same period. Cord blood transplant recipients have been suggested to be at high risk for posttransplant HHV-6B encephalitis[72] and should be monitored for active HHV-6B infection carefully. Typical clinical features of posttransplant HHV-6B encephalitis are consistent with acute limbic encephalitis that demonstrates memory loss and abnormal findings in limbic area by brain MRI.[24,73] Thus, HHV-6B has been considered to be main etiologic agent for posttransplant acute limbic encephalitis. Although most of the cases of posttransplant HHV-6B encephalitis have been adult transplant recipients, it has been suggested that HHV-6B infection may be associated with mild cognitive dysfunction in pediatric transplant recipients.[74]

As described previously, our group reported significantly higher amounts of HHV-6 DNA in the CSF collected from posttransplant acute limbic encephalitis patients than those from HHV-6 encephalitis patients at the time of primary viral infection.[67] Taken together, these in vivo findings indicate that HHV-6 latently infects brain tissues after primary infection and reactivates in brain tissues, particularly in the limbic area in patients with posttransplant HHV-6B encephalitis. Additionally, these findings have also suggested that administration of antiviral drugs may be reasonable for patient treatment.

Although no randomized placebo control study has been carried out to date, efficacy of either ganciclovir or foscarnet has been demonstrated by clinical improvement and reduction in viral DNA load in CSF.[75–77] Various types of clinical trials have been attempted to prevent posttransplant HHV-6 encephalitis, which can result in fatal outcome in some cases. Plasma HHV-6 DNA-guided preemptive approaches have been demonstrated to be inadequate in preventing the development of HHV-6 encephalitis.[78,79] Furthermore, prophylactic administration of anti-HHV-6 antivirals will suppress HHV-6 replication and may effectively prevent the development of HHV-6 encephalitis.[80,81] However, the toxicity of currently applicable antivirals limits the practical application for prophylaxis. A study evaluating the effects of prophylactic foscarnet administration (PFA) showed that 50 mg/kg/day of PFA for 10 days was safe but failed to effectively suppress HHV-6 reactivation and could not prevent HHV-6 encephalitis. Thus, although clinical characteristics and diagnosis and treatment strategies for posttransplant HHV-6B encephalitis have been developed, indeed, no prophylactic treatment strategy has been successful to date. Therefore, it is important to establish reliable prophylactic treatment protocol for prevention of HHV-6B reactivation in the CNS in the future.

CONCLUSION

In vivo and in vitro evidences clearly suggest neurovirulence of HHV-6B. Complex type of febrile seizure and encephalitis are important complications at the time of primary viral infection. Primary HHV-6B infection has been associated with various types of encephalitis, indeed, recently, patients with AESD has been dominant. According to the previous studies, the host immune response may play an important role in the pathogenesis of HHV-6B encephalitis at the time of primary viral infection.

REFERENCES

1. Santoro F, Kennedy PE, Locatelli G, Malnati MS, Berger EA, Lusso P. CD46 is a cellular receptor for human herpesvirus 6. *Cell.* 1999;99(7):817–827.
2. Tang H, Serada S, Kawabata A, et al. CD134 is a cellular receptor specific for human herpesvirus-6B entry. *Proc Natl Acad Sci USA.* 2013;110(22):9096–9099.
3. Cassiani-Ingoni R, Greenstone HL, Donati D, et al. CD46 on glial cells can function as a receptor for viral glycoprotein-mediated cell-cell fusion. *Glia.* 2005;52(3):252–258.
4. Yamanishi K, Okuno T, Shiraki K, et al. Identification of human herpesvirus-6 as a causal agent for exanthem subitum. *Lancet.* 1988;1(8594):1065–1067.
5. Yoshikawa T, Suga S, Asano Y, Yazaki T, Kodama H, Ozaki T. Distribution of antibodies to a causative agent of exanthem subitum (human herpesvirus-6) in healthy individuals. *Pediatrics.* 1989;84(4):675–677.
6. Bates M, Monze M, Bima H, et al. Predominant human herpesvirus 6 variant A infant infections in an HIV-1 endemic region of Sub-Saharan Africa. *J Med Virol.* 2009;81(5):779–789.
7. Caserta MT, Hall CB, Schnabel K, Long CE, D'Heron N. Primary human herpesvirus 7 infection: a comparison of human herpesvirus 7 and human herpesvirus 6 infections in children. *J Pediatr.* 1998;133(3):386–389.
8. Hall CB, Long CE, Schnabel KC, et al. Human herpesvirus-6 infection in children. A prospective study of complications and reactivation. *N Engl J Med.* 1994;331(7):432–438.
9. Suga S, Yoshikawa T, Asano Y, et al. Clinical and virological analyses of 21 infants with exanthem subitum (roseola infantum) and central nervous system complications. *Ann Neurol.* 1993;33(6):597–603.
10. Suga S, Suzuki K, Ihira M, et al. Clinical characteristics of febrile convulsions during primary HHV-6 infection. *Arch Dis Child.* 2000;82(1):62–66.
11. Yoshikawa T, Ohashi M, Miyake F, et al. Exanthem subitum-associated encephalitis: nationwide survey in Japan. *Pediatr Neurol.* 2009;41(5):353–358.
12. Asano Y, Yoshikawa T, Kajita Y, et al. Fatal encephalitis/encephalopathy in primary human herpesvirus-6 infection. *Arch Dis Child.* 1992;67(12):1484–1485.
13. Yoshikawa T, Nakashima T, Suga S, et al. Human herpesvirus-6 DNA in cerebrospinal fluid of a child with exanthem subitum and meningoencephalitis. *Pediatrics.* 1992;89(5 Pt 1):888–890.
14. Kondo K, Hayakawa Y, Mori H, et al. Detection by polymerase chain reaction amplification of human herpesvirus 6 DNA in peripheral blood of patients with exanthem subitum. *J Clin Microbiol.* 1990;28(5):970–974.
15. Kondo K, Kondo T, Okuno T, Takahashi M, Yamanishi K. Latent human herpesvirus 6 infection of human monocytes/macrophages. *J Gen Virol.* 1991;72(Pt 6):1401–1408.
16. Yoshikawa T, Ihira M, Taguchi H, Yoshida S, Asano Y. Analysis of shedding of 3 beta-herpesviruses in saliva from patients with connective tissue diseases. *J Infect Dis.* 2005;192(9):1530–1536.
17. Suga S, Yoshikawa T, Kajita Y, Ozaki T, Asano Y. Prospective study of persistence and excretion of human herpesvirus-6 in patients with exanthem subitum and their parents. *Pediatrics.* 1998;102(4 Pt 1):900–904.
18. Chan PK, Ng HK, Hui M, Cheng AF. Prevalence and distribution of human herpesvirus 6 variants A and B in adult human brain. *J Med Virol.* 2001;64(1):42–46.
19. Kondo K, Nagafuji H, Hata A, Tomomori C, Yamanishi K. Association of human herpesvirus 6 infection of the central nervous system with recurrence of febrile convulsions. *J Infect Dis.* 1993;167(5):1197–1200.
20. Zerr DM. Human herpesvirus 6 (HHV-6) disease in the setting of transplantation. *Curr Opin Infect Dis.* 2012;25(4):438–444.
21. Yoshikawa T. Human herpesvirus 6 infection in hematopoietic stem cell transplant patients. *Br J Haematol.* 2004;124(4):421–432.
22. Descamps V, Ranger-Rogez S. DRESS syndrome. *Jt Bone Spine.* 2014;81(1):15–21.
23. Kano Y, Shiohara T. The variable clinical picture of drug-induced hypersensitivity syndrome/drug rash with eosinophilia and systemic symptoms in relation to the eliciting drug. *Immunol Allergy Clin N Am.* 2009;29(3):481–501.
24. Wainwright MS, Martin PL, Morse RP, et al. Human herpesvirus 6 limbic encephalitis after stem cell transplantation. *Ann Neurol.* 2001;50(5):612–619.
25. Seeley WW, Marty FM, Holmes TM, et al. Post-transplant acute limbic encephalitis: clinical features and relationship to HHV6. *Neurology.* 2007;69(2):156–165.
26. Ogata M, Fukuda T, Teshima T. Human herpesvirus-6 encephalitis after allogeneic hematopoietic cell transplantation: what we do and do not know. *Bone Marrow Transpl.* 2015;50(8):1030–1036.
27. Arbuckle JH, Medveczky PG. The molecular biology of human herpesvirus-6 latency and telomere integration. *Microbes Infect.* 2011;13(8–9):731–741.
28. Clark DA. Clinical and laboratory features of human herpesvirus 6 chromosomal integration. *Clin Microbiol Infect.* 2016;22(4):333–339.
29. Pellett PE, Ablashi DV, Ambros PF, et al. Chromosomally integrated human herpesvirus 6: questions and answers. *Rev Med Virol.* 2012;22(3):144–155.
30. Luppi M, Barozzi P, Morris CM, Merelli E, Torelli G. Integration of human herpesvirus 6 genome in human chromosomes. *Lancet.* 1998;352(9141):1707–1708.
31. Tanaka-Taya K, Sashihara J, Kurahashi H, et al. Human herpesvirus 6 (HHV-6) is transmitted from parent to child in an integrated form and characterization of cases with chromosomally integrated HHV-6 DNA. *J Med Virol.* 2004;73(3):465–473.
32. Leong HN, Tuke PW, Tedder RS, et al. The prevalence of chromosomally integrated human herpesvirus 6 genomes in the blood of UK blood donors. *J Med Virol.* 2007;79(1):45–51.
33. Arbuckle JH, Medveczky MM, Luka J, et al. The latent human herpesvirus-6A genome specifically integrates in telomeres of human chromosomes in vivo and in vitro. *Proc Natl Acad Sci USA.* 2010;107(12):5563–5568.

34. Ohye T, Inagaki H, Ihira M, et al. Dual roles for the telomeric repeats in chromosomally integrated human herpesvirus-6. *Sci Rep*. 2014;4:4559.

35. Boutolleau D, Agut H, Gautheret-Dejean A. Human herpesvirus 6 genome integration: a possible cause of misdiagnosis of active viral infection? *J Infect Dis*. 2006;194(7):1019–1020. Author reply 21–23.

36. Ward KN, Leong HN, Thiruchelvam AD, Atkinson CE, Clark DA. Human herpesvirus 6 DNA levels in cerebrospinal fluid due to primary infection differ from those due to chromosomal viral integration and have implications for diagnosis of encephalitis. *J Clin Microbiol*. 2007;45(4):1298–1304.

37. Oikawa J, Tanaka J, Yoshikawa T, et al. An immunocompetent child with chromosomally integrated human herpesvirus 6B accidentally identified during the care of Mycoplasma pneumoniae infection. *J Infect Chemother*. 2014;20(1):65–67.

38. Saito Y, Sharer LR, Dewhurst S, Blumberg BM, Hall CB, Epstein LG. Cellular localization of human herpesvirus-6 in the brains of children with AIDS encephalopathy. *J Neurovirol*. 1995;1(1):30–39.

39. Cuomo L, Trivedi P, Cardillo MR, et al. Human herpesvirus 6 infection in neoplastic and normal brain tissue. *J Med Virol*. 2001;63(1):45–51.

40. Ogata M, Satou T, Kawano R, et al. Correlations of HHV-6 viral load and plasma IL-6 concentration with HHV-6 encephalitis in allogeneic stem cell transplant recipients. *Bone Marrow Transpl*. 2010;45(1):129–136.

41. Bhanushali MJ, Kranick SM, Freeman AF, et al. Human herpes 6 virus encephalitis complicating allogeneic hematopoietic stem cell transplantation. *Neurology*. 2013;80(16):1494–1500.

42. Ablashi DV, Lusso P, Hung CL, et al. Utilization of human hematopoietic cell lines for the propagation and characterization of HBLV (human herpesvirus 6). *Int J Cancer*. 1988;42(5):787–791.

43. Caruso A, Favilli F, Rotola A, et al. Human herpesvirus-6 modulates RANTES production in primary human endothelial cell cultures. *J Med Virol*. 2003;70(3):451–458.

44. Yoshikawa T, Asano Y, Akimoto S, et al. Latent infection of human herpesvirus 6 in astrocytoma cell line and alteration of cytokine synthesis. *J Med Virol*. 2002;66(4):497–505.

45. He J, McCarthy M, Zhou Y, Chandran B, Wood C. Infection of primary human fetal astrocytes by human herpesvirus 6. *J Virol*. 1996;70(2):1296–1300.

46. Harberts E, Yao K, Wohler JE, et al. Human herpesvirus-6 entry into the central nervous system through the olfactory pathway. *Proc Natl Acad Sci USA*. 2011;108(33): 13734–13739.

47. Challoner PB, Smith KT, Parker JD, et al. Plaque-associated expression of human herpesvirus 6 in multiple sclerosis. *Proc Natl Acad Sci USA*. 1995;92(16):7440–7444.

48. Soldan SS, Berti R, Salem N, et al. Association of human herpes virus 6 (HHV-6) with multiple sclerosis: increased IgM response to HHV-6 early antigen and detection of serum HHV-6 DNA. *Nat Med*. 1997;3(12): 1394–1397.

49. Tejada-Simon MV, Zang YC, Hong J, Rivera VM, Zhang JZ. Cross-reactivity with myelin basic protein and human herpesvirus-6 in multiple sclerosis. *Ann Neurol*. 2003;53(2):189–197.

50. Fotheringham J, Donati D, Akhyani N, et al. Association of human herpesvirus-6B with mesial temporal lobe epilepsy. *PLoS Med*. 2007;4(5):e180.

51. Cermelli C, Berti R, Soldan SS, et al. High frequency of human herpesvirus 6 DNA in multiple sclerosis plaques isolated by laser microdissection. *J Infect Dis*. 2003;187(9):1377–1387.

52. Donati D, Akhyani N, Fogdell-Hahn A, et al. Detection of human herpesvirus-6 in mesial temporal lobe epilepsy surgical brain resections. *Neurology*. 2003;61(10): 1405–1411.

53. Soldan SS, Leist TP, Juhng KN, McFarland HF, Jacobson S. Increased lymphoproliferative response to human herpesvirus type 6A variant in multiple sclerosis patients. *Ann Neurol*. 2000;47(3):306–313.

54. Ortega-Madueno I, Garcia-Montojo M, Dominguez-Mozo MI, et al. Anti-human herpesvirus 6A/B IgG correlates with relapses and progression in multiple sclerosis. *PLoS One*. 2014;9(8):e104836.

55. Mirandola P, Stefan A, Brambilla E, Campadelli-Fiume G, Grimaldi LM. Absence of human herpesvirus 6 and 7 from spinal fluid and serum of multiple sclerosis patients. *Neurology*. 1999;53(6):1367–1368.

56. Mayne M, Krishnan J, Metz L, et al. Infrequent detection of human herpesvirus 6 DNA in peripheral blood mononuclear cells from multiple sclerosis patients. *Ann Neurol*. 1998;44(3):391–394.

57. Kawamura Y, Nakayama A, Kato T, et al. Pathogenic role of human herpesvirus 6B infection in mesial temporal lobe epilepsy. *J Infect Dis*. 2015;212(7):1014–1021.

58. Posson DD. Exanthem subitum (roseola infantum) complicated by prolonged convulsions and hemiplegia. *J Pediatr*. 1949;35(2):235.

59. Friedman JH, Golomb J, Aronson L. Hemiplegia associated with roseola infantum (exanthum subitum). *N Y State J Med*. 1950;50(14):1749–1750.

60. Del Mundo F, Cordero LS, Rodriguez S. Pre-eruptive roseola encephalitis; a report of 2 cases. *J Philipp Med Assoc*. 1955;31(11):622–626.

61. Epstein LG, Shinnar S, Hesdorffer DC, et al. Human herpesvirus 6 and 7 in febrile status epilepticus: the FEBSTAT study. *Epilepsia*. 2012;53(9):1481–1488.

62. Ohsaka M, Houkin K, Takigami M, Koyanagi I. Acute necrotizing encephalopathy associated with human herpesvirus-6 infection. *Pediatr Neurol*. 2006;34(2):160–163.

63. Yoshinari S, Hamano S, Minamitani M, Tanaka M, Eto Y. Human herpesvirus 6 encephalopathy predominantly affecting the frontal lobes. *Pediatr Neurol*. 2007;36(1):13–16.

64. Hoshino A, Saitoh M, Oka A, et al. Epidemiology of acute encephalopathy in Japan, with emphasis on the association of viruses and syndromes. *Brain Dev*. 2012;34(5):337–343.

65. Nagasawa T, Kimura I, Abe Y, Oka A. HHV-6 encephalopathy with cluster of convulsions during eruptive stage. *Pediatr Neurol*. 2007;36(1):61–63.

66. Hatanaka M, Kashiwagi M, Tanabe T, Nakahara H, Ohta K, Tamai H. Overlapping MERS and mild AESD caused by HHV-6 infection. *Brain Dev*. 2015;37(3):334–338.

67. Kawamura Y, Sugata K, Ihira M, et al. Different characteristics of human herpesvirus 6 encephalitis between primary infection and viral reactivation. *J Clin Virol*. 2011;51(1):12–19.

68. Ichiyama T, Ito Y, Kubota M, Yamazaki T, Nakamura K, Furukawa S. Serum and cerebrospinal fluid levels of cytokines in acute encephalopathy associated with human herpesvirus-6 infection. *Brain Dev*. 2009;31(10): 731–738.

69. Kawabe S, Ito Y, Ohta R, et al. Comparison of the levels of human herpesvirus 6 (HHV-6) DNA and cytokines in the cerebrospinal fluid and serum of children with HHV-6 encephalopathy. *J Med Virol*. 2010;82(8):1410–1415.

70. Kawamura Y, Yamazaki Y, Ohashi M, Ihira M, Yoshikawa T. Cytokine and chemokine responses in the blood and cerebrospinal fluid of patients with human herpesvirus 6B-associated acute encephalopathy with biphasic seizures and late reduced diffusion. *J Med Virol*. 2014;86(3):512–518.

71. Kawamura Y, Nakai H, Sugata K, Asano Y, Yoshikawa T. Serum biomarker kinetics with three different courses of HHV-6B encephalitis. *Brain Dev*. 2013;35(6):590–595.

72. Mori Y, Miyamoto T, Nagafuji K, et al. High incidence of human herpes virus 6-associated encephalitis/myelitis following a second unrelated cord blood transplantation. *Biol Blood Marrow Transpl*. 2010;16(11):1596–1602.

73. Noguchi T, Mihara F, Yoshiura T, et al. MR imaging of human herpesvirus-6 encephalopathy after hematopoietic stem cell transplantation in adults. *AJNR Am J Neuroradiol*. 2006;27(10):2191–2195.

74. Zerr DM, Fann JR, Breiger D, et al. HHV-6 reactivation and its effect on delirium and cognitive functioning in hematopoietic cell transplantation recipients. *Blood*. 2011; 117(19):5243–5249.

75. Mookerjee BP, Vogelsang G. Human herpes virus-6 encephalitis after bone marrow transplantation: successful treatment with ganciclovir. *Bone Marrow Transpl*. 1997;20(10):905–906.

76. Cole PD, Stiles J, Boulad F, et al. Successful treatment of human herpesvirus 6 encephalitis in a bone marrow transplant recipient. *Clin Infect Dis*. 1998;27(3):653–654.

77. Bethge W, Beck R, Jahn G, Mundinger P, Kanz L, Einsele H. Successful treatment of human herpesvirus-6 encephalitis after bone marrow transplantation. *Bone Marrow Transpl*. 1999;24(11):1245–1248.

78. Ogata M, Satou T, Kawano R, et al. Plasma HHV-6 viral load-guided preemptive therapy against HHV-6 encephalopathy after allogeneic stem cell transplantation: a prospective evaluation. *Bone Marrow Transpl*. 2008;41(3):279–285.

79. Ishiyama K, Katagiri T, Hoshino T, Yoshida T, Yamaguchi M, Nakao S. Preemptive therapy of human herpesvirus-6 encephalitis with foscarnet sodium for high-risk patients after hematopoietic SCT. *Bone Marrow Transpl*. 2011;46(6):863–869.

80. Ishiyama K, Katagiri T, Ohata K, et al. Safety of pre-engraftment prophylactic foscarnet administration after allogeneic stem cell transplantation. *Transpl Infect Dis*. 2012;14(1):33–39.

81. Ogata M, Satou T, Inoue Y, et al. Foscarnet against human herpesvirus (HHV)-6 reactivation after allo-SCT: breakthrough HHV-6 encephalitis following antiviral prophylaxis. *Bone Marrow Transpl*. 2013;48(2):257–264.

CHAPTER 22

Bacterial, Fungal, and Parasitic Encephalitis

PRATIBHA SINGHI, MD, FIAP, FNAMS •
DR. ARUSHI G. SAINI, MD, DM (PEDIATRIC NEUROLOGY)

INTRODUCTION

Encephalitis/encephalopathy can be caused by several bacteria, fungi, and protozoa, but the relative importance of the organisms varies with the region. Bacterial meningitis caused by *Neisseria meningitides*, *Streptococcus pneumoniae*, and *Haemophilus influenza* remains the best characterized central nervous system (CNS) infections in children[1]; rarely they may have an encephalitic presentation and will not be discussed here. Many uncommon bacterial infections present with encephalitis or encephalopathy to the emergency room and contribute significantly to the burden of acute neurologic disorders, especially in developing countries. We discuss here briefly the encephalitic presentations of few uncommon bacterial, fungal, and parasitic CNS infections in children.

BACTERIAL INFECTIONS

Scrub Typhus

Scrub typhus is a common reemerging, zoonotic, bacterial disease endemic in the "tsutsugamushi triangle" of Southeast Asia, the Asian Pacific rim, and Northern Australia.[2] The disease is caused by a Gram-negative, obligate intracellular bacterium *Orientia tsutsugamushi* of the Rickettsiaceae family. It is transmitted to humans by the bite of larval stage (chigger) of the trombiculid mites, most commonly *Leptotrombidium deliense* during forest activities or agricultural work.[3] It is an emergent public health problem in many developing countries such as India due to rapid urbanization of rural and forested areas. The greatest degree of CNS involvement in rickettsial diseases occurs in Rocky Mountain spotted fever and epidemic typhus, followed by scrub typhus. The meninges are more commonly involved by *O. tsutsugamushi* than by other rickettsial infections, and the overall histologic picture in the CNS has been best described as a meningoencephalitis.[4]

Clinical features

Clinical features emerge after an incubation period of 9–12 days. The initial manifestations are nonspecific and include fever, headache, generalized skin-rash, myalgia, arthralgia, lymphadenopathy, malaise, and cough.[5] In severe forms, pneumonia, myocarditis, azotemia, shock, gastrointestinal bleed, and meningoencephalitis are known to occur. An eschar at the inoculation site (Fig. 22.1) is considered a pathognomonic sign of scrub typhus. It is reported variably in 10%–92% of patients; it may be missed when the bite is in uncommon locations such as scalp, back of pinna, axilla, groin, inguinal region, and genitalia, unless thoroughly searched for.[6] The clinical presentation has been broadly classified into mild disease, respiratory-predominant disease, CNS-predominant disease (meningoencephalitis), or sepsis syndrome.[7] Although several features of CNS involvement such as meningismus, neurologic weakness, seizures, delirium, and

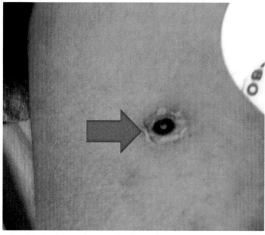

FIG. 22.1 An eschar at the inoculation site is considered a pathognomonic sign of scrub typhus.

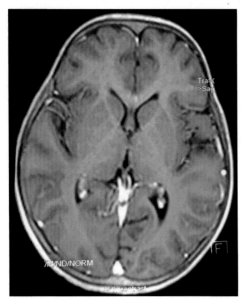

FIG. 22.2 T1-weighted magnetic resonance imaging axial section showing diffuse leptomeningeal enhancement in a child with scrub typhus infection.

coma have been reported, focal neurologic signs are rare. Meningitis or meningoencephalitis has been variably reported in 10%–18% patients in India and 5.7%–13.5% patients in other Southeast Asian regions.[4,8]

Diagnosis

Cerebrospinal fluid (CSF) may show features mimicking viral meningitis; at times there may be associated hypoglycorrhachia that may suggest subacute meningitis, such as tubercular meningitis. There is limited literature on the neuroimaging finding of scrub encephalitis; in most cases the neuroimaging is normal; however, diffuse leptomeningeal enhancement (Fig. 22.2) or cerebral edema along with nonspecific parenchymal hyper intensities may be seen in some cases, indicating primary involvement of the brain parenchyma.

The diagnostic methods available for laboratory confirmation include isolation of the organism in cell-culture, antigen detection by immunohistochemical methods, or the antibodies (IgM) by the indirect immunofluorescence assay and molecular methods.[9] Many of these tests require trained personnel and standardized laboratories. As antigen detection tests have low sensitivity and specificity and require biopsy specimens, serological assays are the mainstay of diagnosis in the clinical setting. The enzyme-linked immunosorbent assay (ELISA) for detection of IgM antibodies in scrub typhus is currently the most

widely used serological test with sensitivity similar to indirect immunofluorescence assay. The Weil-Felix test based on nonspecific agglutination of anti-rickettsial antibodies in patient's serum is a commonly used test in many developing countries although it has low sensitivity and specificity.[10]

Treatment

Supportive treatment includes antipyretics and organ support depending on the nature and extent of organ dysfunction. Commonly used drugs include doxycycline, chloramphenicol, azithromycin, rifampicin, roxithromycin, and tetracycline.[11] Oral doxycycline (100 mg twice a day for 7 days) is the preferred drug in the treatment of scrub typhus and a therapeutic response may be used as a diagnostic test. For critically ill patients or in patients with cytopenias, oral or intravenous azithromycin is a safer choice. Rifampicin may be used when doxycycline resistance is suspected, albeit with caution in tuberculosis-endemic areas.[9]

Future directions

Development of point-of-care diagnostics can help early diagnosis and treatment. Strain-based specific vaccines may help in prevention.

Shigella

Shigellosis or acute bacillary dysentery, caused by the Gram-negative, facultative anaerobic bacilli of the genus *Shigella* in the family Enterobacteriaceae, is a common invasive, gastrointestinal infection that occurs mostly in children living in developing countries.[12] Four species of *Shigella*, i.e., *Shigella dysenteriae*, *Shigella flexneri*, *Shigella boydii*, and *Shigella sonnei*, cause the disease. The morbidity and mortality are predominantly related to the serious neurologic extraintestinal complications that occur in 12%–45% of cases.[13] *S. flexneri*, *S. sonnei*, and *S. dysenteriae* have been implicated in causation of the neurologic syndrome.[14]

The pathogenesis of lethal encephalopathy due to shigellosis or Ekiri syndrome remains unknown. Production of Shiga toxin was initially thought to play a role, but this toxin is only produced by *S. dysenteriae* type 1.[15] Because other *Shigella* species have also been isolated from cases of encephalopathy, production of Shiga toxin may be not be essential for this lethal complication.[16] Acute metabolic derangements such as hypocalcemia and hyponatremia have been associated with the ensuing brain edema or hemorrhage, but no definite causation has been established.

Clinical features

Shigellosis presents with diarrhea and/or dysentery with frequent mucoid bloody stools, tenesmus, and abdominal cramps. *Shigella* encephalopathy is a serious neurologic complication that presents with altered consciousness, seizures (5%–45%), and coma.[17,18] However, febrile seizures may commonly occur even in the absence of associated encephalopathy. A particular form of lethal "toxic encephalopathy" due to shigellosis characterized by rapid onset of neurologic abnormalities with only mild colitis has been named Ekiri syndrome as it was first described in Japan.

Diagnosis

Diagnosis is based on the isolation of organism from fecal specimens and rectal swabs. Sensitive and rapid techniques for detecting *Shigella* based on probes or polymerase chain reaction (PCR) have been developed.

Treatment

Treatment includes rehydration therapy, antimicrobials, and supportive care. An effective oral antimicrobial, most commonly an oral quinolone (ciprofloxacin, levofloxacin, or norfloxacin) for proven or suspected shigellosis, leads to marked symptomatic improvement within 48 h in uncomplicated shigellosis and reduces the average duration of illness. Complications such as seizures, encephalopathy, and intestinal perforation require specific therapy in addition to antimicrobials and fluids.[12] The ability of antibiotic treatment to prevent serious complications due to shigellosis has not been proven. Cerebral edema can result in rapid neurologic deterioration and fatal outcome despite intensive treatment; hence early recognition of encephalopathy and measures to prevent brain edema are important.[18]

Future research

A safe and effective vaccine against shigellosis would be a potentially important public health tool.

Salmonella

Enteric fever due to *Salmonella typhi* and *Salmonella paratyphi A, B, and C* is an acute systemic febrile illness characterized by hectic rise of fever, bacteremia, delirium, and a wide accompaniment of systemic manifestations. Neurologic manifestations constitute an important but often underdiagnosed component of the entire spectrum of salmonella infection, and the encephalitic/encephalopathic presentations are less commonly described.[19] Up to 75% of patients hospitalized with typhoid fever may have neuropsychiatric manifestations, mostly characterized as "stupor," "delirium," or a "confusional state," and have been associated with increased mortality. The exact pathogenesis of these complications is not known. Metabolic disturbances, toxemia, hyperpyrexia, and nonspecific cerebral changes such as edema and hemorrhage have been hypothesized as the possible mechanisms.

Clinical features

The common clinical features include fever, delirium, seizures, meningismus, aggressive behavior, and progressive coma. Typhoid delirium state or "typhoid toxemia" is one of the earliest and perhaps the commonest (42%–57%) neurologic complication in enteric fever but is often underdiagnosed because of its lack of specificity. It is considered to be an acute brain syndrome commonly seen concomitantly with the height of pyrexia and improves quickly following the commencement of treatment.

Treatment

Although antibiotics remain the mainstay of treatment, concurrent high-dose dexamethasone therapy has been suggested to have substantial benefits in reducing mortality and morbidity in patients with typhoid encephalopathy.[20] Prompt recognition of typhoid encephalopathy before availability of culture results is important for initiation of appropriate therapy.

FUNGAL CENTRAL NERVOUS SYSTEM INFECTIONS

Fungal organisms commonly affecting the CNS include yeasts (*Candida*, *Cryptococcus*), molds (*Aspergillus* spp., *Fusarium* spp.), zygomycetes (*Mucor* spp., *Rhizopus* spp.), and dematiaceous fungi (*Pseudallescheria* [Scedosporium] spp.). Certain fungi such as *Coccidioides*, *Histoplasma*, and *Blastomyces* have been reported only from specific geographical areas of the United States and rarely cause disease in children.[21] Conditions that predispose to fungal infections include malnutrition, neutropenia, acquired immunodeficiency syndrome, diabetes mellitus, renal failure, solid-organ transplantation, hematologic and lymphoreticular malignancies, use of immunosuppressive drugs, corticosteroid therapy, and potent broad-spectrum antibiotic therapy.[22,23]

In majority of cases, the primary site of infection is the lungs and rarely skin, followed by hematogenous spread to the CNS. Additionally, *Mucor* and *Aspergillus* may spread contiguously from paranasal sinuses, the ear, or the orbit through tissue planes and blood vessels to the CNS. Less commonly, direct inoculation during head injury or neurosurgic procedures and

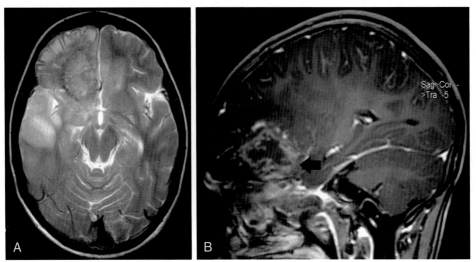

FIG. 22.3 **(A)** T2-weighted axial section and **(B)** T1-weighted contrast enhanced sagittal section of the brain on magnetic resonance imaging showing evolving fungal abscess in the right frontal lobe in a child with fever, altered sensorium, and seizures.

contiguous spread from osteomyelitis of skull or vertebrae can cause CNS infection in children. Once inside the nervous system, the pathology is determined by the size of the fungus. Yeast forms, being small in size, cause a diffuse disease via cerebral microcirculation, while the hyphal forms and molds cause focal lesions with angioinvasion, resulting in hemorrhagic necrosis. The pathologic findings vary from meningitis and meningoencephalitis to microabscesses, focal necrosis, granulomatous inflammation, large abscesses, angioinvasion, and infarction.[23]

Clinical Features

The common clinical syndromes associated with CNS fungal infections in children include altered sensorium with seizures, meningitis/meningoencephalitis, brain abscess (Fig. 22.3), and rhinocerebral syndrome consisting of orbital pain and proptosis, serosanguineous or blackish nasal discharge, and facial edema.[24,25] Although there are no specific clinical features, fungal CNS infections should be suspected in children with underlying predisposing conditions who present with fever and headache with or without CNS signs, orbital pain, or serosanguineous nasal discharge and in all children with a subacute or chronic meningitis syndrome. A combination of fever, headache, lethargy, nausea, vomiting, neck rigidity, impaired consciousness, convulsions, and focal neurologic deficits with or without raised intracranial pressure is often present.[26] Spinal-cord involvement is rare but may occur in the form of

myelopathy, myeloradiculopathy, intramedullary granuloma or epidural abscess, and frank myelitis.[22]

Diagnosis

CSF examination by lumbar puncture and neuroimaging form the mainstay of diagnosis in the correct clinical context in children (Table 22.1).

Treatment

Optimal management of fungal CNS infections includes specific antifungal therapy (Table 22.2) and supportive measures to control raised intracranial pressure, metabolic derangements such as hyperglycemia and acidosis, surgical intervention, management of risk factors, and amelioration of underlying immunosuppression.[22] Clinical guidelines for treatment of fungal infections of the CNS by the Infectious Diseases Society of America are available and should be looked into, in light of local epidemiology and susceptibility testing to guide the choice of appropriate therapy.[37-40]

Outcome and Future Research

The outcome of fungal CNS infections depends primarily on the causative fungus and the underlying immune status of the patient. Mortality is 20%–50% and higher for angioinvasive fungi; outcome of cryptococcal CNS infection is generally better than that of other forms of fungal meningitis. Prophylactic preventive therapy is mainly recommended for immunocompromised children.

TABLE 22.1	
Diagnostic Tests for Common Central Nervous System Infections	
DIAGNOSTIC TESTS FOR FUNGAL INFECTIONS	
Cerebrospinal fluid (CSF) examination	Commonly shows high proteins, low glucose, and mononuclear (lymphocytic or monocytic) leukocytosis (20–500 cells/mm³) Direct microscopic examination of India ink preparation: encapsulated *Cryptococcus* Culture yield is low and takes a long time to grow
Methenamine silver stain	Direct aspirate or biopsy for identification of *Aspergillus* and *Zygomycetes*
Immunologic tests[27]	Latex agglutination test in CSF • Positive in 90% cases of cryptococcal meningitisLateral-flow immunoassay for detection of cryptococcal antigen[28] Complement fixating antibody (CFA) titer of ≥1:32 for coccidioidomycosis Serum or CSF galactomannan assay: aspergillosis[29] 1,3-β-D-glucan assay Specific antibodies in CSF or blood
Other tests	Fungal polymerase chain reaction tests Tissue biopsy for histopathology and culture
Neuroimaging	Nonspecific features: basal involvement, discrete mass lesions with or without contrast enhancement, associated abscess, and areas of infarction. Fungal brain abscesses are T1-hypointense, T2-hyperintense with well-defined contrast enhancement, and high apparent diffusion coefficient. Proton magnetic resonance spectroscopy shows lipids, lactate, amino acids, and trechlose Specific findings: • Cryptococcomas: small enhancing lesions in intraventricular or intraparenchymal locations. Pseudocysts are seen as well-circumscribed, low-density lesions on CT and show CSF attenuation on both T1- and T2-weighted images • Rhinocerebral mucormycosis: opacification of paranasal sinuses, variable mucosal thickening, bony erosion. Intracranial findings include vascular thrombosis and infarct, mycotic emboli, frontal lobe abscess, and involvement of cavernous sinus[30] • *Candida*: multiple punctate enhancing nodules on contrast CT. On MRI, T2-hypointense granuloma and microabscesses and ring enhancement on contrast administration, meningitis, vasculitis, and infarction[30]
DIAGNOSTIC TESTS FOR AMOEBIC MENINGOENCEPHALITIS	
Cerebrospinal fluid	PAM: purulent with neutrophilic predominance, low glucose and elevated proteins, few red blood cells, direct light microscopic examination of a fresh, wet-mount of the CSF to identify motile amoebae, Giemsa or Wright stains for identification of trophozoites GAE: normal to low glucose levels, mild to severely elevated proteins and lymphocytic pleocytosis. Unlike *Naegleria*, *Acanthamoeba*, and *Balamuthia* are generally not found in the CSF
Tissue identification	Wright's, Giemsa, or hematoxylin and eosin stains on fixed preparations Specific histopathologic features Transmission electron microscopy Isoenzyme analyses Polyclonal antibodies by immunofluorescence technique or commercially available ELISA
Culture methods	*Naegleria*, *Acanthamoeba*, and *Sappinia*: by inoculating onto tissue culture cells (Vero or fibroblasts) or nonnutrient agar, in the presence of antibiotics or bacteria such as *Escherichia coli* or *Enterobacter aerogenes*[31] Tissue culture is not a recommended method of diagnosis of *Balamuthia*
Serology (indirect IFA, Western immunoblot analysis, or ELISA)	Nonspecific for *Naegleria* *Acanthamoeba*: high (1:256 to 1:1024) or increasing antibody titers diagnostic[32] *Balamuthia*: diagnostic[33,34]

Continued

TABLE 22.1

Diagnostic Tests for Common Central Nervous System Infections—cont'd

Molecular diagnosis by PCR	PCR and real-time PCR assays for diagnosis and species identification available
Neuroimaging	MRI is the imaging of choice **PAM**: CE-CT shows obliteration of cisterns around the midbrain and the subarachnoid space due to extensive exudates with diffuse meningeal enhancement. MRI features may be nonspecific; vary from normal in early disease to diffuse brain edema, basilar meningeal enhancement, hydrocephalus or infarctions[35] **GAE**: predilection for diencephalon, thalamus, brainstem, and posterior fossa structures, two types of patterns with variable necrotizing angitis and hemorrhages 1. Multifocal pattern: ring-enhancing lesions with perilesional edema seen randomly at the corticomedullary junction 2. Pseudotumor pattern: large solitary masslike lesion *Sappinia*: single reported case with tumourlike mass lesion without an abscess-wall[36]

GAE, granulomatous amebic encephalitis; *PAM*, primary amoebic meningoencephalitis.
Data from Redmond A, Dancer C, Woods ML. Fungal infections of the central nervous system: a review of fungal pathogens and treatment. *Neurol India*. 2007;55:251–259 and Singhi P, Nallaswamy K, Singhi S, eds. *Fungal Infections of the Central Nervous System*. 2nd ed. New York: Oxford University Press; 2016.

TABLE 22.2

Specific Treatment Recommendations for Common Pediatric Fungal and Parasitic Infections of the Central Nervous System

SPECIFIC ANTIFUNGAL AGENTS	

Candidiasis[37]	*First-line treatment*
	    Liposomal amphotericin B (3–5 mg/kg/day) ± flucytosine (100 mg/kg/day in four divided doses) PO
	Second-line treatment
	    Fluconazole (6–12 mg/kg/day) or voriconazole (6 mg/kg/day in two divided doses followed by 3 mg/kg/day) IV for patients unable to tolerate amphotericin B

Cryptococcus[38]	*First-line treatment*
	    Induction: amphotericin B (1 mg/kg/day) IV plus flucytosine (100 mg/kg/day PO in four divided doses)
	    Consolidation: fluconazole (10–12 mg/kg/day in two divided doses) PO
	    Maintenance: fluconazole (6 mg/kg/day) PO
	Second-line treatment
	    Liposomal amphotericin B (5 mg/kg/day) *or* lipid complex (5 mg/kg/day) plus flucytosine (100 mg/kg/day PO in four divided doses)

Aspergillosis[39]	*First-line treatment*
	    Voriconazole (5–7 mg/kg IV every 12 h)
	Second-line treatment
	    Lipid formulations of amphotericin B (3–5 mg/kg/day) IV *or* caspofungin (50 mg/m²/day)

Mucormycosis[40]	*First-line treatment*
	    Amphotericin B 1.5 mg/kg/day IV by continuous infusion *or* lipid formulations of amphotericin B (3–5 mg/kg/day) IV
	Second-line treatment
	    Posaconazole (200 mg PO four times a day or 400 mg PO twice a day) (data for pediatric dosing not available)

PAM[41]	Amphotericin B (intravenous and intrathecal) and rifampin, combined with other agents The optimal duration of therapy is uncertain (9–30 days) ±Miltefosine (<45 kg: 50 mg orally twice daily; >45 kg: 50 mg orally three times daily) OR Triple regimen: low-dose IV amphotericin B, oral rifampicin, and oral ketoconazole[42]

TABLE 22.2 Specific Treatment Recommendations for Common Pediatric Fungal and Parasitic Infections of the Central Nervous System—cont'd	
SPECIFIC ANTIFUNGAL AGENTS	
GAE[41]	Trimethoprim-sulfamethoxazole + rifampin + ketoconazole OR Fluconazole + sulfadiazine + pyrimethamine

Balamuthia[41]	Pentamidine + macrolide (azithromycin or clarithromycin), fluconazole, sulfadiazine, flucytosine, and phenothiazine
	Amebistatic drugs: amphotericin B, sulfadiazine, phenothiazine compounds, pentamidine isethionate, macrolides, and azoles
	Amebicidal drugs: miltefosine, propamidine, and gramicidin S
	Adjunctive therapies
	    Miltefosine-containing treatment regimen
	    Surgical removal of granulomatous mass lesions

Sappinia[43]	The single patient described of encephalitis recovered completely after surgical excision of the tumourlike mass in the brain and treatment using azithromycin, IV pentamidine, itraconazole, and flucytosine

GAE, granulomatous amebic encephalitis; *PAM*, primary amoebic meningoencephalitis.

Future areas of research include development of a cryptococcal vaccine and prophylactic use of azoles to prevent histoplasmosis and coccidioidomycosis in HIV-infected patients.

PARASITIC CENTRAL NERVOUS SYSTEM INFECTIONS

Several parasitic infections can cause CNS infections in children (Table 22.3). Some of them may cause encephalopathy and/or meningoencephalitis. Of these, we briefly discuss cerebral malaria, neurocysticercosis, and amoebic meningoencephalitis. Treatment of these infections varies greatly, from symptomatic management to surgical extraction. Choice of appropriate therapy can be difficult and when possible should be guided by expert opinion.

Cerebral Malaria

Malaria is an important tropical infection caused by four *Plasmodium* species—*Plasmodium vivax, Plasmodium ovale, Plasmodium malariae,* and *Plasmodium. falciparum* and transmitted to humans by the bite of female *Anopheles* mosquitoes. In humans, although the parasite undergoes developmental stages in the liver, it is the erythrocytic cycle that is responsible for disease.[44] Cerebral malaria is a life-threatening neurologic complication and is perhaps the most common cause of nontraumatic encephalopathy in many endemic areas of the world. Most cases of cerebral malaria occur in children with falciparum infection,

TABLE 22.3 Common Parasitic Pathogens Affecting the Central Nervous System (CNS)	
PROTOZOAN DISEASES	
Plasmodium falciparum	Cerebral malaria
Toxoplasma gondii	Associated with congenital defects and AIDS
Entamoeba histolytica	Rare invasion of the brain
Free-living amoeba • Naegleria fowleri (freshwater) • Acanthamoeba species (soil and water) • Balamuthia mandrillaris (soil)	• Fulminant acute primary amoebic meningoencephalitis • Chronic granulomatous amebic encephalitis; skin or lung lesions; amebic keratitis • Subacute or chronic granulomatous amebic encephalitis; skin or lung lesions
African trypanosomes	African sleeping sickness
HELMINTHS AFFECTING THE CNS	
Taenia solium (pork tapeworm)	Cysticercosis: muscle and brain
Echinococcus species	Hydatid disease: liver (75%) and lungs (15%), rarely brain
Schistosoma species	Schistosomiasis of liver and bladder, rarely CNS

rarely with other species. The sequestration of red cells containing mature forms of the parasite (trophozoites and meronts) in the microvasculature in organs, especially the brain, excessive proinflammatory cytokine production,[45] microvascular thrombosis,[46] loss of endothelial barrier function,[47] and endothelial dysregulation[48] are thought to cause the major complication of falciparum malaria including cerebral malaria.[49]

Clinical features

Cerebral malaria is characterized by fever, headache, irritability, restlessness, agitation, seizures, vomiting, meningismus, drowsiness, and rapid-onset coma in untreated patients. In endemic areas, any child presenting with fever and altered sensorium should be investigated and treated for cerebral malaria. The presence of distinctive retinopathy including retinal hemorrhages, retinal whitening, blood vessel color changes, and/or papilledema helps differentiate cerebral malaria from other causes of encephalopathy.[50] Other systemic manifestations include hepatosplenomegaly, gastrointestinal bleeding, anemia, severe acidosis, hypoglycemia, shock, and multiorgan dysfunction.

Diagnosis

Diagnosis of cerebral malaria requires demonstration of asexual form of *P. falciparum* in thick and thin peripheral blood smears, stained by Giemsa stain. CSF examination should be done to exclude other causes of febrile encephalopathy. The rapid diagnostic tests (antigen detection test) such as *P. falciparum* histidine rich protein 2 and lactate dehydrogenase are helpful for rapid detection at the bedside in the emergency area. Additionally, m-RNA-based or DNA-based PCRs may be helpful in species identification but take time and are not routinely available.[51] Neuroimaging may be normal or may show diffuse cerebral edema, cortical or subcortical infarcts in watershed zone, or rarely bilateral thalamic necrosis.

Treatment

Management includes specific antimalarial therapy, supportive treatment for multiorgan dysfunction, and management of associated complications particularly hypoglycemia, anemia, and fluid balance. Cerebral malaria is a neurologic emergency requiring urgent intervention and may need empirical antimalarial drugs in endemic areas. Specific parenteral antimalarial treatment is the only intervention that unequivocally affects the outcome of cerebral malaria.[44] Parenteral

artemisinin derivatives or quinine are drugs of choice for treatment of severe malaria including cerebral malaria.[52] Artesunate (2.4 mg/kg, repeated after 8 h as a loading dose) is preferred over artemether (3.2 mg/kg followed by 1.6 mg/kg/day for 5 days or until oral acceptance) because it can be administered both intravenously and intramuscularly. Both drugs are advantageous over quinidine because of their low toxicity. In patients with hyperparasitemia (>20%), exchange transfusion is recommended. Corticosteroids are not beneficial. Intensive care management, artificial ventilation, hemofiltration, or hemodialysis may significantly improve the outcome.

Cysticercal Encephalitis

Neurocysticercosis caused by the larval tapeworm *Taenia solium* is a major public health problem, in resource-poor countries, but is also seen in developed countries.[53,54] It is the single most common cause of epilepsy in endemic regions of the world including most of South and Central America, India, Southeast Asia, China, and sub-Saharan Africa. Hospital-based studies from North India have shown neurocysticercosis as the cause in >50% of children with partial seizures.[55] Humans get neurocysticercosis by ingestion of *T. solium* eggs, via intake of contaminated food, through infected food handlers, or by autoinfection through fecal-oral route in the carriers. The eggs hatch in the human intestine and the larvae penetrate the intestinal mucosa and migrate through the body. They commonly lodge in the nervous system, skeletal muscles, subcutaneous tissues, and the eyes to form mature cysts. Cysticercal encephalitis is a distinct and rare presentation of neurocysticercosis because of a severe inflammatory response around the dying cysts.

Clinical features

Children commonly present with headache, severe acute raised intracranial pressure, seizures, papilledema, hyperreflexia, and altered sensorium due to the massive cyst burden and diffuse cerebral edema. Encephalitis due to neurocysticercosis should be included in differential diagnosis of acute encephalitic cases especially in endemic countries.[54]

Diagnosis

MRI shows the classic "starry-sky" pattern (Fig. 22.4) due to innumerable cysts with extensive edema. Positive CSF-ELISA for detection of anticysticercal antibodies or cysticercal antigens may provide corroborative evidence. Eyes should be thoroughly examined for intraocular dissemination of neurocysticercosis. The

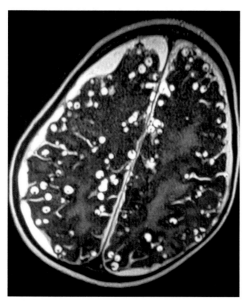

FIG. 22.4 T2-weighted magnetic resonance imaging axial sections showing the classic "starry-sky" pattern due to innumerable cysts with scolices.

disease is often mistaken for tubercular meningitis with tuberculomas and children often receive antitubercular therapy before hospitalization.

Treatment

Use of corticosteroids is the mainstay of management in children with cysticercal encephalitis for the reduction of cerebral edema and raised intracranial pressure. Treatment with albendazole (15 mg/kg/day in two to three divided doses for 28 days) for cyst destruction may be considered once the acute inflammatory state has subsided and intra-ocular cysticercosis has been excluded. Response is usually monitored by repeat neuroimaging at 3–6 months posttreatment. Some cases require repeated administration of steroids. Prognosis of these patients remains poor.

Amoebic Meningoencephalitis

Free-living amoebae are mitochondria-bearing, aerobic, single-celled organisms that are ubiquitous, environmental protozoa found in freshwater lakes, thermally polluted waters, sediments, thermal springs, swimming pools, air conditioning vents, and domestic water supplies.[56] Four genera are associated with human disease: *Naegleria (only Naegleria fowleri)*, *Acanthamoeba (several species)*, *Balamuthia (only Balamuthia mandrillaris)*, *Sappinia (only Sappinia pedata)*. Amoebic meningoencephalitis refers to the infection of the brain parenchyma and meninges caused by these organisms. Primary amoebic meningoencephalitis

(PAM) is caused by *N. fowleri* that usually occurs during the summer months with high ambient temperatures. Granulomatous amebic encephalitis (GAE) caused by *Acanthamoeba* spp. and *B. mandrillaris* occurs round the year with no seasonal variation. Majority of CNS infections by free-living amoebae are fatal.

Trophozoites of *N. fowleri* (commonly referred to as the "brain-eating amoeba") enter the host via the nasal passage, attach to the olfactory mucosa, and reach the olfactory bulbs of the brain via the olfactory nerves in approximately 72 h postinoculation.[57] They cause fulminating hemorrhagic necrotizing meningoencephalitis with fibrinopurulent leptomeningeal reaction leading to death within 7–10 days. *Acanthamoeba* enters the body through nasal passage or skin-breaks and reaches the lungs and brain by hematogenous dissemination. It causes granuloma formation with multinucleated giant cells and severe, fibrinoid, necrotizing angitis in the brain.[57] The source and mode of infection of *Balamuthia* and *Sappinia* are less characterized, with possible hematogenous spread to the brain.[36,43]

Clinical features

Clinical features in PAM resemble bacterial meningoencephalitis with sudden-onset rhinitis, change in taste or smell, acute severe headache, fever, nausea, vomiting, irritability, seizures, diplopia, anosmia, meningeal signs, and raised intracranial pressure. Course is progressive with death within 7–10 days.[31] GAE presents as a chronic CNS infection with prolonged headaches, low-grade fever and seizures, focal CNS deficits, cranial nerve palsies, meningismus, and encephalopathy followed by coma. *Balamuthia* infection may be additionally associated with previous granulomatous lesions of the skin. *Sappinia* infection may produce acute-onset nausea, vomiting, bifrontal headache, photophobia, and visual blurring following a sinus infection, followed by rapid alteration in sensorium.[36] Common differential diagnoses include acute bacterial or viral meningoencephalitis or cerebral malaria in PAM and other chronic CNS infections such as tuberculosis, toxoplasmosis, NCC, bacterial leptomeningitis, fungal infections, and brain tumors in GAE.[57,58]

Diagnosis

A high degree of clinical suspicion, history of contact with water and soil habitats of the amoebae, and familiarity of the pathologist with the appearance of amoebae in tissue samples form the cornerstone of diagnosis of amoebic meningoencephalitis in children (Table 22.1). PAM should be considered in any patient presenting as pyogenic meningitis/encephalitis in whom no organisms are identified.

Treatment

PAM is a serious CNS infection with very few survivors. There are no standard treatment regimens or guidelines.[59] The optimal approach to treatment in *Acanthamoeba* infection is uncertain as these organisms are not inhibited in vitro by amphotericin B. No specific treatment is recommended for *Balamuthia* infection.

Careful maintenance of swimming pools and adequate chlorination (1–2 ppm), blowing the nose after swimming or using nose-plugs, and avoidance of swimming in water bodies and hot springs epidemiologically associated with the disease may reduce the risk of meningoencephalitis. The organism does not spread by drinking contaminated water. Prevention of *Acanthamoeba* can be done by proper care and use of contact lenses and periodic inspection of water supplies and ventilation units. Areas of future research include evaluation of role of azithromycin in humans for PAM and enhancement of early diagnosis with universal availability of rapid ELISA-based assay for CSF testing.[60]

REFERENCES

1. Murray PR, Masur H. Current approaches to the diagnosis of bacterial and fungal bloodstream infections in the intensive care unit. *Crit Care Med.* 2012;40:3277–3282.
2. Kelly DJ, Fuerst PA, Ching WM, Richards AL. Scrub typhus: the geographic distribution of phenotypic and genotypic variants of *Orientia tsutsugamushi*. *Clin Infect Dis.* 2009;48(suppl 3):S203–S230.
3. Lai CH, Huang CK, Chen YH, et al. Epidemiology of acute Q fever, scrub typhus, and murine typhus, and identification of their clinical characteristics compared to patients with acute febrile illness in Southern Taiwan. *J Formos Med Assoc.* 2009;108:367–376.
4. Drevets DA, Leenen PJ, Greenfield RA. Invasion of the central nervous system by intracellular bacteria. *Clin Microbiol Rev.* 2004;17:323–347.
5. Basnyat B, Belbase RH, Zimmerman MD, Woods CW, Reller LB, Murdoch DR. Clinical features of scrub typhus. *Clin Infect Dis.* 2006;42:1505–1506.
6. Kim DM, Won KJ, Park CY, et al. Distribution of eschars on the body of scrub typhus patients: a prospective study. *Am J Trop Med Hyg.* 2007;76:806–809.
7. Chrispal A, Boorugu H, Gopinath KG, et al. Scrub typhus: an unrecognized threat in South India – clinical profile and predictors of mortality. *Trop Doct.* 2010;40:129–133.
8. Mahajan SK, Rolain JM, Kashyap R, et al. Scrub typhus in Himalayas. *Emerg Infect Dis.* 2006;12:1590–1592.
9. Peter JV, Sudarsan TI, Prakash JA, Varghese GM. Severe scrub typhus infection: clinical features, diagnostic challenges and management. *World J Crit Care Med.* 2015;4:244–250.
10. Mahajan SK, Kashyap R, Kanga A, Sharma V, Prasher BS, Pal LS. Relevance of Weil-Felix test in diagnosis of scrub typhus in India. *J Assoc Phys India.* 2006;54:619–621.
11. Fang Y, Huang Z, Tu C, Zhang L, Ye D, Zhu BP. Meta-analysis of drug treatment for scrub typhus in Asia. *Intern Med.* 2012;51:2313–2320.
12. Niyogi SK. Shigellosis. *J Microbiol.* 2005;43:133–143.
13. Ashkenazi S, Dinari G, Weitz R, Nitzan M. Convulsions in shigellosis. Evaluation of possible risk factors. *Am J Dis Child.* 1983;137:985–987.
14. Pourakbari B, Mamishi S, Mashoori N, et al. Frequency and antimicrobial susceptibility of Shigella species isolated in Children Medical Center Hospital, Tehran, Iran, 2001-2006. *Braz J Infect Dis.* 2010;14:153–157.
15. Yuhas Y, Weizman A, Dinari G, Ashkenazi S. An animal model for the study of neurotoxicity of bacterial products and application of the model to demonstrate that Shiga toxin and lipopolysaccharide cooperate in inducing neurologic disorders. *J Infect Dis.* 1995;171:1244–1249.
16. Ashkenazi S, Cleary KR, Pickering LK, Murray BE, Cleary TG. The association of Shiga toxin and other cytotoxins with the neurologic manifestations of shigellosis. *J Infect Dis.* 1990;161:961–965.
17. Goren A, Freier S, Passwell JH. Lethal toxic encephalopathy due to childhood shigellosis in a developed country. *Pediatrics.* 1992;89:1189–1193.
18. Pourakbari B, Mamishi S, Kohan L, et al. Lethal toxic encephalopathy due to childhood shigellosis or Ekiri syndrome. *J Microbiol Immunol Infect.* 2012;45:147–150.
19. Huang DB, DuPont HL. Problem pathogens: extra-intestinal complications of *Salmonella enterica* serotype Typhi infection. *Lancet Infect Dis.* 2005;5:341–348.
20. Chisti MJ, Bardhan PK, Huq S, et al. High-dose intravenous dexamethasone in the management of diarrheal patients with enteric fever and encephalopathy. *Southeast Asian J Trop Med Public Health.* 2009;40:1065–1073.
21. Redmond A, Dancer C, Woods ML. Fungal infections of the central nervous system: a review of fungal pathogens and treatment. *Neurol India.* 2007;55:251–259.
22. Singhi P, Nallaswamy K, Singhi S, eds. *Fungal Infections of the Central Nervous System.* 2nd ed. New York: Oxford University Press; 2016.
23. Singhi S, ed. *Fungal Infections.* 1st ed. London: Mac Keith Press; 2014.
24. Teive H, Carsten AL, Iwamoto FM, et al. Fungal encephalitis following bone marrow transplantation: clinical findings and prognosis. *J Postgrad Med.* 2008;54:203–205.
25. Zaoutis TE, Roilides E, Chiou CC, et al. Zygomycosis in children: a systematic review and analysis of reported cases. *Pediatr Infect Dis J.* 2007;26:723–727.
26. Gumbo T, Chemaly RF, Isada CM, Hall GS, Gordon SM. Late complications of Candida (Torulopsis) glabrata fungemia: description of a phenomenon. *Scand J Infect Dis.* 2002;34:817–818.
27. Likasitwattanakul S, Poneprasert B, Sirisanthana V. Cryptococcosis in HIV-infected children. *Southeast Asian J Trop Med Public Health.* 2004;35:935–939.

28. Lindsley MD, Mekha N, Baggett HC, et al. Evaluation of a newly developed lateral flow immunoassay for the diagnosis of cryptococcosis. *Clin Infect Dis*. 2011;53: 321–325.

29. Wheat LJ. Rapid diagnosis of invasive aspergillosis by antigen detection. *Transpl Infect Dis*. 2003;5:158–166.

30. Jain KK, Mittal SK, Kumar S, Gupta RK. Imaging features of central nervous system fungal infections. *Neurol India*. 2007;55:241–250.

31. Visvesvara GS, Booton GC, Kelley DJ, et al. In vitro culture, serologic and molecular analysis of *Acanthamoeba* isolated from the liver of a keel-billed toucan (*Ramphastos sulfuratus*). *Vet Parasitol*. 2007;143:74–78.

32. Brindley N, Matin A, Khan NA. *Acanthamoeba castellanii*: high antibody prevalence in racially and ethnically diverse populations. *Exp Parasitol*. 2009;121:254–256.

33. Schuster FL, Honarmand S, Visvesvara GS, Glaser CA. Detection of antibodies against free-living amoebae *Balamuthia mandrillaris* and *Acanthamoeba* species in a population of patients with encephalitis. *Clin Infect Dis*. 2006;42:1260–1265.

34. Kiderlen AF, Radam E, Tata PS. Assessment of *Balamuthia mandrillaris*-specific serum antibody concentrations by flow cytometry. *Parasitol Res*. 2009;104:663–670.

35. Singh P, Kochhar R, Vashishta RK, et al. Amebic meningoencephalitis: spectrum of imaging findings. *AJNR Am J Neuroradiol*. 2006;27:1217–1221.

36. Gelman BB, Rauf SJ, Nader R, et al. Amoebic encephalitis due to *Sappinia diploidea*. *JAMA*. 2001;285:2450–2451.

37. Pappas PG, Kauffman CA, Andes D, et al. Clinical practice guidelines for the management of candidiasis: 2009 update by the Infectious Diseases Society of America. *Clin Infect Dis*. 2009;48:503–535.

38. Perfect JR, Dismukes WE, Dromer F, et al. Clinical practice guidelines for the management of cryptococcal disease: 2010 update by the Infectious Diseases Society of America. *Clin Infect Dis*. 2010;50:291–322.

39. Walsh R, Ortiz J, Foster P, Palma-Vargas J, Rosenblatt S, Wright F. Fungal and mycobacterial infections after Campath (alemtuzumab) induction for renal transplantation. *Transpl Infect Dis*. 2008;10:236–239.

40. Spellberg B, Walsh TJ, Kontoyiannis DP, Edwards Jr J, Ibrahim AS. Recent advances in the management of mucormycosis: from bench to bedside. *Clin Infect Dis*. 2009;48:1743–1751.

41. Tunkel AR, Glaser CA, Bloch KC, et al. The management of encephalitis: clinical practice guidelines by the Infectious Diseases Society of America. *Clin Infect Dis*. 2008;47: 303–327.

42. Poungvarin N, Jariya P. The fifth nonlethal case of primary amoebic meningoencephalitis. *J Med Assoc Thail*. 1991;74:112–115.

43. Gelman BB, Popov V, Chaljub G, et al. Neuropathological and ultrastructural features of amebic encephalitis caused by *Sappinia diploidea*. *J Neuropathol Exp Neurol*. 2003;62:990–998.

44. Newton CR, Hien TT, White N. Cerebral malaria. *J Neurol Neurosurg Psychiatry*. 2000;69:433–441.

45. Clark IA, Rockett KA. Sequestration, cytokines, and malaria pathology. *Int J Parasitol*. 1994;24:165–166.

46. Moxon CA, Heyderman RS, Wassmer SC. Dysregulation of coagulation in cerebral malaria. *Mol Biochem Parasitol*. 2009;166:99–108.

47. Dorovini-Zis K, Schmidt K, Huynh H, et al. The neuropathology of fatal cerebral malaria in malawian children. *Am J Pathol*. 2011;178:2146–2158.

48. Wassmer SC, Moxon CA, Taylor T, Grau GE, Molyneux ME, Craig AG. Vascular endothelial cells cultured from patients with cerebral or uncomplicated malaria exhibit differential reactivity to TNF. *Cell Microbiol*. 2011;13:198–209.

49. White NJ, Ho M. The pathophysiology of malaria. *Adv Parasitol*. 1992;31:83–173.

50. Kariuki SM, Newton CR. Retinopathy, histidine-rich protein-2 and perfusion pressure in cerebral malaria. *Brain*. 2014;137:e298.

51. Kariuki SM, Gitau E, Gwer S, et al. Value of *Plasmodium falciparum* histidine-rich protein 2 level and malaria retinopathy in distinguishing cerebral malaria from other acute encephalopathies in Kenyan children. *J Infect Dis*. 2014;209:600–609.

52. White NJ, Pukrittayakamee S, Hien TT, Faiz MA, Mokuolu OA, Dondorp AM. Malaria. *Lancet*. 2014;383:723–735.

53. Singhi P, Ray M, Singhi S, Khandelwal N. Clinical spectrum of 500 children with neurocysticercosis and response to albendazole therapy. *J Child Neurol*. 2000;15:207–213.

54. Singhi P. Neurocysticercosis. *Ther Adv Neurol Disord*. 2011;4:67–81.

55. Singhi P, Singhi S. Neurocysticercosis in children. *J Child Neurol*. 2004;19:482–492.

56. Shoff ME, Rogerson A, Kessler K, Schatz S, Seal DV. Prevalence of *Acanthamoeba* and other naked amoebae in South Florida domestic water. *J Water Health*. 2008;6:99–104.

57. Visvesvara G, Maguire J. Pathogenic and Opportunistic Free-Living Amebas. *Acanthamoeba spp., Balamuthia mandrillaris, Naegleria fowleri, and Sappinia diploidea*. Churchill Livingstone; 2006.

58. Visvesvara GS, Moura H, Schuster FL. Pathogenic and opportunistic free-living amoebae: *Acanthamoeba* spp., *Balamuthia mandrillaris*, *Naegleria fowleri*, and *Sappinia diploidea*. *FEMS Immunol Med Microbiol*. 2007;50:1–26.

59. Martinez AJ, Visvesvara GS. Free-living, amphizoic and opportunistic amebas. *Brain Pathol*. 1997;7:583–598.

60. Schuster FL, Visvesvara GS. Opportunistic amoebae: challenges in prophylaxis and treatment. *Drug Resist Updat*. 2004;7:41–51.

CHAPTER 23

Febrile Infection–Related Epilepsy Syndrome

NICOLA SPECCHIO, MD, PHD • NICOLA PIETRAFUSA, MD

INTRODUCTION

Febrile infection–related epilepsy syndrome (FIRES) is a catastrophic epileptic encephalopathy with refractory status epilepticus (SE) in developmentally normal children[1] without a diagnostic biologic marker.

In 1986 Awaya and Fukuyama first described an encephalitis-like entity occurring in previously normal children.[2]

Since then, multiple cases and case series have been reported in the literature of children and adults who developed refractory SE due to an unidentified agent or immune encephalopathy.[1,3–11]

FIRES is characterized by the development of seizures in healthy children few days after a short febrile illness[6] that rapidly exacerbated into an SE or a cluster of seizures, followed by a chronic drug-resistant epilepsy and cognitive function deficit.[4,6]

Several different names have been proposed in this condition when reporting series of children and adults despite their similarities. Some of them emphasized the characteristics of acute refractory partial epilepsy, others, the presumed pathogenesis: "acute encephalitis with refractory, repetitive partial seizures" (AERRPS),[8] "severe refractory status epilepticus due to presumed encephalitis,"[12] "idiopathic catastrophic epileptic encephalopathy,"[3] "new-onset refractory status epilepticus" (NORSE),[13] "devastating epileptic encephalopathy in school-aged children" (DESC),[4] and FIRES.[1]

However, some differences exist among these entities: AERRPS is associated with higher and longer fever unlike FIRES.[8] NORSE occurs in young adults, not always with a preceding febrile illness, has a clear female predominance, and responds to immunotherapy.[14]

Nabbout suggested the concept of "acute encephalopathy with inflammation-mediated status epilepticus" to put together FIRES (and AERRPS, DESC, NORSE) with "idiopathic hemiconvulsion-hemiplegia and epilepsy" in infants (AEIMSE) based on their similar characteristics.[15]

The exact pathogenesis of this clinical syndrome remains unclear. FIRES is likely to represent an immune-inflammatory-mediated epileptic encephalopathy.[16]

PATHOGENESIS OF FEBRILE INFECTION–RELATED EPILEPSY SYNDROME

Because most of the patients presented with seizures immediately following a febrile episode, an autoimmune mechanism has been considered. Different antibodies have been investigated in patients with FIRES with negative results; therefore, up to now there is no evidence to support that autoantibodies are the etiology of FIRES. Furthermore, poor response to immunotherapy has been reported.[11]

FIRES is likely to represent an immune-inflammatory-mediated epileptic encephalopathy rather than an autoimmune process.[16]

The release of inflammatory molecules (cytokines and other effector molecules released by brain cells) following systemic infection might trigger the activation of innate immunity mechanisms in glial cells, neurons, and cells of the blood-brain barrier activating a neuroinflammatory cascade, which plays a key role in epileptogenesis.[17–20]

An imbalance between proinflammatory and anti-inflammatory molecules can explain the delay between the insult (e.g., infection) that give rise to neuroinflammation and the onset of the disease. Epileptic activity itself might contribute to perpetuate innate immunity processes, activating the process of neuroinflammation that might bring to hyperexcitability in seizure-exposed brain areas and generate a prolonged condition of ongoing seizures. Neuroinflammation might lower the seizures threshold through modifications of brain excitability including posttranslational changes in neuronal voltage-gated and receptor-coupled ion channels, alteration of glutamate and GABA release as well as their cellular reuptake, modifications in glutamate and GABA receptor trafficking at neuronal membranes, and deficient buffering capacity of astrocytes for rapid removal of extracellular K+ and glutamate.[16]

CLINICAL PRESENTATION

FIRES cases seem to be sporadic and very rare: van Baalen et al. (2010) estimated the annual incidence in children and adolescents by a prospective hospital-based German-wide surveillance as 1 in 1,000,000.[1] The real incidence and prevalence of FIRES could be higher, because a certain amount of patients with FIRES could be misdiagnosed as encephalitis because of their similar features.

No familial cases have been published to date. There is no ethnic predisposition, but a male predominance (4:3 male/female) has been reported.[10,16]

FIRES is not observed in infancy and mostly occurs in school age.[21] In Kramer et al. (2011), the largest case series, median age at the onset of FIRES was 8 years (range 2–17 years).[10]

The syndrome almost invariably begins with a febrile illness, most commonly a minor upper respiratory tract infection or a gastroenteritis[10]; fever during the infectious illness is sometimes low grade or absent (with a median duration of 4 days): in about half of the patients it disappeared at the time of first seizures occurrence[1–10] in contrast to febrile seizures and febrile status epilepticus. The clinical course of this disorder is typically biphasic with an initial acute catastrophic phase followed by a chronic refractory epilepsy phase.

After the onset, seizures rapidly became frequent or exacerbated into SE showing resistant to treatment with a variety of antiepileptic drugs (AEDs). It is not uncommon for children with FIRES to have hundreds of seizures a day during the acute phase. Seizures are focal (simple motor with facial twitching or complex partial seizures with lateral deviation of the head, chewing movements, and some autonomous features, suggesting a mesial temporal lobe involvement) with a strong tendency to the secondary generalization. In addition, myoclonic seizures of facial and orobuccal muscles have been reported. Consciousness is decreased, including the interictal period. The duration of this acute phase is variable. It can last from a few days to several months. Usually no patient had neurologic features other than seizures during the acute phase of illness.[1,3,8,10,11,13,15]

INSTRUMENTAL AND LABORATORY INVESTIGATION

Ictal and interictal electroencephalography (EEG) studies revealed focal, generalized or more frequently bilateral, multifocal pattern, and the location of the epileptic foci was predominantly frontotemporal.[10] Background focal or generalized slowing is common.

The EEG between seizures shows slow waves resembling an "encephalitis" pattern.[1,4]

Brain MRI (magnetic resonance imaging) performed in the first weeks of the diseases is normal in most cases. Forty-four patients in the series reported by Kramer showed abnormalities including signal hyperintensities in hippocampi or in the peri-insular region or both. Leptomeningeal or ependymal enhancement was seen.[10] Basal ganglia also could be involved during the acute phase.[22] A second follow-up brain MRI performed later in the disease revealed generalized atrophy in half of patients; signal hyperintensity located bilaterally in the hippocampal region persisted in a minority of them.[10] Timing of the neuroimaging follow-up, however, was not documented; bilateral hippocampal atrophy and sclerosis was also documented.[9]

The chronologic evolution of MRI findings might help to estimate prognosis. In Rivas-Coppola et al. (2016), consistent and persistent hippocampal signal abnormality has been reported within a week after the onset of the illness, with rapid evolution to hippocampal sclerosis and generalized cerebral brain atrophy in 3–4 weeks. Evolution of brain atrophy from mild to severe and development of hippocampal sclerosis occurred in most patients with FIRES a month after seizure onset. Different stages of brain atrophy were appreciated over the next 6–12 months. Hippocampal sclerosis, therefore, occurred in a majority of patients 1 month after seizure onset, resulting in reduced cognitive level and chronic epilepsy. Follow-up MRI performed up to 2 years after disease onset showed significant progression of brain atrophy; cerebellar atrophy was appreciated during the chronic phase, giving rise to a rapid and early neuronal death during the acute phase involving not only the brain but also the cerebellum.[22] Meletti et al. reported six patients with reversible bilateral claustrum MRI hyperintensity on T2-weighted sequences, without restricted diffusion, time-related with SE, supporting a role of the claustrum in postfebrile de novo SE.[23] Positron emission tomography scan identified a very large area of hypometabolism involving bilaterally orbitofrontal and temporoparietal regions, with a good correspondence to the specific cognitive troubles that each child exhibited.[24]

As this is a not yet etiologically defined condition, no specific laboratory test is available to prove the diagnosis.

Cerebrospinal fluid (CSF) was normal or show a pleocytosis (57% of patients in Kramer), usually mild in the initial sample, with normal protein concentration and no oligoclonal bands.[10,16]

In Kramer et al. (2011), investigation for infectious agents (including polymerase chain reaction for virus on CSF), metabolic and immunologic evaluation were negative in all patients. Furthermore, autoantibody tests were performed in 27 patients (35%); the search for autoantibodies revealed the following positive findings: oligoclonal bands in the CSF of 4 of 12 patients, anti-GAD antibodies in 2 of 5 patients, and anti-GluR3 antibodies in 1 of 4 patients.[10]

Genes involved in epilepsy with fever sensitivity (SCN1A, PCDH19) or in refractory status epilepticus did not show any mutation or rare copy number variations.[25]

DIAGNOSIS AND DIFFERENTIAL DIAGNOSES

The diagnosis is usually made on clinical findings in children who develop superrefractory SE, "in temporal association with a febrile illness", after most causes of SE have been carefully excluded.

Patients must undergo extensive investigations to exclude infectious, toxic, metabolic, or genetic causes that may be specifically treatable.[26]

Brain MRI is required to rule out conditions with a characteristic appearance on imaging (e.g., high T2 or FLAIR signal in encephalitis, cortical dysplasia). EEG and continuous EEG monitoring are often required to detect seizures, because they frequently increase during the course of the disease (e.g., to recognize nonconvulsive status), and to monitor therapeutic response.[27]

CSF studies and blood tests should be performed to rule out infectious and known inflammatory (including oligoclonal bands) and autoimmune conditions (limbic encephalitis and other neuronal antibody-associated epileptic encephalopathies, e.g., with VGKC antibodies, AMPA, and GABA-B or NMDA receptor antibodies). In selected cases, additional tests can be performed to identify other rare causes of SE, such as genetic (POLG1, SCN1A, and PCDH19) or metabolic disorders (e.g., biotin-responsive basal ganglia disease, citrullinemia).[16]

TREATMENT (SEE TABLE 23.1)

There is currently no specific therapy for FIRES, and studies are urgently needed to evaluate the best therapeutic options. The traditional antiseizure management has very limited success in patients with FIRES.[16]

Barbiturates at high doses are the only anticonvulsants able to reduce seizure activity in the acute phase[9]; however, this success is limited because seizures tend to recur and there has been no evidence that long-term outcomes are improved.

There have been reports of a dramatic response to the ketogenic diet (KD) in some children with FIRES, but this needs to be confirmed in controlled studies. Following a first attempt with favorable outcome[4] and the impressive improvement for patients with focal epilepsy,[28] Nabbout et al. (2010) reported the data of nine patients with FIRES (with SE refractory to conventional antiepileptic treatment) who received a 4:1 ratio of fat to combined protein and carbohydrate KD: in seven patients KD was effective within 2–4 days following the onset of ketonuria and 4–6 days following the onset of the diet.[7] KD could also be used for its antiinflammatory mechanism in the context of FIRES.[29] KD should be considered early in the course of treatment, perhaps even as first-line therapy.

Cannabidiol is one such potential alternative therapy. In a recent paper, after starting cannabidiol, 6 of 7 patients with FIRES improved in frequency and duration of seizures.[30]

Given the putative causal role of inflammation in FIRES, different approaches have been tried. First-line immunotherapy (steroids and immunoglobulins, plasma exchange) and second-line immunotherapy (e.g., tacrolimus, rituximab, cyclophosphamide) in patients with FIRES[31,32] were reported with inconstant results.

Burst suppression coma (BCS) should be considered with caution in FIRES because it is associated with a worse cognitive outcome.[33]

During the chronic epilepsy most AEDs are ineffective and there are no clear-cut evidences for a superiority of one drug. However, KD, clobazam, phenobarbital, and cannabidiol could be used as first-line therapy.

PROGNOSIS

In Kramer et al., the largest series of patients with FIRES, the outcome was predominantly poor.[10]

Approximately 10% died during the acute phase because of intensive care complications. Ninety-three percent of survivors developed refractory epilepsy.

Regarding neuropsychological outcome, only one-third of the surviving patients had normal or borderline cognitive level (with or without behavioral and learning difficulties), 14% had mild mental retardation, 24% had

TABLE 23.1
Immunotherapies in Febrile Infection–Related Epilepsy Syndrome (FIRES) Series

Author	No. of Patients	Age	Therapy	Efficacy	Outcome
Baxter et al.[3]	6	0–6y	Steroids (5), IVIG (2)	No response	NA
Kramer et al.[34]	7	2.5–15y	IVIG (7), steroids (5)	Seizures gradually disappeared in all patients with no clear correlation with any treatment	2 mild delay, 1 normal, 1 ADHD, 2 still in rehabilitation
Mikaeloff et al.[4]	14	4–11y	Steroids (7), KD (2)	Steroids: 1/7 transient KD: 1/2 seizure cessation	All children had cognitive major sequelae with frontotemporal impairment
Villeneuve et al.[28]	2	8–10y	KD (2)	Effective	NA
Van Baalen et al.[1]	22	3–15y	IVIG (6), steroids (8), plasmapheresis (1)	Poor efficacy	5pts in vegetative state, 2 pts with refractory epilepsy, 1 dead
Nabbout et al.[7]	10	4.5–8.2y	10pts KD	7/10 responders	After few months, isolated weekly seizures
Kramer et al.[10]	77	2–17y	IVIG (30), KD (7), lidocaine (2), plasmapheresis (2)	IVIG: 2/30 KD: 1/7	93% of survivors has refractory epilepsy, only 18% cognitive normal
Howell[9]	7	5–17y	4 steroids, 2 IVIG, 1 plasmapheresis+rituximab, 1 VNS	VNS: no efficacy in acute phase; 30%–40% of seizure reduction in chronic phase. IVIG and plasmapheresis+rituximab: no efficacy. Steroids: mild but not sustained improvement	1 died, 4 pts with moderate to severe IT, 2 patient with borderline intellectual abilities
Van Baalen et al.[11]	12	2–12y	IVIG (6), steroids (6), plasmapheresis (2), anti-IL2 receptor antibodies	Unclear because of multidrug therapy or poor	NA
Caraballo et al.[35]	12	2–13.5y	Acute phase: IVIG (10), steroids (9), rituximab (1), KD (2), plasmapheresis (1). Chronic phase: IVIG (3), KD (3), VNS (1)	Rituximab: partial and transient response (<50% seizure reduction) plasmapheresis: no response. KD: 50%–70% seizure reduction	7/12 refractory epilepsy, 10/12 behavioral disturbances, 9/12 cognitive disability
Byler et al.[36]	1	5y	KD and IVIG	Good response to KD and IVIG	Regained independent walking after a year. SE has not recurred. Resistant epilepsy. Chronic immunomodulation therapy with IVIG
Singh et al.[37]	2	7–10y	KD	2/2 responders	Follow-up 1 month: rare seizures, still on AEDs, learning or attention difficulties
Rivas-Coppola et al.[22]	7	3m–9y	IVIG (5), steroids (4), KD (4), hypothermia (3)	IVIG and steroids: no response. KD: no clinical response. Hypothermia: transient improvement on seizures	Refractory partial-onset epilepsy

AEDs, antiepileptic drugs; *IT*, immunotherapies; *IVIG*, intravenous immunoglobulin; *KD*, ketogenic diet; *m*, months; *No.*, number; *NA*, not applicable; *pts*, patients; *VNS*, vagus nerve stimulation; *y*, years.

moderate mental retardation, 12% had severe mental retardation, and 16% were in a vegetative state.

Poor cognitive outcome has been significantly associated with younger age at onset and longer duration of BSC.[33] Behavior and cognition should be assessment at the end of the acute phase.

Early KD treatment might optimize both seizure control and cognitive outcome after FIRES.

As this is a rare condition, more multicentric studies are needed to improve diagnosis and treatment and to clarify the pathogenesis of this condition.

REFERENCES

1. van Baalen A, Häusler M, Boor R, et al. Febrile infection-related epilepsy syndrome (FIRES): a nonencephalitic encephalopathy in childhood. *Epilepsia.* 2010;51(7):1323–1328.
2. Awaya Y, Fukuyama Y. Epilepsy sequelae of acute encephalitis or encephalopathy (3rd report). *Jpn J Psychiatry Neurol.* 1986;40:385–387.
3. Baxter P, Clarke A, Cross H, et al. Idiopathic catastrophic epileptic encephalopathy presenting with acute onset intractable status. *Seizure.* 2003;12:379–387.
4. Mikaeloff Y, Jambaqué I, Hertz-Pannier L, et al. Devastating epileptic encephalopathy in school-aged children (DESC): a pseudoencephalitis. *Epilepsy Res.* 2006;69:67–79.
5. Shyu CS, Lee HF, Chi CS, Chen CH. Acute encephalitis with refractory, repetitive partial seizures. *Brain Dev.* 2008;30(5):356–361.
6. van Baalen A, Stephani U, Kluger G, Häusler M, Dulac O. FIRES: febrile infection responsive epileptic (FIRE) encephalopathies of school age. *Brain Dev.* 2009;31(1):91.
7. Nabbout R, Mazzuca M, Hubert P, et al. Efficacy of ketogenic diet in severe refractory status epilepticus initiating fever induced refractory epileptic encephalopathy in school age children (FIRES). *Epilepsia.* 2010;51:2033–2037.
8. Sakuma H, Awaya Y, Shiomi M, et al. Acute encephalitis with refractory, repetitive partial seizures (AERRPS): a peculiar form of childhood encephalitis. *Acta Neurol Scand.* 2010;121:251–256.
9. Howell KB, Katanyuwong K, Mackay MT, et al. Long-term follow- up of febrile infection-related epilepsy syndrome. *Epilepsia.* 2012;53(1):101–110.
10. Kramer U, Chi CS, Lin KL, et al. Febrile infection-related epilepsy syndrome (FIRES): pathogenesis, treatment, and outcome: a multicenter study on 77 children. *Epilepsia.* 2011;52(11):1956–1965.
11. van Baalen A, Häusler M, Plecko-Startinig B, et al. Febrile infection-related epilepsy syndrome without detectable autoantibodies and response to immunotherapy: a case series and discussion of epileptogenesis in FIRES. *Neuropediatrics.* 2012;43(4):209–216.
12. Sahin M, Menache CC, Holmes GL, Riviello JJ. Outcome of severe refractory status epilepticus in children. *Epilepsia.* 2001;42:1461–1467.
13. Wilder-Smith EPV, Lim ECH, Teoh HL, et al. The NORSE (new-onset refractory status epilepticus) syndrome: defining a disease entity. *Ann Acad Med Singap.* 2005;34:417–420.
14. Körtvelyessy P, Lerche H, Weber Y. FIRES and NORSE are distinct entities. *Epilepsia.* 2012;53(7):1276.
15. Nabbout R. FIRES and IHHE: delineation of the syndromes. *Epilepsia.* 2013;54(suppl 6):54–56.
16. van Baalen A, Vezzani A, Häusler M, Kluger G. Febrile infection-related epilepsy syndrome: clinical review and hypotheses of epileptogenesis. *Neuropediatrics.* 2017;48(1):5–18.
17. Vezzani A, French J, Bartfai T, Baram TZ. The role of inflammation in epilepsy. *Nat Rev Neurol.* 2011;7(1):31–40.
18. Vezzani A, Maroso M, Balosso S, Sanchez MA, Bartfai T. IL-1 receptor/Toll-like receptor signaling in infection, inflammation, stress and neurodegeneration couples hyperexcitability and seizures. *Brain Behav Immun.* 2011;25(7):1281–1289.
19. Miskin C, Hasbani DM. Status epilepticus: immunologic and inflammatory mechanisms. *Semin Pediatr Neurol.* 2014;21(3):221–225.
20. Varadkar S, Cross JH. Rasmussen syndrome and other inflammatory epilepsies. *Semin Neurol.* 2015;35(3):259–268.
21. Nabbout R, Vezzani A, Dulac O, Chiron C. Acute encephalopathy with inflammation-mediated status epilepticus. *Lancet Neurol.* 2011;10(1):99–108.
22. Rivas-Coppola MS, Shah N, Choudhri AF, Morgan R, Wheless JW. Chronological evolution of magnetic resonance imaging findings in children with febrile infection-related epilepsy syndrome. *Pediatr Neurol.* 2016;55:22–29.
23. Meletti S, Slonkova J, Mareckova I, et al. Claustrum damage and refractory status epilepticus following febrile illness. *Neurology.* 2015;85(14):1224–1232.
24. Mazzuca M, Jambaque I, Hertz-Pannier L, et al. 18F-FDG PET reveals frontotemporal dysfunction in children with fever-induced refractory epileptic encephalopathy. *J Nucl Med.* 2011;52(1):40–47.
25. Appenzeller S, Helbig I, Stephani U, et al. Febrile infection-related epilepsy syndrome (FIRES) is not caused by SCN1A, POLG, PCDH19 mutations or rare copy number variations. *Dev Med Child Neurol.* 2012;54(12):1144–1148.
26. Benson LA, Olson H, Gorman MP. Evaluation and treatment of autoimmune neurologic disorders in the pediatric intensive care unit. *Semin Pediatr Neurol.* 2014;21(4):284–290.
27. Baysal-Kirac L, Tuzun E, Altindag E, et al. Are there any specific EEG findings in autoimmune encephalitis? *Clin EEG Neurosci.* 2016;47(3):224–234.
28. Villeneuve N, Pinton F, Bahi-Buisson N, Dulac O, Chiron C, Nabbout R. The ketogenic diet improves recently worsened focal epilepsy. *Dev Med Child Neurol.* 2009;51(4):276–281.
29. Dupuis N, Curatolo N, Benoist JF, Auvin S. Ketogenic diet exhibits anti-inflammatory properties. *Epilepsia.* 2015;56(7):95–98.

30. Gofshteyn JS, Wilfong A, Devinsky O, et al. Cannabidiol as a Potential Treatment for Febrile Infection-Related Epilepsy Syndrome (FIRES) in the Acute and Chronic Phases. *J Child Neurol.* 2017;32(1):35–40.

31. Sato Y, Numata-Uematsu Y, Uematsu M, et al. Acute encephalitis with refractory, repetitive partial seizures: pathological findings and a new therapeutic approach using tacrolimus. *Brain Dev.* 2016;38(8):772–776.

32. Melvin JJ, Huntley Hardison H. Immunomodulatory treatments in epilepsy. *Semin Pediatr Neurol.* 2014;21(3): 232–237.

33. Kramer U, Chi CS, Lin KL, et al. Febrile infection-related epilepsy syndrome (FIRES): does duration of anesthesia affect outcome? *Epilepsia.* 2011;52(suppl 8):28–30.

34. Kramer U, Shorer Z, Ben-Zeev B, Lerman-Sagie T, Goldberg-Stern H, Lahat E. Severe refractory status epilepticus owing to presumed encephalitis. *J Child Neurol.* 2005;20(3):184–187.

35. Caraballo RH, Reyes G, Avaria MF, et al. Febrile infection-related epilepsy syndrome: a study of 12 patients. *Seizure.* 2013;22(7):553–559.

36. Byler DL, Grageda MR, Halstead ES, Kanekar S. Rapid onset of hippocampal atrophy in febrile-infection related epilepsy syndrome (FIRES). *J Child Neurol.* 2014;29(4):545–549.

37. Singh RK, Joshi SM, Potter DM, Leber SM, Carlson MD, Shellhaas RA. Cognitive outcomes in febrile infection-related epilepsy syndrome treated with the ketogenic diet. *Pediatrics.* 2014;134(5):1431–1435.

Acute Encephalitis With Refractory, Repetitive Partial Seizures

HIROSHI SAKUMA, MD, PHD

INTRODUCTION

Acute encephalitis with refractory, repetitive partial seizures (AERRPS) is a disease that exhibits a peculiar clinical picture that primarily involves a cluster of refractory seizures associated with fever.[1] Although the cause of AERRPS has not been identified, recent research suggests that genetic background and inflammation of the central nervous system are involved. This article, based primarily on findings from multicenter studies in Japan, presents an overview of the clinical characteristics and presumed clinical conditions comprising this disease.

HISTORY

A description of AERRPS was first reported by Awaya and Fukuyama in Japan in 1986.[2] They suggested that there are cases of epilepsy after encephalitis/encephalopathy that show the symptoms of refractory, repetitive, complex partial seizures where seizures of the same type persist, recur, and progress from the acute phase to the convalescent phase and chronic phase. Since then, this disease has been known in Japan as "a group of peculiar epilepsies after encephalitis/encephalopathy." Shiomi et al. reported a similar disease, defined as "encephalitis associated with repetitive seizures." With the goal of unifying these names, we proposed in 2001 to use the name AERRPS to define the disease.[3]

Subsequently, similar concepts of the disease were proposed from various countries. Kramer et al. reported a case of encephalitis, with a poor prognosis involving refractory status epilepticus accompanied by fever requiring burst-suppression coma, as "severe refractory status epilepticus due to presumed encephalitis."[4] For adult cases, "new-onset refractory status epilepticus" (NORSE) syndrome, proposed by Wilder-Smith et al., has often been used.[5] The characteristics of NORSE closely match those of AERRPS except that the former has been observed mostly in women. "Devastating epileptic encephalopathy in school-aged children" (DESC) was proposed by Michaelof et al. in 2006.[6] DESC primarily develops in school-aged children, with the focal areas of convulsion seizures around the Sylvian fissure and temporal cortex. In 2010, a novel concept of FIRES was proposed.[7] FIRES is an acronym used for various other disease names such as "febrile infection–related refractory epilepsy syndrome" and "fever-induced refractory epileptic encephalopathy in school-aged children." As discussed later in this review, AERRPS, NORSE syndrome, and FIRES are currently considered the same disease.[8]

CLINICAL CHARACTERISTICS

AERRPS generally occurs in healthy children with no apparent neurologic abnormality. The age of onset peaks at 4–5 years of age and is observed in school-aged children in relatively large numbers. It tends to be more common in males, with a male-to-female ratio of 2:1 to 3:2. The rate of this disease among acute childhood encephalitis patients in Japan is 0.6%,[9] with a predicted onset of at least three to five cases a year. If epilepsy or developmental retardation is observed in a patient, or if the patient has suffered a neurologic disorder in the past, the patient will not be diagnosed with AERRPS. However, if the patient suffers only simple febrile seizures or is a borderline case of language development delay, a diagnosis of AERRPS would not necessarily be denied.

The disease is necessarily accompanied by fever at its onset. In general, fever is an antecedent of the infection by 2–10 days (5 days on average) before the development of neurologic symptoms. There are cases where fever persists for several weeks in the acute phase during which convulsions recur. If this is the case, there is a possibility that the fever is not simply a symptom of an antecedent infection, but a symptom of the disease itself. The etiology of the antecedent infection varies, and a causal relationship with specific pathogens has not been proven.

The initial neurologic symptom of AERRPS, in nearly every case, is seizure. There are a variety of neurologic diseases in children characterized by seizures that are accompanied by fever at seizure onset. However, seizures observed in AERRPS have several distinctive features, and these are of diagnostic value. First, seizures are, without exception, focal seizures. Eye deviation and clonic facial movements are predominant, and clonic lateral limb seizures are less frequent. During the acute phase, secondary generalization is often observed, but if primarily generalized tonic-clonic convulsion is the main seizure type, it is difficult to consider a diagnosis of AERRPS. In addition, the frequency of tonic seizures is relatively low. Second, although each seizure naturally ends within a few minutes, it occurs frequently, every 5–15 min in a far advanced period. In typical cases, seizures consistently recur with a period of several minutes. In other words, AERRPS is characterized by cluster status epilepticus and less by continuous status epilepticus. Third, seizures are extremely recalcitrant and exhibit strong resistance to ordinal antiepileptic drugs. This trend is especially strong in the acute phase. It is necessary to keep the electroencephalogram to a state of burst suppression, or complete suppression, by continuous, intravenous administration of barbiturates at high doses to suppress seizures. In mild cases, a benzodiazepine-type intravenous drug such as midazolam may produce a response. However, it must be administered at high doses in many cases. The acute phase generally persists for several weeks to several months, requiring an extended period of ICU management.

In AERRPS, the degree of disturbance of consciousness is relatively mild, and cases leading to coma are rare. In addition, transient, involuntary movements or psychologic symptoms may be observed in some cases during the convalescent phase. These symptoms, however, are contingent on seizures and do not constitute the primary symptoms of the disease.

Epilepsy must be developed as sequelae of AERRPS and change to refractory epilepsy after the acute phase without going through the incubation period. The seizure type of epilepsy in its chronic phase is generally the same as the type found in the acute phase. However, with the emergence of new antiepileptic drugs, cases have been observed that completely suppress seizures. Furthermore, AERRPS has a high rate of comorbidity with intellectual disability and the prognosis is poor, with nearly half of cases requiring prolonged bed rest. However, there are cases, albeit small in number, where patients return to a normal social life. Cases leading to sudden and unexplained death have also been reported.

EXAMINATION FINDINGS
Examination of Cerebrospinal Fluid
Pleocytosis is found in ~40% of cases. In general, the increase is mild, less than 100/μL, and occurs predominantly in mononuclear cells. It is often observed transiently at an early phase of the disease. Levels return to normal during examination of the cerebrospinal fluid (CSF), even if refractory convulsions persist, producing a gap between the diagnosis and the clinical course. Levels of neopterin in the CSF also increase. No pathogens are detected in the CSF.

Electroencephalographic Examination
Electroencephalographic (EEG) examination is extremely important for the diagnosis of AERRPS. Although diffuse high-amplitude slow waves are observed in the earliest phase of the disease, epileptic discharges often emerge in a comparatively earlier course of the disease. Regions that surround the Sylvian fissure are suspected of being AERRPS-affected regions. However, the distribution of epileptic discharges is not limited to these regions and it varies according to each case. Multifocal abnormalities or bilateral abnormalities are exhibited in most cases. Periodic discharges are often observed at nadir, when seizures occur frequently. These discharges can be related to high epileptogenesis, and it is often hard to end treatment of continuous, intravenous-injection of barbiturates by the time this pattern arises.[10] Periodic discharges often sequentially evolve into ictal discharges.

Ictal EEG of AERRPS are usually a sharp wave or spike burst that normally centers on θ area, representing a focal origin and secondary generalization, followed by convergence to an originated region. To reflect the seizures that emerge in a periodic manner, a brain wave at the time of a seizure consistently and recurrently emerges and disappears, and when recorded using an amplitude integrated EEG, a saw tooth–shaped wave will be obtained.[11] Many cases have been observed that are of multiple seizure origin and where the seizure wave has migrated to a contralateral region.

Neuroimaging Diagnosis
Although neuroimaging is necessary, it only plays a subsidiary role in the diagnosis of AERRPS. It is rare to discover abnormalities using CT; MRI is superior at

detecting lesions. Lesions observed in a relatively high frequency include hyperintensity on T2-weighted images in the hippocampus. Note, however, that these lesions may be secondary because of continuous status convulsion. T2 hyperintensity in the periventricular white matter is also often observed. On the other hand, lesions that are highly peculiar to AERRPS are T2 hyperintensities in the claustrum and in the insular cortex.[10] Lesions are also sometimes observed in the basal ganglia and thalamus in critical cases. In others cases, multifocal T2 prolongation may be observed in the cortex.[12]

ARE ACUTE ENCEPHALITIS WITH REFRACTORY, REPETITIVE PARTIAL SEIZURES AND FEBRILE INFECTION–RELATED REFRACTORY EPILEPSY SYNDROME THE SAME DISEASE?

AERRPS, NORSE syndrome, and FIRES are all characterized by severe refractory epilepsy, accompanied by fever; all three are considered to be the same disease.[8] We compared cases of AERRPS and FIRES reported in the literature to assess similarities in clinical features.[13,14] Disease characteristics were comparable in many respects, including male-female ratio, incubation period after an antecedent infection, CSF pleocytosis, and the rate of onset of lesions in the hippocampus. Although age of onset was slightly higher with FIRES, cases of school-age children might have been biased because FIRES was previously described as Devastating epileptic encephalopathy in school-aged children (DESC). However, some differences were also observed. AERRPS was defined as cases exhibiting focal seizures and its secondary generalization, whereas FIRES included many cases of only secondary generalization, or of only generalized seizures. Furthermore, regarding treatment, the duration of burst-suppression coma was longer with AERRPS than with FIRES, and the intellectual prognosis tended to be worse in AERRPS. These findings suggest that FIRES includes more mild cases than AERRPS.

ETIOLOGY

The etiology of AERRPS is unknown. Although the hypotheses described below have been proposed, a consensus has not been reached.

Epilepsy Hypothesis

The idea that AERRPS is a part of the epilepsies is based on the fact that there are cases where abnormalities are observed in the epilepsy-causing gene.

In a male with a history of AERRPS, a point mutation (R1575T) was identified in the *SCN1A* gene that causes Dravet syndrome.[15] More recently, a point mutation of *SCN2A* was identified in a separate case.[16] These findings suggest that ion channel defects are associated with AERRPS. On the other hand, there is a report that of 15 FIRES cases, not a single case of *SCN1A* mutations or a copy number variation was found.[17] Therefore, not all cases of AERRPS possess these mutations. Therefore, although these ion channel defects are not a direct cause of AERRPS, they can be involved in the onset of AERRPS as its predisposing causes.

Inflammation Hypothesis

The idea that AERRPS is an inflammatory disease can be supported by several of its clinical characteristics. The disease is, without exception, accompanied by fever, and fever not only serves as a trigger of the disease but also often persists during the acute phase. Moreover, the disease is sometimes accompanied by complications such as high CRP values of unknown etiology, hemophagocytic syndrome during the acute phase, and inflammation that may spread beyond the central nervous system. Transient pleocytosis is observed in CSF, and a characteristic high-amplitude slow wave, typical of encephalitis, emerges in the EEG. However, the cause of the inflammation is not clear.

Previously, the idea that AERRPS is an autoimmune disease caused by an autoantibody was a promising hypothesis. Autoantibodies against voltage-gated potassium channel complex, glutamic acid decarboxylase, and GABA-A receptors are detected in cases of autoimmune encephalitis characterized by seizures. In FIRES case studies, however, autoantibodies for neuronal antigens have not been detected, and currently, this hypothesis is deemed suspect.[18]

We have demonstrated that inflammatory cytokines and chemokines within the CSF are prominently increased in AERRPS.[19] Among others, elevation of CXCL-10, IL-8, and IL-6 levels was the most prominent. In addition, the levels were higher even when compared with other inflammatory neurologic diseases as when compared with noninflammatory neurologic diseases. This shows that strong inflammation is occurring in the central nervous system in AERRPS. However, even though these inflammatory cytokines and chemokines within the CSF increase transiently at an earlier stage of the onset of the disease, levels quickly decline and return to normal within 2 weeks. Therefore, inflammation in the central nervous system, although a predisposing cause of AERRPS, is presumably not a direct cause of refractory seizures. The challenge henceforth is to reveal the mechanism of how inflammation in the central nervous system causes intractable status epilepticus.

TREATMENT

The characteristics of seizures in AERRPS show that AERRPS is extremely refractory. This is the predominant trait that makes the disease difficult to treat. In the past, we have argued that continuous, intravenous administration of high-dose barbiturates is the most effective, as well as a necessary treatment, for prevention of secondary brain damage due to recurrent seizures. In fact, barbiturate-induced burst-suppression coma is used as a standard treatment of AERRPS. However, a recent report suggested that this method of treatment might be harmful. Kramer et al. reported that patients who were diagnosed with FIRES and received treatment by means of burst-suppression coma for a long period exhibited poor intellectual prognosis compared with the group that received the same treatment for a short period.[14] However, it is possible that the group that received treatment for an extended period was severely diseased and that the difference in the intellectual prognosis simply reflected the severity of the disease. For this reason, reconsidering treatment strategy based on a prospective study is required. Regardless, continuous, intravenous administration of high-dose barbiturates causes inhibition of cardiorespiratory function, functional ileus, and thrombophlebitis, and it is thus desirable to withdraw from this treatment as quickly as possible.

Several alternative treatment methods have been proposed. Levetiracetam, zonisamide, clonazepam, and bromide are relatively effective during the chronic phase.[20] There is also a report that combined administration of high-dose lidocaine and topiramate was effective.[21] What has attracted the most attention in recent years is a ketogenic diet. The ketogenic diet has been utilized in FIRES cases primarily in European countries, and it has been reported that the seizure can be suppressed for a relatively shorter period, even during the acute phase.[22]

Although immunomodulation therapies have been implemented based on the hypothesis that AERRPS is an inflammatory disease, the outcome is less than satisfactory. Methylprednisolone pulse therapy and intravenous immunoglobulin therapy are the main therapies that have been applied. Overall, however, a short-term effect of the immunomodulation has not been observed. The effects of immunosuppressive drugs such as cyclophosphamide or rituximab are unknown. There is opportunity, henceforth, for examining the long-term effect of immunoregulation therapies (Table 24.1).

TABLE 24.1
Acute Encephalitis With Refractory, Repetitive Partial Seizures Diagnostic Criteria

A: SYMPTOMS

Fever at the onset of the disease (at the time of worsening seizure)

Focal seizures that center on the face (eye deviation, clonic facial movements, apnea, etc.)

Cluster status epilepticus (more than once in 15 min)

Severe refractory seizures (requiring high doses of barbiturates or benzodiazepine-type drugs)

Epilepsy in the chronic phase (seizures that persist more than 6 months after onset)

B: EXAMINATION FINDINGS

Cerebrospinal fluid pleocytosis

High levels of inflammatory markers such as neopterin and IL-6 in the CSF

Periodic discharge on EEG during interictal state

A cyclic pattern of emerging seizures observed on an EEG

Abnormal signals in hippocampus, insula neighboring cortices, thalamus, claustrum, and basal ganglia

Atrophy of cerebral cortex during the chronic period

C: DIFFERENTIAL DIAGNOSIS

The following diseases have been differentiated: Viral encephalitis, other virus-related acute encephalopathy (acute encephalopathy with biphasic seizures and late reduced diffusion, etc.), autoimmune encephalitis (acute limbic encephalitis, anti-NMDA receptor encephalitis), metabolic disease, cerebral vasculitis, other epilepsies (Dravet syndrome, PCDH19 related epilepsies, etc.)

Category of Diagnosis
    Definite: All four items satisfied from A, at least two items satisfied from B, and all diseases in C excluded
    Probable: At least four items satisfied from A, at least two items satisfied from B, and all diseases in C excluded
    Possible: At least four items satisfied from A and at least one item satisfied from B

REFERENCES

1. Sakuma H. Acute encephalitis with refractory, repetitive partial seizures. *Brain Dev.* 2009;31:510–514.
2. Awaya Y, Fukuyama Y. Epilepsy sequelae of acute encephalitis or encephalopathy (3rd report). *Jpn J Psychiatr Neurol.* 1986;40:385–387.
3. Sakuma H, Fukumizu M, Kohyama J. Efficacy of anticonvulsants on acute encephalitis with refractory, repetitive partial seizures (AERRPS). *No To Hattatsu.* 2001;33:385–390.

4. Kramer U, Shorer Z, Ben-Zeev B, Lerman-Sagie T, Goldberg-Stern H, Lahat E. Severe refractory status epilepticus owing to presumed encephalitis. *J Child Neurol.* 2005;20:184–187.

5. Wilder-Smith EP, Lim EC, Teoh HL, et al. The NORSE (new-onset refractory status epilepticus) syndrome: defining a disease entity. *Ann Acad Med Singap.* 2005;34:417–420.

6. Mikaeloff Y, Jambaque I, Hertz-Pannier L, et al. Devastating epileptic encephalopathy in school-aged children (DESC): a pseudo encephalitis. *Epilepsy Res.* 2006;69: 67–79.

7. van Baalen A, Hausler M, Boor R, et al. Febrile infection-related epilepsy syndrome (FIRES): a nonencephalitic encephalopathy in childhood. *Epilepsia.* 2010;51:1323–1328.

8. Ismail FY, Kossoff EH. AERRPS, DESC, NORSE, FIRES: multi-labeling or distinct epileptic entities? *Epilepsia.* 2011;52:e185–e189.

9. Hoshino A, Saitoh M, Oka A, et al. Epidemiology of acute encephalopathy in Japan, with emphasis on the association of viruses and syndromes. *Brain Dev.* 2012;34:337–343.

10. Saito Y, Maegaki Y, Okamoto R, et al. Acute encephalitis with refractory, repetitive partial seizures: case reports of this unusual post-encephalitic epilepsy. *Brain Dev.* 2007;29:147–156.

11. Okumura A, Komatsu M, Abe S, et al. Amplitude-integrated electroencephalography in patients with acute encephalopathy with refractory, repetitive partial seizures. *Brain Dev.* 2011;33:77–82.

12. Okanishi T, Mori Y, Kibe T, et al. Refractory epilepsy accompanying acute encephalitis with multifocal cortical lesions: possible autoimmune etiology. *Brain Dev.* 2007;29:590–594.

13. Sakuma H, Awaya Y, Shiomi M, et al. Acute encephalitis with refractory, repetitive partial seizures (AERRPS): a peculiar form of childhood encephalitis. *Acta Neurol Scand.* 2010;121:251–256.

14. Kramer U, Chi CS, Lin KL, et al. Febrile infection-related epilepsy syndrome (FIRES): pathogenesis, treatment, and outcome: a multicenter study on 77 children. *Epilepsia.* 2011;52:1956–1965.

15. Kobayashi K, Ouchida M, Okumura A, et al. Genetic seizure susceptibility underlying acute encephalopathies in childhood. *Epilepsy Res.* 2010;91:143–152.

16. Kobayashi K, Ohzono H, Shinohara M, et al. Acute encephalopathy with a novel point mutation in the SCN2A gene. *Epilepsy Res.* 2012;102:109–112.

17. Appenzeller S, Helbig I, Stephani U, et al. Febrile infection-related epilepsy syndrome (FIRES) is not caused by SCN1A, POLG, PCDH19 mutations or rare copy number variations. *Dev Med Child Neurol.* 2012;54:1144–1148.

18. van Baalen A, Hausler M, Plecko-Startinig B, et al. Febrile infection-related epilepsy syndrome without detectable autoantibodies and response to immunotherapy: a case series and discussion of epileptogenesis in FIRES. *Neuropediatrics.* 2012;43:209–216.

19. Sakuma H, Tanuma N, Kuki I, Takahashi Y, Shiomi M, Hayashi M. Intrathecal overproduction of proinflammatory cytokines and chemokines in febrile infection-related refractory status epilepticus. *J Neurol Neurosurg Psychiatry.* 2015;86:820–822.

20. Ueda R, Saito Y, Ohno K, et al. Effect of levetiracetam in acute encephalitis with refractory, repetitive partial seizures during acute and chronic phase. *Brain Dev.* 2015;37: 471–477.

21. Lin JJ, Lin KL, Wang HS, Hsia SH, Wu CT. Effect of topiramate, in combination with lidocaine, and phenobarbital, in acute encephalitis with refractory repetitive partial seizures. *Brain Dev.* 2009;31:605–611.

22. Nabbout R, Mazzuca M, Hubert P, et al. Efficacy of ketogenic diet in severe refractory status epilepticus initiating fever induced refractory epileptic encephalopathy in school age children (FIRES). *Epilepsia.* 2010;51:2033–2037.

Children With Encephalitis/ Encephalopathy-Related Status Epilepticus and Epilepsy—A Global View of Postencephalitic Epilepsy

KUANG-LIN LIN, MD • I-JUN CHOU, MD • JAINN-JIM LIN, MD • HUEI-SHYONG WANG, MD • CHEESE STUDY GROUP

INTRODUCTION

Acute encephalitis is a relatively common disease in childhood with potentially devastating clinical complications. It refers to inflammation and swelling of the brain, and it is often caused by either a direct viral infection or an immune-mediated process. Acute encephalitis can result in the development of neurologic sequelae and represents an important cause of acute seizures and subsequent epilepsy in previously healthy children.[1,2] Epidemiologic studies have reported that 2.7%–27% of epilepsies are secondary to previous central nervous system infections.[3–5] Encephalitis-related seizures may present as a single seizure, repetitive seizures, refractory status epilepticus, or even drug-resistant epilepsy.

Acute encephalitis is most often identified during the first episode of status epilepticus and appears to be associated with morbidity and mortality.[5,6] In addition, postencephalitic epilepsy has been reported to become intractable in 15%–50% of children.[1,5,7] Therefore, based on the underlying risk factors, children with encephalitis have a high rate of postencephalitic epilepsy and are likely to develop drug-resistant epilepsy. Adequate antiepileptic drugs, a multimodal approach and management, may minimize brain damage in the acute stage and improve the outcomes of postencephalitic epilepsy.[5]

ACUTE SYMPTOMATIC SEIZURES IN THE ACUTE STAGE OF ENCEPHALITIS

Central nervous system infections are a known risk factor for the development of acute symptomatic

seizures and represent a major risk factor for acquired epilepsy.[5] In a study on seizures caused by central nervous system infections by Kim et al., 23% of the patients had acute seizures and 73% had encephalitis, which is a significantly more frequent etiology than meningitis. Viral encephalitis has been shown to result in a 14-fold increase in the risk of acute seizures.[8] In the CHEESE study of 1038 pediatric patients, 463 (44.6%) with encephalitis had seizures in the acute phase, suggesting that encephalitis leads to a high rate of acute seizures, especially in pediatric encephalitis. In this cohort, 153 (33%) patients with acute seizures had status epilepticus, including 53 (34.6%) who then developed refractory status epilepticus.[5] Thus, once seizures develop in the acute phase of pediatric encephalitis, clinicians should be aware of the possible development of refractory status epilepticus. The patterns and frequency of acute seizures in the acute stage of encephalitis have been reported to be a single seizure (18%–21%), repetitive seizures (39%–58%), status epilepticus (20%–25%), and refractory status epilepticus (11%–15%).[1,5,7]

The mechanisms of the generation of acute symptomatic seizures after infections vary with the type of infection and are often multifactorial. Triggering of the inflammatory cascade with the release of inflammatory cytokines appears to be a common underlying factor in most central nervous system infections and has been well studied in both meningitis and encephalitis.[9]

HOW TO APPROACH A PATIENT WITH FEBRILE STATUS EPILEPTICUS—ROLE OF INFECTIOUS PATHOGENS AND ANTINEURONAL ANTIBODIES IN CHILDREN WITH ENCEPHALITIS

Detection of the Underlying Etiology

Central nervous infections are usually presumed to be the cause of febrile refractory status epilepticus. Many aspects of the pathogenesis of acute encephalitis and acute febrile encephalopathy with status epilepticus have been clarified in the past 10 years, and it can be classified into direct pathogen invasion or immune-mediated mechanisms (Fig. 25.1).[10] Over the past 20 years, the number of antineuronal antibodies to ion channels, receptors, and other synaptic proteins described in association with central nervous system disorders has increased dramatically, and especially their role in pediatric encephalitis and status epilepticus. These antineuronal antibodies are classified according to the location of their respective antigens: (1) intracellular antigens, including glutamic acid decarboxylase (GAD), and classical onconeural antigens, such as Hu (antineuronal nuclear antibody 1, ANNA1), Ma2, Yo (Purkinje cell autoantibody, PCA1), Ri (antineuronal nuclear antibody 2, ANNA2), CV2/CRMP5, and amphiphysin, and (2) cell membrane ion channels or surface antigens, including voltage-gated potassium channel (VGKC) receptor, N-methyl-D-aspartate (NMDA) receptor, amino-3-hydroxy-5-methyl-4-isoxazolepropionic acid (AMPA) receptor, g-aminobutyric acid-B (GABA$_B$) receptor, leucine-rich glioma-inactivated protein 1 (LGI1), and contactin-associated protein-like 2 (CASPR2).[10,11] The outcome of status epilepticus generally depends on the underlying cause. Therefore, identifying the possible infectious pathogens and clarifying the underlying immunologic pathogenic entity (such as a treatable viral infection, antineuronal antibodies, or a combination of viral infection and immune-mediated process) is very important in the management of febrile status epilepticus (Fig. 25.2).

Coexistence of Infectious Pathogens and Antineuronal Antibodies in a Patient With Encephalitis and Status Epilepticus

Children with febrile status epilepticus usually have a catastrophic course and are resistant to many antiepileptic drugs. The mechanism of disease in these patients remains unknown, although the clinical features and experimental models point to a likely vicious cycle involving inflammation and seizure activity.[12-14] Approximately one-third of acute cases of encephalitis are considered to be immune mediated.[15]

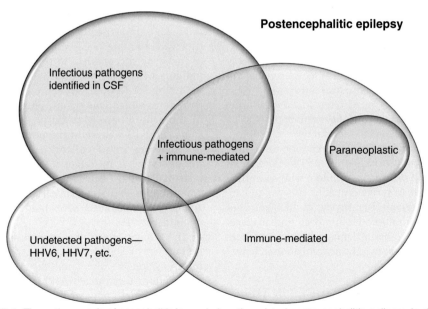

FIG. 25.1 The pathogenesis of encephalitis/encephalopathy-related postencephalitic epilepsy is classified into direct infectious pathogen invasion or immune-mediated mechanisms. Some of the infectious pathogens may be as yet undiscovered. Some infectious pathogens and antineuronal antibodies coexisted. *CSF*, cerebrospinal fluid.

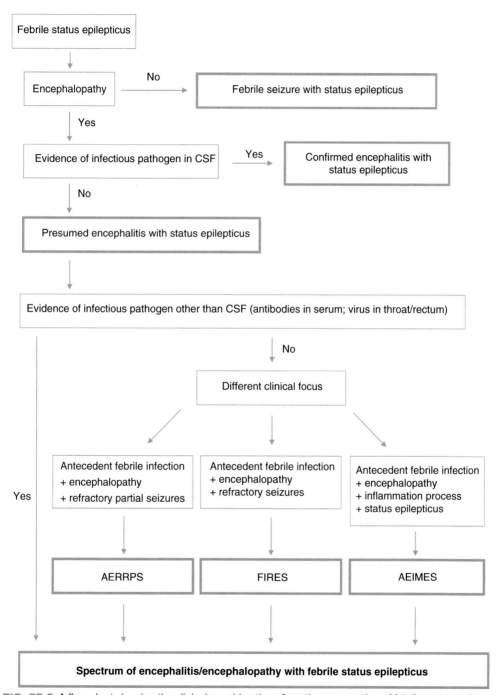

FIG. 25.2 A flow chart showing the clinical considerations from the presentation of febrile status epilepticus to the spectrum of related conditions of children with encephalitis/encephalopathy and febrile status epilepticus. The abbreviated medical terms used in different areas and study groups describe these similar conditions, all of which represent the unique characteristics as a part of this condition. *AEIMSE*, acute encephalopathy with inflammation-mediated status epilepticus; *AERRPS*, acute encephalitis with refractory, repetitive partial seizures; *CSF*, cerebrospinal fluid; *FIRES*, febrile infection-related epilepsy syndrome. (From Lin KL, Wang HS. Role of antineuronal antibodies in children with encephalopathy and febrile status epilepticus. *Pediatr Neonatol*. 2014;55:161–167; with permission.)

Furthermore, many studies have reported that infectious pathogens can coexist with antineuronal antibodies in patients with encephalitis.[16–21] These findings may suggest that infectious pathogens are potential triggers of inflammation and that they are not always involved in direct invasion into the central nervous system.

In the California Encephalitis Project, 10 patients with antibodies to the NMDA receptor were possibly associated with *Mycoplasma* infection but not with cancer.[16] In addition, Lin et al. reported that of 16 children with presumed causative infectious pathogens in 7 (43.8%) also had anti-GAD antibodies and 1 also had anti-GAD antibodies and VGKC antibodies.[17]

The association between positive VGKC-complex antibodies and *Mycoplasma pneumoniae* with respiratory symptoms (five of seven patients) suggests that VGKC-complex antibodies could be induced as part of the immune response to Mycoplasma pneumonia.[18] Takanashi et al. found positive or elevated levels of antibodies against the NMDA receptor in the cerebrospinal fluid or serum of five patients with H1N1 influenza–related encephalitis.[19] Furthermore, Prüss et al. detected anti-NMDA receptor antibodies in the serum or cerebrospinal fluid of 13 of 44 (30%) patients with herpes simplex virus infection.[20] Therefore, the relationship between infectious pathogens and antineuronal antibodies may contribute to the pathogenesis of the disease and affect the choice of treatment.

RISK FACTORS FOR DEVELOPING POSTENCEPHALITIC EPILEPSY

In a study of *Mycoplasma pneumoniae*-related postencephalitic epilepsy by Lin et al., children with seizures during the acute phase of encephalitis had an increased risk of postencephalitic epilepsy (odds ratio [OR] 70.07, 95% confidence interval [CI] 17.76–276.48; $P < .001$).[1] In addition, those with single seizures before or during admission did not have an increased risk of postencephalitic epilepsy. However, the children with recurrent seizures during hospitalization had a 4.85-fold (95% CI 1.61–14.60, $P = .003$) increased risk of developing postencephalitic epilepsy, and all children with status epilepticus during hospitalization, including those with refractory status epilepticus, developed postencephalitic epilepsy ($P < .001$). Therefore, poor seizure control in the acute phase may be a risk factor for postencephalitic epilepsy.

Other risk factors have also been reported in cohort studies of infectious and antibody-associated encephalitis.[22] Status epilepticus, focal seizures, and electroencephalographic epileptiform discharges during acute encephalitis episodes have been reported to be risk factors for drug-resistant epilepsy, along with admission to an intensive care unit and the use of more than three antiepileptic drugs in hospital.[22]

Regarding brain imaging studies, risk factors in brain magnetic resonance imaging for drug-resistant epilepsy include T2/T2-weighted fluid-attenuated inversion recovery hyperintensity involving the hippocampus/amygdala, which may be a manifestation of status epilepticus or represent limbic encephalitis, a recognized precedent of temporal lobe epilepsy and mesial temporal sclerosis in adulthood.[28] Another brain magnetic resonance imaging feature of drug-resistant epilepsy is gadolinium enhancement, which is a typical neuroimaging feature of herpes simplex virus encephalitis.

The risk of drug-resistant epilepsy varies according to its etiology. The herpes simplex virus has been reported to be a high risk factor for drug-resistant epilepsy.[7,22,23] In comparison, enterovirus, acute disseminated encephalomyelitis, and anti-NMDA receptor encephalitis were considered to be low risk in the study by Pillai et al.[22] Mycoplasma pneumonia encephalitis has been reported to be a high risk factor for drug-resistant epilepsy in Taiwan,[1,7] but it has been reported to be rare in Western countries.[22]

A high titer of GAD antibodies is often associated with non-paraneoplastic stiff-person syndrome and cerebellar dysfunction; however, an increasing number of reports have shown that these antibodies are also associated with subtypes of limbic encephalitis and refractory epilepsy.[10,24] The presence of anti-GAD antibodies suggests that the underlying neurologic syndrome may be immune mediated.[10] Lin et al. investigated antibodies to GAD and cell membrane ion channels or surface antigens in acute-phase serum from 17 children with encephalitis and status epilepticus and found that anti-GAD antibody titers were significantly higher in the children with encephalitis and status epilepticus than in those with therapy-resistant epilepsy.[10] In addition, three patients had postencephalitic epilepsy with neurologic deficits, and higher anti-GAD antibody titers were noted in the children with encephalitis and status epilepticus. The potential role of anti-GAD antibodies in children with encephalitis and status epilepticus should therefore be emphasized.

MULTIMODAL MANAGEMENT OF POSTENCEPHALITIC EPILEPSY

Antiepileptic Drugs for Acute Seizures and Chronic Seizures of Postencephalitic Epilepsy

In general, seizures are initially treated with boluses of intravenous lorazepam or diazepam as first-line drugs, followed by intravenous infusions of phenytoin and/ or phenobarbital as second-line drugs. Phenytoin has been reported to be ineffective for febrile status epilepticus.[25] Sugai suggested that pentobarbital is effective for prolonged status epilepticus, whereas phenytoin is effective for cluster convulsive status epilepticus.[26] In the CHEESE study on postencephalitic epilepsy, phenobarbital (97.5%) was more effective than phenytoin (75.4%) in controlling repetitive seizures (P = .009).[9] Therefore, phenobarbital may be a suitable second-line antiepileptic drug for seizures in pediatric encephalitis.[5,27] Nevertheless, in the study of acute encephalitis with refractory, repetitive partial seizures (AERRPS) by Shyu et al., the patients had a high rate of hypersensitivity to antiepileptic drugs (n = 11/14, 78.6%).[28] Therefore, physicians should be aware of complications from hypersensitivity syndrome when using antiepileptic drugs for patients with encephalitis.

Patients who do not respond to the initial antiepileptic drug and develop refractory status epilepticus may respond to high-dose suppressive therapy such as intravenous thiopental, propofol, high-dose topiramate combined with high-dose phenobarbital, or high-dose lidocaine.[5] Nevertheless, in the multicenter study of febrile infection–related epilepsy syndrome by Kramer et al., decreased cognitive levels at follow-up were significantly associated with the duration of a burst-suppression coma (n = 46; P = .005).[13] Therefore, treatment that involves inducing a prolonged burst-suppression coma may be associated with a worse cognitive outcome.[13] Nevertheless, this association should be interpreted cautiously, because a longer burst-suppression coma state can also be due to a longer disease process and thus is likely to reflect a more severe condition. In addition, the adverse effects of thiopental and propofol have been reported in several studies, including mortality, myocardial and respiratory depression, profound hypotension, and propofol infusion syndrome.[5,28,29] Therefore, high-dose topiramate combined with intravenous high-dose phenobarbital or high-dose lidocaine may be considered as an alternative third-line treatment for refractory status epilepticus due to encephalitis.[5]

Regarding the long-term management of postencephalitic epilepsy, it has been reported that high-dose phenobarbital is the most effective agent for seizure control during the recovery phase and chronic phase of acute encephalitis with refractory repetitive focal seizures.[26] Phenobarbital and clonazepam are the most common drugs used alone or in combination for postencephalitic epilepsy, followed by valproic acid and carbamazepine.[5] The role of new antiepileptic drugs in postencephalitic epilepsy warrants further research.

Immunotherapy for Seizures With Encephalitis

Byun et al. analyzed 41 patients with new-onset seizures and autoimmune encephalitis. After the initial immunotherapy (steroids, intravenous immunoglobulin, or a combination), 51.2% of the patients were seizure free at the end of first month, and 73.2% of the patients had seizure remission at 6 months. Rituximab was used as second-line immunotherapy, and seizure remission was achieved in a further 66.6% of the patients.[21] However, when patients present with febrile status epilepticus, the syndromic features of limbic encephalitis are always lacking, and hence the diagnosis of autoimmune epilepsy is often delayed. Therefore, initial immunotherapy may be considered in the treatment of febrile refractory status epilepticus.[21,30] In addition, some seronegative patients may harbor as-yet unidentified autoantibodies targeting plasma membrane antigens. Thus, the absence of an antineuronal antibody in the appropriate clinical context should not preclude consideration of an immunotherapy trial.[30]

OUTCOMES OF POSTENCEPHALITIC EPILEPSY

In the CHEESE study on the long-term management of postencephalitic epilepsy, a total of 990 survivors of encephalitis were discharged from hospital, including 268 (27.1%) who were discharged with antiepileptic drug treatment.[5] Excluding 23 patients who were lost to follow-up, 251 of the remaining 967 (26%) patients developed postencephalitic epilepsy. After 1 year of follow-up (n = 205), 168 (82%) patients with postencephalitic epilepsy had favorable outcomes (including 18% who were seizure free and off antiepileptic drugs) and 37 (15%) had intractable epilepsy. Among them, 138 (54.9%) received a single antiepileptic drug for seizure control, 30 (11.9%) received two antiepileptic drugs, and 37 (14.7%) received more than two antiepileptic drugs.

In the study, 14/53 (26.4%) patients with refractory status epilepticus died, whereas only 19/971 (2.0%) patients with nonrefractory status epilepticus died ($P < .001$). Therefore, mortality is significantly associated with the presence of refractory status epilepticus in pediatric patients with encephalitis.

Etiology is the main factor determining the outcome of postencephalitic epilepsy. Therefore, early interventions for the underlying etiology and seizure management in the encephalitis stage are important to improve the long-term outcomes of postencephalitic epilepsy.[1,5,7,23] Early interventions include antineuronal antibody detection, infectious pathogen detection, prescription of appropriate antiepileptic drugs, and possibly immunotherapy, therapeutic hypothermia, and a ketogenic diet.[5,13] Burst-suppression coma for encephalitis with refractory status epilepticus should be used cautiously because of the associated poor cognitive outcomes.[13]

ACKNOWLEDGMENTS

This work was performed by the Children with Encephalitis/Encephalopathy-Related Status Epilepticus and Epilepsy (CHEESE) Study Group at Chang Gung Children's Hospital in Taoyuan, Taiwan. This study was supported in part by grants from Chang Gung Memorial Hospital (CMRPG4C0022 and CMRPG4C0023) and grants from Ministry of Science and Technology, R.O.C. (105-2314-B-182A-118).

REFERENCES

1. Lin JJ, Hsia SH, Wu CT, et al. Mycoplasma pneumoniae-related postencephalitic epilepsy in children. *Epilepsia.* 2011;52:1979–1985.
2. Misra UK, Tan CT, Kalita J. Viral encephalitis and epilepsy. *Epilepsia.* 2008;49(suppl 6):13–18.
3. Awaya Y, Kanematsu S, Fukuyama Y. A follow-up study of children with acute encephalitis or encephalopathy (II): from the viewpoint of epileptogenesis. *Folia Psychiatr Neurol Jpn.* 1982;36:338–339.
4. Annegers JF, Hauser WA, Beghi E, et al. The risk of unprovoked seizures following encephalitis and meningitis. *Neurology.* 1988;38:1407–1410.
5. Lin KL, Lin JJ, Hsia SH, et al. Effect of antiepileptic drugs for acute and chronic seizures in children with encephalitis. *PLoS One.* 2015;10:e0139974.
6. Lin KL, Lin JJ, Hsia SH, et al. Analysis of convulsive status epilepticus in children of Taiwan. *Pediatr Neurol.* 2009;41:413–418.
7. Lee WT, Yu TW, Chang WC, et al. Risk factors for postencephalitic epilepsy in children: a hospital-based study in Taiwan. *Eur J Paediatr Neurol.* 2007;11:302–309.
8. Kim MA, Park KM, Kim SE, et al. Acute symptomatic seizures in CNS infection. *Eur J Neurol.* 2008;15:38–41.
9. Vezzani A, Fujinami RS, White HS, et al. Infections, inflammation and epilepsy. *Acta Neuropathol.* 2016;131:211–234.
10. Lin KL, Wang HS. Role of antineuronal antibodies in children with encephalopathy and febrile status epilepticus. *Pediatr Neonatol.* 2014;55:161–167.
11. Vincent A, Bien CG, Irani SR, et al. Autoantibodies associated with diseases of the CNS: new developments and future challenges. *Lancet Neurol.* 2011;10:759–772.
12. Nabbout R, Vezzani A, Dulac O, et al. Acute encephalopathy with inflammation-mediated status epilepticus. *Lancet Neurol.* 2011;10:99–108.
13. Kramer U, Chi CS, Lin KL, et al. Febrile infection-related epilepsy syndrome (FIRES): pathogenesis, treatment, and outcome: a multicenter study on 77 children. *Epilepsia.* 2011;52:1956–1965.
14. Sakuma H, Awaya Y, Shiomi M, et al. Acute encephalitis with refractory, repetitive partial seizures (AERRPS): a peculiar form of childhood encephalitis. *Acta Neurol Scand.* 2010;121:251–256.
15. Granerod J, Tam CC, Crowcroft NS, et al. Challenge of the unknown. A systematic review of acute encephalitis in non-outbreak situations. *Neurology.* 2010;75:924–932.
16. Gable MS, Gavali S, Radner A, et al. Anti-NMDA receptor encephalitis: report of ten cases and comparison with viral encephalitis. *Eur J Clin Microbiol Infect Dis.* 2009;28:1421–1429.
17. Lin JJ, Lin KL, Chiu CH, et al. Antineuronal antibodies and infectious pathogens in severe acute pediatric encephalitis. *J Child Neurol.* 2014;29:11–16.
18. Pillai SC, Hacohen Y, Tantsis E, et al. Infectious and autoantibody-associated encephalitis: clinical features and long-term outcome. *Pediatrics.* 2015;135:e974–e984.
19. Takanashi J, Takahashi Y, Imamura A, et al. Late delirious behavior with 2009 H1N1 influenza: mild autoimmune-mediated encephalitis? *Pediatrics.* 2012;129:e1068–e1071.
20. Prüss H, Finke C, Höltje M, et al. N-methyl-D-aspartate receptor antibodies in herpes simplex encephalitis. *Ann Neurol.* 2012;72:902–911.
21. Byun JI, Lee ST, Jung KH, et al. Effect of immunotherapy on seizure outcome in patients with autoimmune encephalitis: a prospective observational registry study. *PLoS One.* 2016;11:e0146455.
22. Pillai SC, Mohammad SS, Hacohen Y, et al. Postencephalitic epilepsy and drug-resistant epilepsy after infectious and antibody-associated encephalitis in childhood: clinical and etiologic risk factors. *Epilepsia.* 2016;57:e7–e11.
23. Chen YJ, Fang PC, Chow JC. Clinical characteristics and prognostic factors of postencephalitic epilepsy in children. *J Child Neurol.* 2006;21:1047–1051.
24. Saiz A, Blanco Y, Sabater L, et al. Spectrum of neurological syndromes associated with glutamic acid decarboxylase antibodies: diagnostic clues for this association. *Brain.* 2008;131:2553–2563.

25. Ismail S, Lévy A, Tikkanen H, et al. Lack of efficacy of phenytoin in children presenting with febrile status epilepticus. *Am J Emerg Med.* 2012;30:2000–2004.

26. Sugai K. Treatment of convulsive status epilepticus in infants and young children in Japan. *Acta Neurol Scand.* 2007;115(suppl 186):62–70.

27. Saito Y, Maegaki Y, Okamoto R, et al. Acute encephalitis with refractory, repetitive partial seizures: case reports of this unusual post-encephalitic epilepsy. *Brain Dev.* 2007;29:147–156.

28. Shyu CS, Lee HF, Chi CS, et al. Acute encephalitis with refractory, repetitive partial seizures. *Brain Dev.* 2008;30:356–361.

29. Shorvon S, Ferlisi M. The treatment of super-refractory status epilepticus: a critical review of available therapies and a clinical treatment protocol. *Brain.* 2011;134:2802–2818.

30. Toledano M, Britton JW, McKeon A, et al. Utility of an immunotherapy trial in evaluating patients with presumed autoimmune epilepsy. *Neurology.* 2014;82:1578–1586.

CHAPTER 26

Intensive Care Management of Acute Encephalopathy and Encephalitis

SUNIT SINGHI, MBBS, MD, FIAP, FAMS, FISCCM, FCCM • KARTHI NALLASAMY, MBBS, MD, DM (PED CRIT CARE)

Acute encephalopathy is a clinical syndrome that manifests as reduced consciousness and/or altered cognition or behavior. It results from diverse etiologies including infection, immune mediated, metabolic derangements, toxins, trauma, hypoxia, and vascular disorders. Acute encephalitis literally means inflammation of brain; it may occur in children because of infection of the central nervous system (CNS) by a wide range of microorganisms or noninfectious causes. It is often difficult to discern encephalitis and encephalopathy and various types of encephalitis clinically; only surrogate markers such as the presence of fever and inflammatory changes in cerebrospinal fluid (CSF) or neuroimaging are used to rule in or rule out infections in the initial phase of illness. However, regardless of etiology (Box 26.1), most children with acute encephalitis/encephalopathy syndrome have similar clinical presentations and complications, and therefore the broad principles of management are common.

The goal of intensive care management is not just reduction of mortality but to minimize the long-term neurologic disability in survivors as well. Improved outcomes depend largely on rapid diagnosis, immediate management of life-threatening complications that occur early in the course such as raised intracranial pressure (ICP) and status epilepticus, prompt initiation of appropriate antimicrobials, and supportive and adjunctive therapy. These goals are challenging because of nonspecific initial symptoms, limitation in obtaining CSF for diagnosis, pharmacokinetic barriers in achieving effective concentrations of antimicrobials in the CNS, emerging resistance to available antimicrobials, limited availability of effective antiviral drugs, and lack of adjunctive therapies to block the pathophysiologic mechanisms and prevent complications.

EVALUATION AND DIAGNOSIS

Management of a child with encephalopathy goes hand in hand with clinical evaluation. A detailed history should be obtained as quickly as possible. Focused examination should include spotting systemic signs such as jaundice, rash, and hepatosplenomegaly and then a comprehensive neurologic assessment directed toward localizing brain dysfunction and determining early indicators of prognosis.[1] Recognizing clinical clues from history and examination is crucial for narrowing down the etiology and deciding initial therapy (Table 26.1). Monitoring the subsequent course is equally important because the neurologic status of these children can change rapidly. Complete neurologic examination may be challenging in comatose and sedated children. A quick assessment of essential components must be performed and repeated at the bedside (Box 26.2).

Cerebrospinal Fluid Analysis

CSF analysis is paramount to diagnose encephalitis and its etiology and to differentiate them from other causes of encephalopathy. Lumbar puncture (LP) must be done as early as possible in suspected cases of encephalitis unless contraindicated. Clinical assessment and not cranial computed tomography (CT) should be the guide to determine if it is safe to perform an LP.[2,3]

CSF opening pressure should be documented whenever possible. All CSF samples should be evaluated for white cells with differential counts, glucose and protein concentrations, Gram stain, and cultures. Furthermore,

---

BOX 26.1
Etiology of Acute Encephalopathy and Encephalitis

INFECTIOUS
- Bacterial—Acute bacterial meningitis, brain abscess, enteric encephalopathy, Shigella encephalopathy, tubercular meningitis, leptospirosis, pertussis, mycoplasma, listeria.
- Viral Encephalitis—Japanese B virus, herpes simplex virus, enteroviruses, West Nile virus, dengue, other arboviruses, measles, mumps, rabies
- Cerebral malaria
- Scrub typhus
- Viral-associated encephalopathy—Influenza, rotavirus, varicella zoster, HHV-6, RSV

PARA/POSTINFECTIOUS
- Acute disseminated encephalomyelitis (ADEM)
- Acute hemorrhagic leukoencephalopathy
- Acute necrotizing encephalitis (ANE) in children

IMMUNE MEDIATED
- Anti-NMDA receptor encephalitis
- Paraneoplastic neurologic syndromes
- Other antibody-associated encephalitis (VGKC, GAD 65, AMPAR, GABA B, ANNA-1, ANNA-2, ANNA-3, AGNA, PCA-2, amphiphysin, anti-Ma)

VASCULITIC
- Systemic lupus erythematosus
- Polyarteritis nodosa
- Antiphospholipid antibody syndrome

METABOLIC
- Hepatic encephalopathy, Reye's syndrome
- Diabetic ketoacidosis
- Hypoglycemia, hyponatremia, hyperosmolar states
- Inborn errors of metabolism (mitochondrial disorders, aminoacidopathies, organic acidemias, urea cycle disorders, fat oxidation defects)
- Uremia

OTHERS
- Trauma, intracranial hemorrhage
- Nonconvulsive status epilepticus, postictal
- Hypoxic ischemic encephalopathy
- Stroke
- CNS tumors
- Drugs and toxins
- Post-immunization
- Benign intracranial hypertension
- Heat stroke

---

depending on the suspected etiology, other relevant investigations may be carried out including staining for acid-fast bacilli and fungi such as *Cryptococcus*, antigen assays, and PCR for viruses and atypical organisms and antibodies to detect autoimmune or demyelinating disorders. Routine CT of the head before LP is not necessary and may delay the initiation of antimicrobial therapy.

Normal CSF in children is a clear, colorless fluid containing <20 cells/mm³ (1–4 years age) and <10 cell/mm³ (5 years age to puberty), and lymphocytic predominant; neutrophils are rarely seen. Mild pleocytosis can be found in infants with nonspecific symptoms without CNS infection. CSF absolute neutrophil count above 1000/mm³ is highly suggestive of bacterial meningitis, although sometimes very early in bacterial meningitis CSF may be normal.[4,5] Predominant CSF lymphocytic reaction is seen with viral, tubercular, and fungal infections; demyelinating disease; and autoimmune disorders. CSF pleocytosis may be absent in patients with severe overwhelming sepsis and meningitis or in children who are immunocompromised or

severely undernourished. Typical CSF findings in various forms of CNS infections are shown in Table 26.2.

The presence of erythrocytes in CSF may not always be indicative of a traumatic tap; herpes simplex (HSV-1) encephalitis may be associated with elevated CSF red cell count, typically 10–15 erythrocytes per high-power field.

A lowering of CSF glucose (less than 60% of plasma glucose) is seen in bacterial or tubercular meningitis, metabolic conditions, and subarachnoid hemorrhage. A reduced absolute CSF glucose (<40 mg/dL or <2.2 mmol/L) is highly suggestive of bacterial meningitis.[6] Gram stain of CSF-centrifuged sediment can identify organisms in 60%–90% of cases.[7] Contamination from skin flora or reagent can rarely result in falsely positive Gram stain. CSF culture may be positive in 60%–90% cases of acute bacterial meningitis, although the rates may be lower in developing countries. Polymerase chain reaction (PCR) is now available for rapid etiologic diagnosis of meningoencephalitis. CSF multiplex PCR for detection of common bacterial as well as viral DNA or RNA for suspected encephalitis is effective in the diagnosis of encephalitis caused by several

TABLE 26.1
Diagnostic Clues to Etiology of Encephalopathy and Encephalitis

Clinical Features	Possible Etiology
Acute high-grade fever, neck stiffness, seizures	Bacterial meningitis
Prolonged fever, subacute progression	Tubercular meningitis, enteric encephalopathy
Recent fever with acutely progressing altered consciousness or cognition, new-onset seizures, and/or motor deficits	Acute viral encephalitis (HSV, JE, enterovirus) ADEM, antibody-mediated encephalitis Rarely, mitochondrial disorders
Short history, lower cranial nerve involvement, respiratory drive dysfunction, autonomic disturbances, locked-in syndrome	Brainstem encephalitis (enterovirus, rabies, West Nile virus, JE virus, brucellosis)
Insidious onset, gradually progressive symptoms, headache, vomiting, focal deficits	Expanding mass lesions (tumors, tuberculoma, abscess), hydrocephalus
Abrupt onset of encephalopathy in a healthy child	Stroke, hemorrhage, seizure, toxin exposure, or metabolic cause
Absence of fever, history of previous similar episodes or similar family history, developmental delay, myoclonic seizures, acidotic breathing, fluctuating sensorium	Inborn errors of metabolism
Acute fever with features of systemic illness (rash, respiratory distress, hepatosplenomegaly, edema)	Malaria, scrub typhus, dengue
H/o diarrhea	Electrolyte and hyperosmolar disorders, enteroviral encephalitis, Shigella encephalopathy (dysentery)
Preceding respiratory tract infection	Mycoplasma
H/o recent vaccination	ADEM, adverse event following immunization (DTwP)
Jaundice	Hepatic encephalopathy, leptospirosis, complicated malaria
Petechial rash	Meningococcemia, dengue, scrub typhus, hemorrhagic fevers
Anemia	Cerebral malaria, uremia, intracranial hemorrhage

ADEM, acute disseminated encephalomyelitis.

viruses including herpes simplex virus, VZV, CMV, EBV, JE virus, and enteroviruses. PCR has the advantage of lesser turnaround time (<24 h) and ability to detect pathogens in acute stage of infection, even after short courses of antiviral therapy.

Neuroimaging

Neuroimaging studies are vital for identifying many etiologies, extent of brain involvement, and their complications. Early neuroimaging is indicated in children with encephalitis having clinical contraindications to LP, focal neurological findings, suspected complications, and persistent encephalopathy despite addressing correctable factors.[8,9] CT is widely used in emergency settings because it is readily available and quick. It should be done only after stabilization of the child with raised ICP; the information obtained from CT should be weighed against the risk of transporting a critically ill child. CT will readily identify hemorrhage, mass lesions, cerebral edema, chronic

meningitis including TB, and complications of bacterial meningitis. Initial normal CT, however, does not rule out raised ICP or an evolving lesion.[10] In herpes encephalitis, CT head may be normal in the first week of illness and is abnormal in approximately 50% of cases.

Magnetic resonance imaging (MRI) is sensitive for early detection of parenchymal involvement and differentiating various types of encephalitis that have characteristic neuroimaging patterns as well as the diagnosis of acute disseminated encephalomyelitis (ADEM).[11] MRI findings that suggest specific etiologies are given in Table 26.3. MRI brain with diffusion weighted images should be done as soon as possible, ideally within 48 h in children with unexplained encephalopathy with normal or equivocal CT findings.[12] Spinal MRI is included in children with suspected demyelinating illnesses. Advanced MRI techniques, such as magnetic resonance spectroscopy, compare chemical composition of the lesions and may help in distinguishing different etiologies to a certain extent.

BOX 26.2
Essential Neurologic Assessment in a
Comatose Child

LEVEL OF CONSCIOUSNESS
- Objective assessment using modified Glasgow Coma Score
- Monitoring for subtle alterations in wakefulness

EYE
- Pupil examination for size, shape, symmetry, and response to light
- Look for tonic deviation of eyes or nystagmus
- Fundus examination for papilledema

ASSESSMENT OF BRAINSTEM FUNCTION
- Pattern of breathing
- Posture, response to pain (flexion, extension, or no response)
- Limb tone, deep tendon reflexes, plantars
- Oculocephalic (doll's eye) reflex
- Cough and gag reflex

Magnetic resonance venography is indicated in suspected cerebral venous sinus thrombosis. Familiarity with the clinical course and imaging appearances of various CNS diseases is helpful in making correct differential diagnoses and in prompting timely treatment.

Electroencephalography

EEG is not routinely required as it may show nonspecific changes in most patients with acute encephalitis. In HSV encephalitis, characteristic temporal lobe spike-and-wave activity and periodic lateralized epileptiform discharges may be seen.[13] Bedside continuous EEG monitoring is indicated for 48–72 h in children with status epilepticus and persistent unexplained encephalopathy, in comatose patients with raised ICP, and in those on thiopentone infusion.

IMMEDIATE STABILIZATION
Airway and Breathing

In patients with reduced consciousness, airway patency should be ensured by proper positioning of the head,

TABLE 26.2
Cerebrospinal Fluid Findings in Various Causes of Encephalopathy/Encephalitis

Diagnosis	Opening Pressure (mmH$_2$O)	White Blood Cell Count (Cells/mm^3)	Protein (mg/dL)	Glucose (mg/dL)
Normal	50–80	<5, predominantly lympho-cytes	20–45	>50 (or 60% of plasma glucose)
Bacterial meningitis	Usually high (100–300)	100–10,000 or more, predominantly polymorpho-nuclear (PMN) cells	Usually 100–500	Decreased, usually <40 (<50% of plasma glucose)
Partially treated bacterial meningitis	Normal or high	5–10,000, usually PMN but lymphocytes may be elevated with prolonged antibiotic course	Usually 100–500	Normal or low
Viral meningitis or meningoencephalitis	Normal or high	50–500, lymphocytes predominate, PMNs in early phase	Usually 50–150	Usually normal, may be low (<40) in mumps
Tubercular meningitis	Usually high	May be normal; usually 10–500; predominantly lymphocytes, PMNs may be seen in early phase	100–3000; may be higher in the presence of block	Usually low, reduces further with time
Fungal meningitis	Usually high	5–500; PMNs in early phase, lymphocytes predominate in rest of the course	25–500	Usually low, reduces further with time
ADEM	Normal to mild elevation	10–100; lymphocytes	Normal to mild elevation	Normal
Autoimmune encephalitis	Normal to mild elevation	10–100; lymphocytes	Normal to mild elevation	Normal

ADEM, acute disseminated encephalomyelitis.

TABLE 26.3
Neuroimaging Findings and Possible Etiology

MRI Features	Possible Etiology
Medial temporal lobe hyperintensities, edema of insula, cingulate gyrus	Herpes simplex virus encephalitis
Lesions in thalamus, basal ganglia and midbrain (hypointense on T1 and hyperintense on T2 and FLAIR images)	Japanese encephalitis, West Nile virus, or other flavivirus encephalitis
Bilateral symmetrical thalamic involvement with or without white matter lesions	Inborn errors of metabolism, mitochondrial disorders, Japanese encephalitis, acute necrotizing encephalopathy, acute hemorrhagic encephalitis (associated cavitation, hemorrhage)
Hyperintensities in globus pallidus and putamen	Rabies encephalitis
Lesions in midbrain, pons, and medulla (hyperintense T2 changes)	Enterovirus
Ischemic changes/infarction in white matter, particularly at gray-white junctions	Varicella zoster virus vasculopathy
Multifocal subcortical white matter lesions involving subcortical U fibers with tangential lesions	Acute disseminated encephalomyelitis
Basal exudates, basal ganglia infarcts, hydrocephalus	Tuberculosis

suctioning of oropharyngeal secretions, and use of oropharyngeal or nasopharyngeal airways, if needed. Forceful opening of clenched jaws should be avoided. The stomach should be decompressed by early insertion of nasogastric tube to prevent aspiration. Oxygen by mask can be started in children with a stable airway and spontaneous breathing. Endotracheal intubation is warranted in children with a Glasgow Coma Scale (GCS) score of 8 or lower or those with raised ICP; significant pharyngeal hypotonia, poor gag reflex, and loss of swallowing reflex in them can lead to unstable airway and aspiration. Children with signs of inadequate ventilation and oxygenation, such as irregular respiratory efforts, inadequate chest movements, poor air entry, central cyanosis, or peripheral oxygen saturation of 92% or less, should receive initial bag and mask ventilation followed by endotracheal intubation and mechanical ventilation. Rapid sequence intubation is preferred for emergency intubation to prevent aspiration and sudden surge in ICP. Combinations of thiopental/midazolam, lidocaine, fentanyl, and a short-acting nondepolarizing neuromuscular blocking agent (e.g., vecuronium, atracurium) can be used for induction.

Hemodynamic Stabilization

Vascular access should be immediately established for administration of fluids, anticonvulsants, and antibiotics. Patients with signs of poor perfusion or hypotension should receive a bolus of normal saline

(0.9% saline, 20 mL/kg) before continuing with the rest of the assessment and management.

Hypertension is common in acute CNS infections. The causes include pain, agitation, and Cushing response to raised ICP (i.e., widening of pulse pressure with an increase in systolic blood pressure, bradycardia, and irregular breathing). Systemic hypertension may increase cerebral blood flow (CBF) and ICP when autoregulation is impaired, which may promote cerebral edema. Moderate elevation of blood pressure in the acute stage often resolves with sedation and does not require antihypertensive medication. Treatment is indicated in persistent elevation of BP with worsening cerebral edema and in patients with extreme surge in blood pressure. β-Blockers or central acting α-receptor agonists are preferred because they reduce blood pressure without worsening ICP. Vasodilators, such as nitroprusside and nifedipine, should be avoided as they can increase ICP.

Addressing Correctable Factors

Alterations in blood glucose and electrolytes can cause reversible encephalopathy. More commonly, hypoglycemia and hyponatremia can be accompanying derangements in critically ill children potentiating encephalopathy caused by the underlying disease. Prompt treatment of glucose levels <60 mg/dL with 2 mL/kg of intravenous 25% dextrose generally will reverse the neurologic signs. Plasma sodium <125 meq/L in a symptomatic child requires correction

TABLE 26.4
Indications for ICU Admission

| Glasgow Coma Score ≤ 8 or a rapid fall of 3 or more points |
| Status epilepticus |
| Features of raised intracranial pressure |
| Respiratory failure requiring mechanical ventilation |
| Hemodynamic instability |
| Hepatic encephalopathy |
| Severe hyperammonemia requiring dialysis |
| Children requiring neurosurgical intervention |

with 5 mL/kg of 3% saline to raise the sodium to safer levels.

After stabilization in the emergency room, patients should be assessed and those in need of intensive care should be transferred to an intensive care unit. Clinical signs that suggest the need for admission to an intensive care unit are shown in Table 26.4.

SPECIFIC THERAPY
Antimicrobial Therapy

In children with suspected infectious etiology, antimicrobials should be administered as early as possible without waiting for laboratory confirmation. For suspected bacterial meningitis, ceftriaxone is the initial choice in immunocompetent children beyond neonatal age. All children with suspected viral encephalitis should receive intravenous acyclovir. Because herpes simplex virus (HSV) is among the commonly implicated pathogens in viral encephalitis, treatment with acyclovir is usually started without delay, definitely within 6 h, while waiting for the laboratory reports.[3] Acyclovir exhibits strong antiviral activity against HSV and related herpes viruses, including varicella zoster virus and is shown to improve outcome.[14] The dose for children aged 3 months up to 12 years is 500 mg/m^2 and for >12 years, 10 mg/kg administered 8 hourly. Dose reduction is needed in patients with preexisting renal impairment. No specific treatment is recommended for enterovirus encephalitis; in patients with life-threatening disease, pleconaril has been tried with some benefit. Children from tropical areas where systemic infections such as scrub typhus, rickettsial spotted fevers, and malaria presenting as encephalitis syndrome are common should receive additional doxycycline or artesunate based on clinical assessment and results of point-of-care tests.[15] Antibiotic therapy with azithromycin has been found beneficial in

children with mycoplasma encephalitis. Other rare but treatable CNS infections include CMV, toxoplasma, and *Cryptococcus* that are seen in children with compromised immunity (Table 26.5).

Other Treatable Conditions

Immunomodulation is the mainstay of treatment of demyelinating and autoimmune encephalitis. Pulse methylprednisolone (at 30 mg/kg/day, max 1 g) for 3–5 days is the first-line therapy for ADEM. The treatment approach for autoimmune encephalitis is still evolving.[16] Pulse methylprednisolone, intravenous immunoglobulin, plasma exchange, or a combination of these therapies is the accepted first-line management for antibody-mediated encephalitis. Second-line treatments such as rituximab and cyclophosphamide are typically reserved for patients who remain significantly impaired after first-line agents.

If a metabolic disorder is suspected, it is important to stop or modify feeds and start intravenous dextrose to prevent further damage. Hyperammonemia is treated with sodium benzoate, sodium phenylacetate, and arginine. Dialysis may be required for treating severe hyperammonemia and refractory high anion gap metabolic acidosis.

ADJUNCTIVE THERAPY AND SUPPORTIVE CARE
Corticosteroids

Routine use of corticosteroids in children with acute infectious encephalitis is not indicated. In children from high-income countries with acute bacterial meningitis, dexamethasone at 0.15 mg/kg 6 hourly for 48 h reduced hearing loss and short-term neurologic sequelae without improving mortality. There was no beneficial effect of corticosteroid therapy in low-income countries.[17] The use of adjunctive corticosteroid treatment is recommended for tubercular meningitis. It is shown to reduce the risk of death or disability, although the biologic mechanisms underlying their beneficial effect remain poorly understood. Corticosteroids are also advocated in treating vasogenic edema accompanying tumors, granulomas, and abscesses.

Nursing Care

Changes in neurologic condition in children with encephalitis may be subtle hence require frequent assessment for detection of new neurologic signs, seizures, or agitation. Essential nursing care components include appropriate body positioning; care of skin, eyes, and mouth; handling of monitoring devices; and respiratory care.

TABLE 26.5
Etiology and Specific Treatment of Various Conditions Causing Encephalopathy

Etiology	Drug	Dose/Duration
Acute bacterial meningitis	Ceftriaxone	100 mg/kg/day (IV) in one or two divided doses/7–10 days (10–14 days for *S. pneumoniae*)
	±	
	Vancomycin (in regions with high rates of *Streptococcus pneumoniae* resistance to penicillin)	60 mg/kg/day (IV) in four divided doses/ and (2–3 weeks for gram-negative organisms)
Listeria monocytogenes	Ampicillin	200–300 mg/kg/day (IV) in four divided doses/2–4 weeks
	±	
	Gentamycin	7.5 mg/kg/day (IV)/7 days
Mycoplasma pneumonia	Azithromycin	10 mg/kg/day (PO/IV)/5 days
Scrub typhus Rickettsial spotted fevers	Doxycycline	5 mg/kg/day (IV/PO) in two divided doses/7–14 days
Malaria	Artesunate	2.4 mg/kg/dose (IV)/At 0, 12, 24 h (3 mg/kg for children <20 kg) Followed by 4 mg/kg/day (PO) (as Artesunate Combination Therapy)/3 days
Herpes simplex virus	Acyclovir	500 mg/m^2/day (age 3 months to 12 years)/21 days 30 mg/kg/day (age >12 years) (IV) in three divided doses/(should be continued for longer with weekly CSF-PCR until PCR negative)
Varicella zoster virus	Acyclovir	500 mg/m^2/day (age 3 months to 12 years)/7–10 days 30 mg/kg/day (age >12 years) (IV) in three divided doses
Cytomegalovirus	Ganciclovir	10 mg/kg/day (IV) in two divided doses/3 weeks
	+	
	Foscarnet	60 mg/kg 8 hourly by IV infusion /3 weeks (followed by maintenance therapy in immunocompromised)
Toxoplasma	Pyrimethamine	2 mg/kg/day (PO)/3 days followed by 1 mg/kg/day (25 mg/day max)/4 weeks
	+	
	Sulfadiazine	100–200 mg/kg/day (PO) in four divided doses/4 weeks
	or	
	Clindamycin	5–7.5 mg/kg/day (IV/PO) in three or four divided doses/4 weeks

Continued

TABLE 26.5
Etiology and Specific Treatment of Various Conditions Causing Encephalopathy—cont'd

Etiology	Drug	Dose/Duration
Cryptococcus	Amphotericin B + 5-Flucytosine Followed by fluconazole	3–5 mg/kg/day (IV) of LfAmB/2 weeks 100 mg/kg/day (PO) in four divided doses/2 weeks 6–12 mg/kg/day (PO)/6 months to 1 year In HIV patients: indefinite
Mycobacterium tuberculosis	Isoniazid Rifampicin Pyrazinamide Ethambutol + Dexamethasone	10 mg/kg/day (PO)/12 months 15 mg/kg/day (PO)/12 months 35 mg/kg/day (PO)/2–12 months 20 mg/kg/day (PO)/2 months 0.6 mg/kg/day (IV) in four divided doses/4 weeks (or prednisolone 1–2 mg/kg/day [PO])/Then tapered
Naegleria	Amphotericin B + Rifampicin	1.5 mg/kg/day (IV) in two divided doses/3 days Then 1 mg/kg/day (IV) (±0.5 mg/day intraventricular)/11 days 10 mg/kg/day (PO)/4 weeks
Acute disseminated encephalomyelitis	Methylprednisolone	30 mg/kg/day, maximum 1 g/day (IV)/3–5 days Followed by prednisolone 1–2 mg/kg/day (PO)/4 weeks
Autoimmune encephalitis (antibody mediated)	Methylprednisolone ± IVIg or Plasma exchange	30 mg/kg/day (IV) (maximum 1 g/day)/3–5 days 2 g/kg divided over 2–5 days (IV) 5 exchanges over 10 days

Positioning of comatose patients

In side-lying position, a pillow is placed between the legs to prevent internal rotation, adduction, and inversion of the upper leg. It is important to guard against compression at the elbows to protect the ulnar nerve. If supine position is adopted, the head is placed in neutral position and arms flexed at the elbow with the hands resting at the side of the abdomen. Knees are slightly flexed with rolls of padding folded under the greater trochanter-hip joint area to reduce pressure on the perineal nerve at the fibula head, the feet at right angle to the legs, and the toes pointing upward. In patients with hemiparesis, paralyzed arm is supported on a pillow with the elbow partially flexed. Trochanter rolls are used to prevent external rotation at the hip joint. In the lateral position, patients should be turned on the unaffected side without flexion of the trunk/spine.

Eye care

Comatose and sedated children in intensive care units are at risk of exposure keratopathy. Various eye care protocols are being used including ocular lubricants, horizontal lid taping, and creating a moisture chamber to prevent corneal dryness.[18]

Sedation, Analgesia, and Paralysis

Children with acute encephalitis are often uncomfortable or agitated. Pain, anxiety, and paroxysmal sympathetic activity increase the cerebral metabolic rate and ICP and should be prevented with appropriate sedation and adequate analgesia. Additionally, mechanically ventilated neurologically ill children may require sedation to blunt central hyperventilation and improve patient-ventilator synchrony. There are no specific protocols or controlled studies to indicate the best choice of medication or dosing in children with acute encephalitis. Nonsteroidal antiinflammatory agents are useful in awake patients with severe headaches. Opioid analgesics (morphine 0.1 mg/kg, 4–6 hourly or fentanyl 1–2 µg/kg/h infusion) remain the mainstay of pain management in ventilated children. For sedation, the favored drug should have minimum effect on blood pressure and ICP, and recovery should be rapid to facilitate neurologic assessment. Benzodiazepines are commonly used sedatives. Selection of shorter-acting agents such as midazolam (0.2 mg/kg bolus followed by infusion at a rate of 2–3 µg/kg/min) is preferred. Propofol (0.1 mg/kg/min with incremental doses until reasonable sedation) may have the advantage of rapid onset, shorter duration of action, and favorable CNS effect in patients with raised ICP. However, drug accumulation and risk of propofol infusion syndrome at high doses preclude its prolonged

use in ICU. There is a renewed interest in ketamine for sedation of neurologically ill patients ever since the concern of ICP elevation by the drug has been refuted in the recent studies. Dexmedetomidine is an attractive option because it allows reliable neurologic examination; however, the data are limited. Hypovolemia should be corrected before administering sedatives. Cisatracurium or vecuronium as a muscle relaxant is sometimes used in children with refractory raised ICP. The major problem with this therapy is that the neurologic examination cannot be monitored closely because the neuromuscular block eliminates motor activity. These children should have continuous EEG monitoring.

Fluid, Electrolytes, and Nutrition

Children with encephalitis often have alteration in their fluid and electrolyte homeostasis. The goals of fluid therapy are to maintain euvolemia and normoglycemia and to prevent hyponatremia. Fever, diminished intake, and vomiting may lead to dehydration and hypovolemia; sepsis-induced capillary leak can further worsen the situation. Hypovolemia often manifests with a sudden fall in blood pressure when patients are intubated and subjected to positive pressure ventilation. Empirical fluid restriction under the assumption that hyponatremia may result from syndrome of inappropriate secretion of antidiuretichormone (SIADH) is not supported by available evidence. In a prospective study in children with acute meningitis, high ADH levels returned to normal on fluid administration, suggesting that elevation of ADH is an appropriate response to hypovolemia.[19] In randomized controlled clinical trials, fluid restriction did not improve the outcome of acute meningitis in children.[20,21] Therefore, daily maintenance plus replacement fluids aimed at maintaining euvolemia, normal urine output (>1 mL/kg/h) and normal blood pressure, and thereby adequate cerebral perfusion are recommended. All fluids should be isotonic; hypotonic fluids should be avoided.

Enteral feeding is encouraged and should be initiated as early as possible, preferably within 24–48 h of admission. Early enteral feeding is associated with reduced intensive care stay and complications.

About 25% of patients with meningitis and encephalitis may develop hyponatremia. The etiology can be multifactorial, such as salt wasting, SIADH, hypotonic fluid therapy, or adrenal insufficiency. Hyponatremia should be identified early and corrected gradually to maintain serum sodium at 135–145 mmol/L or higher (145–155 mmol/L) in the presence of raised ICP. Both hyperglycemia and hypoglycemia should be avoided. Rarely, children with acute encephalitis may develop diabetes insipidus because of hypothalamic and/or pituitary involvement; it is generally associated with poor prognosis.

Seizures and Status Epilepticus

Acute seizures are common in patients with CNS infections. They can be focal or generalized and may progress into status epilepticus in substantial proportion of children. Acute encephalitis is one of the most common cause of refractory status epilepticus in PICU. Seizures can also be subtle and, less commonly, may present as nonconvulsive status epilepticus. Seizure activity can adversely affect the already compromised brain by increasing the metabolic demand and CBF, thereby worsening raised ICP.

Prompt and energetic control of seizures and status epilepticus is essential for prevention of secondary brain injury. A protocolized management is useful in timely achievement of endpoints. Immediate termination of seizures is achieved with intravenous administration of benzodiazepines. Intravenous lorazepam, diazepam, or midazolam can be used; all three drugs have onset of action within 1–3 min and they are equally effective. The dose can be repeated after 5–10 min if seizures persist. If seizures continue, phenytoin or fosphenytoin infusion is commonly used with cardiac monitoring to guard against hypotension and cardiac arrhythmia. Phenobarbital (loading dose 15–20 mg/kg) is generally preferred over phenytoin in neonates. Intravenous valproate (40 mg/kg) and intravenous levetiracetam (40–60 mg/kg) are used as second-line agents. However, there is no evidence to substantiate the preference of one over the other. Persistence of seizures even after adequate treatment with benzodiazepines and a second-line agent is referred to as refractory status epilepticus. There is little consensus regarding the standard protocol for management of refractory status epilepticus.[22] A repeat minidose of second-line agents have been tried. Midazolam infusion (2–12 µg/kg/min at incremental doses), anesthetic doses of thiopental, or propofol are other available options. All children with refractory status epilepticus require admission to PICU. Continuous EEG monitoring is indicated in children with status epilepticus and those with persistent unexplained encephalopathy even after complete control of clinical convulsions. Facilities for mechanical ventilation and invasive arterial blood pressure monitoring should be available if thiopental infusion is planned. The initial bolus dose is 3–4 mg/kg IV over 2 min, followed by infusion of 1-5 mg/kg/h, in some cases upto 12 mg/kg/h. The rate is increased every 3–5 min until status epilepticus is controlled or a burst-suppression EEG recording is obtained.

Raised Intracranial Pressure

Substantial proportion of hospitalized children with encephalitis have intracranial hypertension at initial presentation or develop it within 48 h. Raised ICP is an important cause of mortality. The pathogenesis is multifactorial. Early increase in ICP is primarily due to inflammatory cytotoxic edema, infarction, and increased capillary permeability in brain parenchyma (vasogenic edema) and subarachnoid space. Raised ICP that manifests later in the course, especially in purulent meningitis and tubercular meningitis, may be due to ventriculitis, subdural effusion, and basal exudates and obstructed or communicating hydrocephalus. Raised ICP compromises CBF and causes ischemic damage to the brain, leading to progressive brain injury. With impaired autoregulation, CBF becomes a direct function of cerebral perfusion pressure (CPP) and highly sensitive to rise in ICP or fall in mean arterial blood pressure. The management goals to break the vicious cycle of raised ICP and cerebral ischemia at the earliest and maintain an adequate CPP simply by manipulating the blood pressure up to 90th to 95th centile with judicious use of fluids and vasopressors such as dopamine and norepinephrine.[23] A CPP-targeted therapy, which relied on more frequent use of vasopressors and lesser use of hyperventilation and osmotherapy, was superior to ICP-targeted therapy for management of raised ICP in children with meningitis and encephalitis in reducing mortality and morbidity. Although normal CPP values for children are not clearly established, but generally accepted, minimum CPP values are 50–60 mmHg in older children and 40–50 mmHg in infants and toddlers. Protocols for the management of raised ICP are presented in Fig. 26.1.

Intracranial pressure monitoring

Early clinical features of increased ICP are difficult to elicit in comatose patients. Signs that strongly correlate with raised ICP such as abnormal posturing, pupillary dilatation, fluctuating heart rate (bradycardia) and hypertension, abnormal respiratory pattern (periodic breathing, hyperventilation), and a GCS score below 8 are late manifestations. Papilledema is uncommon in acute stages of encephalitis. CT findings of brain swelling and compressed basal cisterns are predictive of increased ICP, but intracranial hypertension can occur without these findings. Therefore, ICP monitoring for the initial 72 h, where feasible, can be helpful in guiding therapy to maintain ICP below 20 mmHg, adequate CBF, and CPP above 50–60 mmHg in comatose (GCS score of 8 or less) children with encephalitis. Pediatric intensivists can safely and successfully perform burr

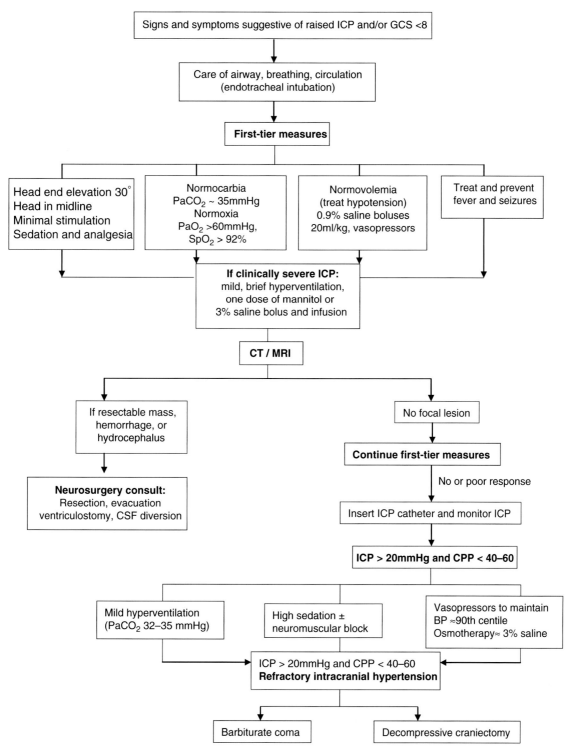

FIG. 26.1 Algorithm for management of raised intracranial pressure (ICP). *CPP*, cerebral perfusion pressure; *CT*, computed tomography; *GCS*, Glasgow Coma Scale; *MRI*, magnetic resonance imaging.

holes at bedside for establishing intraparenchymal ICP monitoring if a neurosurgeon is not available.[24]

General measures

Positioning: Patients with raised ICP should be nursed in supine position with head in midline and head end elevated to 30 degrees to promote venous drainage.

Treatment of precipitating factors: Control of factors that can aggravate raised ICP is important. These include pain, agitation, hypoxia, hypercapnia, fever, seizures, hypoglycemia, hyponatremia, and anemia. Fever increases metabolic rate by 10%–13% per degree Celsius and induces dilation of cerebral vessels with increase in CBF and ICP. Fever should be controlled with antipyretics (IV or rectal paracetamol) and tepid sponging. Severe anemia contributes to increase ICP through increase in CBF and relative hypoxia. The common practice is to maintain hemoglobin concentration around 10 g/dL. However, optimal hemoglobin concentration in patients with raised ICP needs further research.[25] Seizures irrespective of underlying etiology worsen the raised ICP. In comatose patients with raised ICP, it is advisable to start continuous EEG monitoring for nonconvulsive seizures; phenytoin prophylaxis (5–8 kg/day) is used by some. In intubated children, suctioning should be done only if necessary, ensuring adequate sedoanalgesia and using a bolus of lidocaine (1 mg/kg IV) to dampen the ICP surge.

Hyperosmolar therapy

Mannitol: Mannitol has been the primary hyperosmolar agent used for many decades for reduction of cerebral edema. The usual dose is 0.25–0.5 g/kg of 20% solution administered over 10–15 min, repeated every 4–6 h for 48–72 h. For urgent reduction of ICP an initial dose up to 1 g/kg may be given. Mannitol creates an ongoing osmotic gradient that reduces cerebral edema and decreases intracranial volume. Mannitol also transiently expands intravascular volume and reduces viscosity, thereby improves CBF. When using mannitol, volume status needs to be carefully monitored because mannitol-induced diuresis can cause profound hypovolemia and can adversely affect the outcome. Serum osmolarity must be kept under 320 mOsm/L for mannitol to be effective. In addition, higher osmolarity increases the risk of acute tubular necrosis and renal failure. Use of mannitol may also lead to rebound intracranial hypertension. Most recent evidence suggests a trend favoring the use of hypertonic saline over mannitol as a hyperosmolar agent for reduction of intracranial hypertension in neurocritical care.[26,27]

Hypertonic (3%) saline: The mechanism of action of hypertonic saline (commonly 3.0%, up to 23.4%) is not fully clear, but it is likely that it has an osmotic effect similar to mannitol. 3% saline is used in a loading dose of 10 mL/kg over 30 min followed by 0.1–1 mL/kg/h as continuous infusion. Serum osmolarity must be monitored and kept under 350 mOsm/L. Hypertonic saline has a distinct advantage in children who are hypovolemic or hypotensive because it is a volume expander and improves mean arterial pressure. Hypertonic saline has been shown to achieve a greater reduction in ICP as compared with other hyperosmolar therapies in CNS infections.[28] In our experience, hypertonic saline as compared with mannitol successfully controlled ICP in higher proportion of children with improved, modified Glasgow Coma Score and overall outcome.[29]

Hyperventilation

Mild hyperventilation ($PaCO_2$ 33–35 mmHg) can be used when other measures to decrease ICP are not effective. This is done mainly by increasing respiratory rate, while maintaining normal tidal volume (8–10 mL/kg). End-tidal CO_2 can be used to monitor CO_2 and to guard against sudden reduction in pCO_2. It reduces CBF by causing vasoconstriction that lasts for 11–20 h before CSF pH equilibrates to new $PaCO_2$ levels. Prolonged hyperventilation can result in vasoconstriction, reduced CBF, and increased risk of ischemia. Weaning from hyperventilation is done gradually to prevent rebound rise of ICP. Brief bursts of hyperventilation ($PaCO_2$ 29–32 mmHg), using bag-valve, is practiced for emergency reduction of raised ICP in children who present with signs of imminent or impending herniation. However, hyperventilation lasting more than an hour has been associated with poor long-term outcome.

Barbiturate coma

Barbiturates reduce the cerebral metabolic rate and lower ICP. However, they can also cause significant hypotension threatening cerebral perfusion. High-dose barbiturate therapy is generally reserved for hemodynamically stable patients with intracranial hypertension refractory to other interventions. Thiopental is given in a loading dose of 5 mg/kg over 30 min followed by infusion of 1–5 mg/kg/h until EEG shows a burst-suppression pattern. There is no evidence to support the use of barbiturates for prophylactic neuroprotection in children with acute neurologic injury.

Cerebrospinal fluid drainage

External ventricular drainage of CSF or ventriculoperitoneal shunt is effective in reducing ICP in patients with hydrocephalus. CSF drainage can also be utilized in others, particularly if a ventriculostomy catheter is present and the basal cisterns are visible on imaging. However, it is of limited value in diffuse cerebral edema with collapsed ventricles.

Decompressive craniectomy

Surgical decompression should be considered in children with encephalitis with intracranial hypertension refractory to medical therapy. It is particularly effective in unilateral lesions and is performed in patients with clinical and imaging evidence of brainstem compression. Better prognosis can be expected in patients with herpes simplex viral encephalitis, and results are favorable even after clinical signs of brainstem dysfunction.[30,31]

Mechanical Ventilation

Children with acute encephalopathy or encephalitis may require mechanical ventilation because of impaired mechanics due to neuromuscular failure, impaired respiratory drive, or aspiration pneumonia. However, depressed level of consciousness is not an absolute indication for ventilation. The signs suggestive of imminent neuromuscular failure are restlessness, tachycardia, tachypnea, forehead sweating, paradoxical breathing, and weakness of trapezius and neck muscles. Aspiration occurs frequently in comatose patients and in patients with acute bulbar dysfunction, repeated seizures, and/or vomiting. Aspiration is rarely witnessed; patients often develop signs of respiratory distress and cough after 4–6 h. Settings of mechanical ventilation depend on the indication and condition of underlying lung. Ventilation is aimed at maintaining normoxia and normocarbia. In a typical patient with encephalopathy, the ventilator is set in synchronized intermittent mandatory ventilation mode with rate and tidal volume (8 mL/kg) that are near-normal for age. Positive end expiratory pressure (PEEP) is maintained at 3–5 mmHg, and the inspiratory:expiratory time ratio at 1:2 to 1:3; FiO_2 is set at 0.4 or more to achieve normoxia (PaO_2 60–80 mmHg). Once the condition improves and spontaneous efforts appear, pressure support mode is appropriate. Patients having spontaneous hyperventilation may be served better by assisted mode of ventilation with mild sedation. High PEEP can worsen ICP by impeding venous return and increasing cerebral venous pressure. PEEP at low-to-moderate levels is used. End-tidal CO_2 monitoring is recommended in all ventilated patients to guard against hypercarbia or inadvertent CO_2 washout; both are detrimental. Weaning from the ventilator should be gradual. Sudden transition may be stressful. Extubation is contemplated when patient shows improvement of sensorium, normal airway protective reflexes, and ability to handle oral secretions.

Isolation Precautions

Viral infections such as varicella and measles need airborne precautions. Patients should be cared for in a separate room having negative-pressure airflow or laminar flow. Precautions to be observed include the use of N95 respirators, gowns, and gloves. Droplet precautions are indicated in meningococcal and mycoplasma infections and hemorrhagic fevers. A single-patient room is preferred, but if not available, spatial separation of >3 ft with curtains between beds is advocated. Healthcare personnel should wear mask, gowns, and gloves. Patients requiring contact isolation include those with adenovirus, herpes simplex (disseminated), and CNS infections with cutaneous draining lesions. Strict handwashing should be observed between visits to patients. Gloves should be worn for anticipated contact with blood, secretions, and any moist body substances.

Family Support

Most children with encephalitis are comatose or need to be in induced coma and may rapidly worsen in the first 24 h. The physician should anticipate a very complex physician-family relationship in the first 24–48 h. The main goals are (1) clarification and explanation of the acute neurologic disease; (2) discussion of the level of responsiveness of the patient; and (3) the expected progression or improvement in the first few days. It is often difficult to ascertain the long-term prognosis based on clinical or imaging findings during the acute stage. One should avoid a discussion on possible long-term functional outcome. Initially the family's assessment of prognosis can be more optimistic than that of the physician. It is ill-advised to express an exaggerated sense of hope and optimism in the first 24 h. Any stress reaction in the family members that accompanies neurologic catastrophe should be handled calmly. When no improvement in the neurologic deficit is seen and the outlook for a meaningful recovery is remote, an honest effort to help parents realize the gravity of the situation should be made. In patients with confirmed brain death, decision of withdrawal of treatment and support must be discussed with the family and it is crucial for them to feel that they were not pressurized.

OUTCOME

Encephalitis requiring intensive care may be associated with significant mortality (5%–30%) and long-term neurologic sequelae. In a systematic review of 934 survivors, incomplete recovery was reported in 42% of children.[32] Apart from major morbidities such as motor impairment, intellectual disability, and epilepsy, a significant proportion also suffered from attention deficit, personality changes, and learning disorders. The presence of seizures at presentation increased the risk of subsequent epilepsy. Children who made a full recovery did so within 1 year.

REFERENCES

1. Solomon T, Hart IJ, Beeching NJ. Viral encephalitis: a clinician's guide. *Pract Neurol.* 2007;7:288–305.
2. Kneen R, Solomon T, Appleton R. The role of lumbar puncture in children with suspected central nervous system infection. *BMC Pediatr.* 2002;2:8.
3. Kneen R, Michael BD, Menson E, et al. Management of suspected viral encephalitis in children – Association of British Neurologists and British Paediatric Allergy, Immunology and Infection Group national guidelines. *J Infect.* 2012;64:449–477.
4. Berkley JA, Mwangi I, Ngetsa CJ, et al. Diagnosis of acute bacterial meningitis in children at a sub-Saharan district hospital. *Lancet.* 2001;357:1753–1757.
5. Lussiana C, Lôa Clemente SV, Pulido Tarquino IA, Paulo I. Predictors of bacterial meningitis in resource-limited contexts: an Angolan case. *PLoS One.* 2011;6:e25706.
6. Nigrovic LE, Kimia AA, Shah SS, Neuman MI. Relationship between cerebrospinal fluid glucose and serum glucose. *N Engl J Med.* 2012;366:576–578.
7. Greenlee JE. Approach to diagnosis of meningitis. Cerebrospinal fluid evaluation. *Infect Dis Clin N Am.* 1990;4:583–598.
8. Raschilas F, Wolff M, Delatour F, et al. Outcome of and prognostic factors for herpes simplex encephalitis in adult patients: results of a multicenter study. *Clin Infect Dis.* 2002;35:254–260.
9. van de Beek D, de Gans J, Spanjaard L, Weisfelt M, Reitsma JB, Vermeulen M. Clinical features and prognostic factors in adults with bacterial meningitis. *N Engl J Med.* 2004;351:1849–1859.
10. Kneen R, Jakka S, Mithyantha R, Riordan A, Solomon T. The management of infants and children treated with acyclovir for suspected viral encephalitis. *Arch Dis Child.* 2010;95:100–106.
11. Marchbank ND, Howlett DC, Sallomi DF, Hughes DV. Magnetic resonance imaging is preferred in diagnosing suspected cerebral infections. *Br Med J.* 2000;320:187–188.
12. McCabe K, Tyler K, Tanabe J. Diffusion-weighted MRI abnormalities as a clue to the diagnosis of herpes simplex encephalitis. *Neurology.* 2003;61:1015–1016.
13. García-Morales I, García MT, Galan-Davila L, et al. Periodic lateralized epileptiform discharges: etiology, clinical aspects, seizures, and evolution in 130 patients. *J Clin Neurophysiol.* 2002;19:172–177.
14. McGrath N, Anderson NE, Croxson MC, Powell KF. Herpes simplex encephalitis treated with acyclovir: diagnosis and long term outcome. *J Neurol Neurosurg Psychiatry.* 1997;63:321–326.
15. Singhi S, Chaudhary D, Varghese GM, et al. Tropical fevers: management guidelines. *Indian J Crit Care Med.* 2014;18:62–69.
16. Brenton JN, Goodkin HP. Antibody-mediated autoimmune encephalitis in childhood. *Pediatr Neurol.* 2016;60:13–23.
17. Brouwer MC, McIntyre P, Prasad K, van de Beek D. Corticosteroids for acute bacterial meningitis. *Cochrane Database Syst Rev.* 2015;12: CD004405.
18. Rosenberg JB, Eisen LA. Eye care in the intensive care unit: narrative review and meta-analysis. *Crit Care Med.* 2008;36:3151–3155.
19. Powell KR, Sugarman LI, Eskenazi AE, et al. Normalization of plasma arginine vasopressin concentrations when children with meningitis are given maintenance plus replacement fluid therapy. *J Pediatr.* 1990;117:515–522.
20. Singhi SC, Singhi PD, Srinivas B, et al. Fluid restriction does not improve the outcome of acute meningitis. *Pediatr Infect Dis J.* 1995;14:495–503.
21. Duke T, Mokela D, Frank D, et al. Management of meningitis in children with oral fluid restriction or intravenous fluid at maintenance volumes: a randomised trial. *Ann Trop Paediatr.* 2002;22:145–157.
22. Glauser T, Shinnar S, Gloss D, et al. Evidence-based guideline: treatment of convulsive status epilepticus in children and adults: report of the Guideline Committee of the American Epilepsy Society. *Epilepsy Curr.* 2016;16:48–61.
23. Kumar R, Singhi S, Singhi P, Jayashree M, Bansal A, Bhatti A. Randomized controlled trial comparing cerebral perfusion pressure-targeted therapy versus intracranial pressure-targeted therapy for raised intracranial pressure due to acute CNS infections in children. *Crit Care Med.* 2014;42:1775–1787.
24. Singhi S, Kumar R, Singhi P, Jayashree M, Bansal A. Bedside burr hole for intracranial pressure monitoring performed by pediatric intensivists in children with CNS infections in a resource-limited setting: 10-year experience at a single center. *Pediatr Crit Care Med.* 2015;16:453–460.
25. Kramer AH, Zygun DA. Anemia and red blood cell transfusion in neurocritical care. *Crit Care.* 2009;13:R89.
26. Rickard AC, Smith JE, Newell P, Bailey A, Kehoe A, Mann C. Salt or sugar for your injured brain? A meta-analysis of randomised controlled trials of mannitol versus hypertonic sodium solutions to manage raised intracranial pressure in traumatic brain injury. *Emerg Med J.* 2014;31:679–683.
27. Burgess S, Abu-Laban RB, Slavik RS, Vu EN, Zed PJ. A systematic review of randomized controlled trials comparing hypertonic sodium solutions and mannitol for traumatic brain injury: implications for emergency department management. *Ann Pharmacother.* 2016;50:291–300.

28. Gwer S, Gatakaa H, Mwai L, et al. The role for osmotic agents in children with acute encephalopathies: a systematic review. *BMC Pediatr.* 2010;10:23.

29. Kumar R, Singhi S, Singhi P, Bansal A. Randomized comparison of 20%-mannitol vs 3%-hypertonic saline in children with raised intracranial pressure due to acute central nervous system infections. *Pediatr Crit Care Med.* 2014;15. suppl-p.82.

30. Singhi P, Saini AG, Sahu JK, et al. Unusual clinical presentation and role of decompressive craniectomy in herpes simplex encephalitis. *J Child Neurol.* 2015;30:1204–1207.

31. Pérez-Bovet J, Garcia-Armengol R, Buxó-Pujolràs M, et al. Decompressive craniectomy for encephalitis with brain herniation: case report and review of the literature. *Acta Neurochir (Wien).* 2012;154:1717–1724.

32. Khandaker G, Jung J, Britton PN, King C, Yin JK, Jones CA. Long-term outcomes of infective encephalitis in children: a systematic review and meta-analysis. *Dev Med Child Neurol.* 2016;58:1108–1115.

FURTHER READING

1. Siegel JD, Rhinehart E, Jackson M, et al. Guideline for isolation precautions: preventing transmission of infectious agents in healthcare settings. Available at: https://www.cdc.gov/hicpac/pdf/isolation/Isolation2007.pdf; 2007.

CHAPTER 27

Strategy for the Treatment of Intractable Epilepsy Secondary to Acute Encephalopathy and Encephalitis

JUDITH HELEN CROSS, MBCHB, PHD

When the phase of an acute encephalopathy or encephalitis has passed, many children are left with residual seizures, often resistant to antiepileptic medication. Long-term follow-up studies are few, however, and outcomes are variable considering the heterogeneity of the diseases presenting as such. A systematic review of studies evaluating long-term outcome of infective encephalitis in children suggested seizure occurrence in 10%.[1,2] However, autoimmune encephalopathy may be as high as 35%. The risk appears to be related to the antigen: lower if located on the cell surface and higher if intracellular.[3] The strategy for treatment then should follow that utilized for any child presenting with drug-resistant epilepsy.

When a child presents with continuing epileptic seizures, several stages of assessment are needed before proceeding as to whether further antiepileptic treatment is required. First, it needs to be considered whether the events continuing are all still consistent with epileptic seizures. As a sequela of acute encephalopathy many children may exhibit movement disorder or nonepileptic staring events, and at times it may be difficult to distinguish from epileptic events. There may always be the presumption that events in a child with an existing diagnosis of epilepsy must always be epileptic in origin. However, should there be certainty that the individual is experiencing epileptic seizures, have we the correct syndrome diagnosis,[4] and if so, have the most appropriate antiepileptic medications be used. Furthermore, what is the likely prognosis? Is it likely seizure freedom will be achieved? There also remains the possibility that seizures may have been aggravated by the treatments used to date. There are well-recognized aggravations, e.g., lamotrigine in Dravet syndrome,[5] or sodium channel blockers in general in the idiopathic generalized epilepsies.[6] However, should all these factors have been taken into consideration, there are further options in management that may be considered.

HAVE WE USED THE CORRECT DRUG?

Once a diagnosis of epilepsy is confirmed, more specifically there should be an attempt to determine whether drugs used have been appropriate for the type of epilepsy, whether an epilepsy syndrome or an epilepsy is characterized by seizure type, and whether it is linked to the underlying etiology. Often in the case of autoimmune encephalopathies, it is difficult to know whether there is residual acute pathology or the ongoing seizures are sequelae to the disorder. The epilepsy syndromes remain a way of determining whether appropriate medication has been utilized, and in addition to outline an overall prognosis, specifically to address expectations with regard to seizure control and long-term remission. The International League Against Epilepsy has recently outlined an updated framework for addressing diagnosis in the epilepsies, whether by seizure type, syndrome, or etiology.[7] There is a wide range of new antiepileptic medication now available, but the relative merits of newer medication over older medication are unclear. There is discussion that the newer medications may be more limited in their side effects and lack of drug interactions, but there remain few randomized controlled trials, specifically addressing efficacy in children. Long-term retention and efficacy also remain undetermined. Regulatory authorities have attempted to address the difficulty through avenues for assessment of medications for orphan status in specific syndromes, e.g., buccal midazolam in prolonged seizures, and have also outlined reduced criteria for assessment of medications in focal seizures where efficacy was demonstrated in adults. However, data and consequently the choice, particularly in infants, remain extremely limited.

WHAT DO WE MEAN BY DRUG RESISTANCE?

Diagnosing the type of epilepsy also highlights the likely prognosis and consequently the expectations for seizure control. The International League Against Epilepsy have also outlined useable definitions for both what may be considered as a response to intervention and drug resistance.[8] They have proposed a rule of three—a response would be demonstrated by a seizure-free duration that is at least three times the longest seizure-free interval before starting a new intervention and a sustained response that is seen over at least 12 months. Furthermore, drug-resistant epilepsy may be defined as a failure of adequate trials of two tolerated and appropriately chosen and used antiepileptic drug (AED) schedules, whether as monotherapies or in combination, to achieve sustained seizure freedom. There is evidence that there appears to be an inherent responsiveness to many of the epilepsies. Consequently, many studies report similar response rate, or indeed not, to antiepileptic drugs. Furthermore, there is evidence repeatedly quoted that after the failure of three AEDs, the likelihood of response to a further medication remains small.[9] Besides, data, from the cases of adults, suggest there may always be a chance of seizure freedom with introduction of a new medication even after repeated failure of previous trials of medication.[10]

SHOULD ALTERNATIVE THERAPY BE CONSIDERED?

The ketogenic diet (KD) is a high-fat, low-carbohydrate, low-protein diet that has been used in the treatment of epilepsy for almost 100 years. A randomized controlled trial has demonstrated significant efficacy when compared with no change in treatment in children aged 2–16 years with drug-resistant epilepsy,[11] and a further study reports similar results utilizing a modified KD— low carbohydrate, unlimited protein.[12] Furthermore, a KD may be administered in a number of ways including the classical and medium-chain triglyceride diets,[13] or the more relaxed forms such as modified KD, or the low-glycemic index diet.[14] There are reports on efficacy

of the diet in both the acute phase of acute encephalopathy, particularly refractory status epilepticus on the intensive care unit,[15,16] and for ongoing seizures as sequelae, although reports on the latter are limited. The type of diet to be used may depend on the eating behaviors of the child, whether gastrostomy fed, and the degree of ketosis required. It is now evident that the KD is utilized in many countries of the world[17] and can therefore be administered utilizing foods from a wide range of cultures.

Whether surgery may be an option in the long-term treatment of epilepsies as sequelae to acute encephalopathy may need individual discussion. In the acute phase even in the presence of an apparent single focus on EEG, surgery is unlikely to play a significant role. In the chronic phase, however, surgery may be considered if a possible single focus is identified through standard presurgical evaluation. This may be the case particularly in children with focal epilepsy following herpes simplex encephalitis. Resective surgery may be successful if seizures are evaluated to come from a single source as in any standard presurgical evaluation. A biphasic nature to the illness may indicate the development of chronic granulomatous encephalitis.[18] Besides, care and consideration should be given to such a procedure, considering the risk benefit, specifically because the likelihood of multifocal pathology, and the fact that surgery may lead to recrudescence of the disease.[19]

TREATING THE UNDERLYING CAUSE

Of course, as increasingly seen with many of the structural and genetic epilepsies, targeting the underlying cause may be an ongoing possibility following acute encephalopathy. In autoimmune disease, there remains the possibility of an ongoing acute autoimmune process that will respond to immunosuppression.[20] The presence of autoantibodies that can be monitored provides some clue, although the possibility of these in lower titers being a marker of ongoing neurologic disease, rather than the cause. It remains unclear as to whether such diseases may be monophasic, or indeed biphasic in their presentation, and may require ongoing discussion as to whether immunosuppression or immunoglobulin is required on an ongoing basis.

Herpes simplex encephalitis may itself pose particular challenges. There have now been several reports of NMDA antibody positive encephalitis occurring following treatment for HSV[21] and may explain and subsequent further acute phase to the illness, requiring a different track in management.

TREATMENTS ON THE HORIZON

New medications are in development and may provide further treatment to consider in drug-resistant epilepsy the sequelae to acute encephalopathy or encephalitis. There has been a long interest in the possible benefits of cannabidiol in epilepsy, with many anecdotal reports suggesting not only seizure control but also improved alertness and quality of life.[22] Cannabidiol as produced by GW Pharma, almost pure cannabidiol with insignificant tetra-hydrocannabidiol (THC), has been evaluated as an add-on therapy in Dravet syndrome and Lennox-Gastaut syndrome, benefits seen over placebo in a randomized controlled trial reported most recently in Dravet syndrome.[23] The mechanism of action and consequently specificity to this syndrome remain unclear; therefore possible utilization in other drug-resistant epilepsies should be considered. However, a definite interaction with clobazam has been documented, with a tendency to raised levels of the clobazam metabolite, norclobazam in children taking cannabidiol concomitantly.[24] Fenfluramine is a further agent undergoing trial in Dravet syndrome; definitive results are awaited. Open label use has suggested an encouraging response in major motor seizures.[25,26] Cardiac side effects, as emerged with previous use, are being evaluated although the dose currently being utilized is far lower than that associated with cardiac side effects with previous use.

ARE SEIZURES THE ONLY CONCERN?

As seizures continue, the focus mainly remains in the attempt to gain control. However, there may be limitations in the response to treatment and, indeed, misperceptions as to the contribution of the seizures to the underlying learning and behavior difficulties. There is no question that epileptic activity may contribute to the neurodevelopmental problems, but the rate of the latter as sequelae to acute encephalopathy remains higher than that of ongoing seizures. Consequently, the latter may be of greater importance to the family and need to be addressed. Appropriate neuropsychological assessment may highlight the specific difficulties as well as the level of functioning and may therefore provide information as to the educational level to be considered. Furthermore, neuropsychiatric assessment, with clinical psychology input, may help to address behavior and social communication difficulties. Specific aims to management, comparing progress over a longer period of time, may need to be negotiated with the family. As many of the children may have been neurodevelopmentally normal before the acute presentation, parents may need to adjust to their expectations and may require a degree of ongoing discussion for them to come to terms with this.

REFERENCES

1. Khandaker G, Jung J, Britton PN, King C, Yin JK, Jones CA. Long-term outcomes of infective encephalitis in children: a systematic review and meta-analysis. *Dev Med Child Neurol.* 2016;58:1108–1115.
2. Pillai SC, Mohammad SS, Hacohen Y, et al. Postencephalitic epilepsy and drug resistant epilepsy after infectious and antibody-associated encephalitis in childhood: clinical and aetiological risk factors. *Epilepsia.* 2016;57:e7–e11.
3. Spatola M, Dalmau J. Seizures and risk of epilepsy in autoimmune and other inflammatory encephalitis. *Curr Opin Neurol.* 2017;30:345–353.
4. Berg AT, Berkovic SF, Brodie MJ, et al. Revised terminology and concepts for organisation of seizures and epilepsies: report of the ILAE Commission on Classification and Terminology, 2005-2009. *Epilepsia.* 2010;51:676–685.
5. Guerrini R, Dravet C, Genton P, Belmonte A, Kaminska A, Dulac O. Lamotrigine and seizure aggravation in severe myoclonic epilepsy. *Epilepsia.* 1998;39:508–512.
6. Genton P. When antiepileptic drugs aggravate epilepsy. *Brain Dev.* 2000;22:75–80.
7. Scheffer IE, Berkovic S, Capovilla G, et al. ILAE classification of the epilepsies: position paper of the ILAE Commission for Classificaiton and Terminology. *Epilepsia.* 2017;58:512–521.
8. Kwan P, Arzimanoglou A, Berg AT, et al. Definition of drug resistant epilepsy: consensus proposal by the ad hoc Task Force of the ILAE Commission on Therpeutic Strategies. *Epilepsia.* 2010;51:1069–1077.
9. Kwan P, Brodie MJ. Early identification of refractory epilepsy. *New Engl J Med.* 2000;342:314–319.
10. Luciano AL, Shorvon S. Results of treatment changes in patients with apparently drug resistant chronic epilepsy. *Ann Neurol.* 2007;62:375–381.
11. Neal EG, Chaffe HM, Schwartz RH, et al. A randomised controlled trial of classical and medium chain triglyceride ketogenic diets in the treatment of childhood epilepsy. *Epilepsia.* 2008;49:9.
12. Sharma S, Sankhyan N, Gulati S, Agarwala A. Use of the modified Atkins diet for the treatment of refractory childhood epilepsy: a randomised controlled trial. *Epilepsia.* 2013;54:481–486.
13. Neal EG, Chaffe HM, Schwartz RH, et al. A randomised controlled trial of classical and medium-chain triglyceride ketogenic diets in the treatment of childhood epilepsy. *Epilepsia.* 2009;50(5):1109–1117.
14. Muzykewicz DA, Lyczkowski DA, Memon N, Conant KD, Pfeifer HH, Thiele EA. Efficacy, safety, and tolerability of the low glycemic index treatment in pediatric epilepsy. *Epilepsia.* 2009;50(5):1118–1126.

15. Amer S, Shah P, Komminenii V. Refractory status epilepticus from NMDA receptor encephalitis successfully treated with an adjunctive ketogenic diet. *Ann Indian Acad Neurol.* 2015;18:56–57.

16. Nabbout R, Mazzuca M, Hubert P, et al. Efficacy of ketogenic diet in severe refractory status epilepticus initiating fever induced refractory epileptic encephalopathy in school age children (FIRES). *Epilepsia.* 2017;51:2033–2037.

17. Kossoff EH, Caraballo RH, du Toit T, et al. Dietary therapies: a worldwide phenomenon. *Epilepsy Res.* 2012;100:205–209.

18. Taskin BD, Tanji K, Feldstein NA, McSwiggan-Hardin M, Akman CI. Epilepsy surgery for epileptic encephalopathy as a sequela of herpes simplex encephalitis: case report. *J Neurosurg (Pediatrics 2).* 2017;28:1–8.

19. Alonso-Vanegas MA, Quintero-Lopez E, Martinez-Albarran AA, Moreiraa-Holguin JC. Recurrent herpes simplex virus encephalitis after neurologic surgery. *World Neurosurg.* 2016;89:e5.

20. Hacohen Y, Wright S, Waters P, et al. Paediatric autoimmune encephalopathies: clinical features, laboratory investigations and outcomes in patients with or without antibodies to known central nervous system autoantigens. *J Neurol Neurosurg Psychiatry.* 2012;0:1–8.

21. Bamford A, Crowe BH, Hacohen Y, et al. Pediatric herpes simplex virus encephalitis complicated by N-methyl-D-aspartate receptor antibody encephalitis. *J Pediatr Infect Dis Soc.* 2015;4:e17–e21.

22. Devinsky O, March E, Friedman D, et al. Cannabidiol in patients with treatment resistant epilepsy: an open label interventional trial. *Lancet Neurol.* 2016;15:270–278.

23. Devinsky O, Cross JH, Laux L, et al. Trial of cannabidiol for drug resistant seizures in the Dravet syndrome. *New Engl J Med.* 2017;376:2011–2020.

24. Geffrey AL, Pollack SF, Bruno PL, Thiele EA. Drug-drug interaction between clobazam and cannabidiol in children with refractory epilepsy. *Epilepsia.* 2015;56:1246–1251.

25. Ceulemans B, Boel M, Leyssens K, et al. Successful use of fenfluramine as an add-on treatment for Dravet syndrome. *Epilepsia.* 2012;53:1131–1139.

26. Scoonjans A, Paelinck BP, Marchau F, et al. Low dose fenfluramine significantly reduces seizures frequency in Dravet syndrome: a prospective study of a new cohort of patients. *Eur J Neurol.* 2017;24:309–314.

CHAPTER 28

The Pros and Cons of Therapeutic Hypothermia for Acute Encephalitis and Refractory Status Epilepticus

JAINN-JIM LIN, MD • KUANG-LIN LIN, MD • CHEESE STUDY GROUP

INTRODUCTION OF ACUTE ENCEPHALITIS AND REFRACTORY STATUS EPILEPTICUS

Refractory status epilepticus is a neurologic emergency associated with high mortality and morbidity rates. Acute encephalitis is one of the most important causes of febrile refractory status epilepticus, and hyperthermia is thought to aggravate epileptic brain damage. Acute central nervous system infections have been reported to be the most common etiology of first episodes of convulsive status epilepticus and appear to be markers for morbidity and mortality.[1]

The intravenous administration of general anesthetics (such as midazolam, propofol, and barbiturates) is currently the mainstay management of refractory status epilepticus.[2] However, treatment with general anesthetics may lead to complications such as cardiovascular instability, respiratory suppression, infections, metabolic disturbances, paralytic ileus, ischemic bowel, and thromboembolic events.[3] Therefore, it is necessary to balance the risks and benefits of rapid seizure control. When general anesthetic treatment fails, several pharmacologic and nonpharmacologic options have been described, including targeted temperature management.

MULTIPLE MECHANISMS OF TARGETED TEMPERATURE MANAGEMENT

Targeted temperature management, previously termed therapeutic hypothermia, exerts multiple antiepileptic and neuroprotective mechanisms. The antiepileptic effect of targeted temperature management remains unclear; however, hypotheses include a reduction in presynaptic excitatory transmitter release, alterations of postsynaptic voltage-gated channels, disturbance of

membrane polarity via ion pumps, and modification of gene expression.[4–6] These actions reduce the neuroexcitatory effect and would be expected to inhibit seizure activity. The potential neuroprotective mechanisms include decreases of calcium overload, glutamate release, free radicals, oxidative stress, mitochondrial dysfunction and also reductions in cerebral metabolism, adenosine triphosphate consumption, inflammatory reactions and an increase in brain-derived neurotrophic factor as a result of inhibition of apoptosis.

CLINICAL APPLICATIONS OF TARGETED TEMPERATURE MANAGEMENT FOR ACUTE ENCEPHALITIS AND REFRACTORY STATUS EPILEPTICUS

Although the benefits of targeted temperature management for patients with acute brain injury have been described, the benefits in the setting of adult postcardiac arrest and neonatal hypoxemic-ischemic encephalopathy are only evidence based. Targeted temperature management has also been shown to be beneficial in a wide variety of other acute neurologic injuries.[7]

Targeted Temperature Management for Acute Encephalitis

Only a few case reports and two retrospective studies have reported the use of targeted temperature management to treat acute encephalitis/encephalopathy in children due to various viral and postviral pathologies (Table 28.1).[8–12] The results of these studies showed that targeted temperature management can effectively improve the neurologic outcomes of acute encephalitis/encephalopathy. However, there are currently no

TABLE 28.1
Published Literature of Targeted Temperature Management (TTM) on Acute Encephalitis/
Encephalopathy

References	No.	Age (y)	Goal Temperature (°C)	Duration of TTM (Days)	Outcome
Yokota et al.[8]	1	5	34	3	Stabilizing the immune activation and the brain edema
Vargas et al.[9]	1	4	34	2	Lacked cognitive deficits Intention tremor
Ichikawa et al.[10]	1	3	34	6	Mild intention tremor
Kawano et al.[11]	43	2–5	33.5–35	2–3	Early hypothermia improved neurologic outcomes (≦12 h)
Nishiyama et al.[12]	57	6.9–14.2	34.5–36	3	Improve outcome in some patients

reports of targeted temperature management for pediatric bacterial meningitis.

Comprehensive guidelines exist for the diagnosis and treatment of pediatric encephalitis and meningitis[13-15]; however, targeted temperature management is only briefly mentioned in these guidelines as a possible adjunctive therapy in bacterial meningitis.[13] Otherwise, high-quality studies with a large number of cases showing the effectiveness and safety of the clinical use of targeted temperature management for acute encephalitis/encephalopathy are lacking.

Targeted Temperature Management for Refractory Status Epilepticus

Targeted temperature management has also been shown to abort seizures in animal models.[5,6] Although no prospective comparative data exist regarding the use of controlled normothermia or targeted temperature management in status epilepticus, many case reports have demonstrated the effectiveness of targeted temperature management in treating refractory status epilepticus. Recently, several case studies have reported the efficacy of targeted temperature management for acute encephalitis and refractory status epilepticus (Table 28.2).[16-23] Nakagawa et al. reported a large retrospective case series of 12 children with febrile refractory status epilepticus treated with a combination of targeted temperature management (34–36°C) and general anesthesia in Japan and showed improved functional outcomes compared with 16 children treated with conventional therapy.[20]

Zeiler et al. performed a systematic review of 13 studies with 10 manuscripts and 3 meeting abstracts on the use of targeted temperature management for refractory status epilepticus and reported a common target

temperature of 33°C for a median of 48 h. The results were promising, with seizure cessation and seizure reduction rates of 62.5% and 15%, respectively, for patients with refractory status epilepticus.[24] Thus targeted temperature management may be a viable option for refractory status epilepticus.

The Neurocritical Care Society (NCS) guidelines for the treatment of status epilepticus in adults state that targeted temperature management is an emerging therapy "with limited data on the safety and effectiveness of these treatments for refractory status epilepticus" and therefore "recommend to reserve these therapies to patients who do not respond to refractory status epilepticus antiepileptic drug treatment."[2] A recent review by the Pediatric Status Epilepticus Research Group stated that targeted temperature management is an emerging therapy for refractory status epilepticus but made no treatment recommendations.[25] Therefore, studies on protocol-based targeted temperature management for refractory status epilepticus are needed.

PROS AND CONS
Pros

The rationale for using targeted temperature management for acute encephalitis/encephalopathy is to reduce cytokine-mediated inflammation that may be exacerbated by fever and sepsis.[8] In addition, the antiepileptic effect of targeted temperature management is based on a variety of changes at the molecular level. Because targeted temperature management activates multiple anticonvulsant and neuroprotective mechanisms in the pathophysiology of acute encephalitis and refractory status epilepticus, it has the potential to

TABLE 28.2
Published English Literature of Targeted Temperature Management (TTM) for Acute Encephalitis With Refractory Status Epilepticus

References	Etiology (No.)	Age (y)	Goal Temperature (°C)	Duration of TTM	Outcome
Vastola et al.[16]	Meningoencephalitis (1)	16	37	24 h	Seizure control
Orlowski et al.[17]	Viral encephalitis (1)	11	30–31	72 h	GOS = 4
Ito et al.[18]	Anti-Glu-Epsilon-2 encephalitis (1)	11	Unknown	10 days	Recurrent Seizures, GOS = 3
Corry et al.[19]	Limbic encephalitis (2)	Case 1: 66 Case 2: 75	Case 1: 32 Case 2: 31	Case 1: 61 h Case 2: 25.5 h	Case 1: died Case 2: seizure-free with rehabilitation
Nakagawa et al.[20]	Febrile RSE (12)	Unknown	34–36	Unknown	Treatment with hypothermia significantly improved outcome
Lin et al.[21]	FIRES (2)	Case 1: 4.5 Case 2: 10	33 in both	Case 1: 5 days Case 2: 3 days	Both mild deficits (GOS = 4)
Missert et al.[22]	CJD (1)	67	32–33	2 days	Complete seizure control
Guilliams et al.[23]	Anti-NMDAR encephalitis (1)	15	33–35	5 days	Mild cognitive and behavioral deficits

CJD, Creutzfeldt-Jakob disease; *FIRES*, febrile infection–related epilepsy syndrome; *GOS*, Glasgow outcome scale; *h*, hours; *NMDAR*, N-methyl-D-aspartate receptor; *RSE*, refractory status epilepticus; *y*, years.

impact seizure control and neuroprotection in the setting of refractory status epilepticus.[4,7]

Recently, several case studies have reported the efficacy of targeted temperature management for acute encephalitis and refractory status epilepticus. Although a small number of studies reported that targeted temperature management may contribute to seizure control in patients with refractory status epilepticus, we believe that targeted temperature management may be beneficial for both adults and children with acute encephalitis and refractory status epilepticus.

Cons

A majority of studies on targeted temperature management for refractory status epilepticus have focused on animal models, and few clinical studies exist. In addition, targeted temperature management may contribute to seizure control. However, the patients in most case studies received a combination of intravenous anesthetic agents and targeted temperature management; thus the seizure response reported may reflect the combination of therapies. Moreover, its efficacy seems to be only transient and rarely allows for sustained control of status epilepticus, and seizures tend

to recur on rewarming. For example, in a review by Zeiler et al., 7.5% of the patients displayed seizure recurrence on rewarming. Therefore, targeted temperature management seems rather to be a bridge to optimize anticonvulsants than to definitively control seizures.[24] Furthermore, the current study shows the heterogeneity of prior treatment, time to implementation of targeted temperature management and variable target temperature, time to target, and duration of therapy at target.

The benefits of targeted temperature management for refractory status epilepticus may be linked to the etiology of the seizures, and further large-scale studies are needed to evaluate refractory status epilepticus from a variety of causes to determine which groups would benefit from targeted temperature management.[26] Finally, the complications of targeted temperature management including arrhythmias, coagulopathy, electrolyte disturbance, increased infection rate, and venous thrombosis also limit its application for patients with acute encephalitis and refractory status epilepticus. Because of the complexity of the critical illness in this patient population, the pros and cons need to be carefully balanced.

CONCLUSION

Targeted temperature management is a potential treatment option for acute encephalitis and refractory status epilepticus. The multiple antiepileptic and neuroprotective mechanisms of targeted temperature management are based on a variety of changes at the molecular level. Although there is currently a lack of clinical evidence, targeted temperature management may represent a therapeutic option. A well-designed, prospective trial is necessary to assess the exact role of targeted temperature management for patients with acute encephalitis and refractory status epilepticus.

ACKNOWLEDGMENT

This work was performed by the Children With Encephalitis/Encephalopathy-Related Status Epilepticus and Epilepsy (CHEESE) Study Group at Chang Gung Children's Hospital in Taoyuan, Taiwan.

REFERENCES

1. Lin KL, Lin JJ, Hsia SH, et al. Analysis of convulsive status epilepticus in children of Taiwan. *Pediatr Neurol.* 2009;41:413–418.
2. Brophy GM, Bell R, Claassen J, et al. Guidelines for the evaluation and management of status epilepticus. *Neurocrit Care.* 2012;17:3–23.
3. Cereda C, Berger MM, Rossetti AO. Bowel ischemia: a rare complication of thiopental treatment for status epilepticus. *Neurocrit Care.* 2009;10:355–358.
4. Motamedi GK, Lesser RP, Vicini S. Therapeutic brain hypothermia, its mechanisms of action, and its prospects as a treatment for epilepsy. *Epilepsia.* 2013;54:959–970.
5. Schmitt FC, Buchheim K, Meierkord H, et al. Anticonvulsant properties of hypothermia in experimental status epilepticus. *Neurobiol Dis.* 2006;23:689–696.
6. Kowski AB, Kanaan H, Schmitt FC, et al. Deep hypothermia terminates status epilepticus–an experimental study. *Brain Res.* 2012;1446:119–126.
7. Rossetti AO. What is the value of hypothermia in acute neurologic diseases and status epilepticus? *Epilepsia.* 2011;52(suppl 8):64–66.
8. Yokota S, Imagawa T, Miyamae T, et al. Hypothetical pathophysiology of acute encephalopathy and encephalitis related to influenza virus infection and hypothermia therapy. *Pediatr Int.* 2000;42:197–203.
9. Vargas WS, Merchant S, Solomon G. Favorable outcomes in acute necrotizing encephalopathy in a child treated with hypothermia. *Pediatr Neurol.* 2012;46:387–389.
10. Ichikawa K, Motoi H, Oyama Y, et al. Fulminant form of acute disseminated encephalomyelitis in a child treated with mild hypothermia. *Pediatr Int.* 2013;55:e149–e151.
11. Kawano G, Iwata O, Iwata S, et al. Determinants of outcomes following acute child encephalopathy and encephalitis: pivotal effect of early and delayed cooling. *Arch Dis Child.* 2011;96:936–941.
12. Nishiyama M, Tanaka T, Fujita K, et al. Targeted temperature management of acute encephalopathy without AST elevation. *Brain Dev.* 2015;37:328–333.
13. Chaudhuri A, Martinez-Martin P, Kennedy PG, et al. EFNS guideline on the management of community-acquired bacterial meningitis: report of an EFNS Task Force on acute bacterial meningitis in older children and adults. *Eur J Neurol.* 2008;15:649–659.
14. Kneen R, Michael BD, Menson E, et al. Management of suspected viral encephalitis in children -Association of British Neurologists and British Paediatric Allergy, Immunology and Infection Group National Guidelines. *J Infect.* 2012;64:449–477.
15. Tunkel AR, Hartman BJ, Kaplan SL, et al. Practice guidelines for the management of bacterial meningitis. *Clin Infect Dis.* 2004;39:1267–1284.
16. Vastola EF, Homan R, Rosen A. Inhibition of focal seizure a clinical and experimental study. *Arch Neurol.* 1969;20:430–439.
17. Orlowski JP, Erenberg G, Lueders H, et al. Hypothermia and barbiturate coma for refractory status epilepticus. *Crit Care Med.* 1984;12:367–372.
18. Ito H, Mori K, Toda Y, et al. A case of acute encephalitis with refractory, repetitive partial seizures, presenting autoantibody to glutamate receptor Glu-epsilon-2. *Brain Dev.* 2005;27:531–534.
19. Corry JJ, Dhar R, Murphy T, et al. Hypothermia for refractory status epilepticus. *Neurocrit Care.* 2008;9:189–197.
20. Nakagawa T, Fujita K, Saji Y, et al. Induced hypothermia/normothermia with general anesthesia prevents neurological damage in febrile refractory status epilepticus in children. *No To Hattatsu.* 2011;43:459–463.
21. Lin JJ, Lin KL, Hsia SH, et al. Therapeutic hypothermia for febrile infection-related epilepsy syndrome in two patients. *Pediatr Neurol.* 2012;47:448–450.
22. Missert MJ, Qazi KJ, Ionita CC. Utilising therapeutic hypothermia in the control of non-convulsive status epilepticus in a patient with Creutzfeldt-Jakob encephalopathy. *BJMP.* 2012;5:a515.
23. Guilliams K, Rosen M, Buttram S, et al. Hypothermia for pediatric refractory status epilepticus. *Epilepsia.* 2013;54:1586–1594.
24. Zeiler FA, Zeiler KJ, Teitelbaum J, et al. Therapeutic hypothermia for refractory status epilepticus. *Can J Neurol Sci.* 2015;42:221–229.
25. Sánchez Fernández I, Abend NS, et al. Gaps and opportunities in refractory status epilepticus research in children: a multi-center approach by the Pediatric Status Epilepticus Research Group (pSERG). *Seizure.* 2014;23:87–97.
26. Hakimi R, Talsania S, Fesler JR, et al. Does the efficacy of therapeutic hypothermia in refractory status epilepticus depend on seizure etiology? *Neurocrit Care.* 2013;19(suppl 1):S218.

CHAPTER 29

Therapeutic Hypothermia as Potential Intervention on Acute Encephalopathy

GEORGE IMATAKA, MD, PHD, BA, PGDBA

INTRODUCTION

The use of brain hypothermic therapy (BHT) for acute encephalopathy occurring in childhood may be very valuable and promising, but to date the medical evidence for efficacy is still very small.[1,2] There are few institutions worldwide where this treatment is currently conducted. However, presently in Japan, this state-of-the-art treatment is actively performed in more than 20 facilities specialized in pediatric emergency center.

HISTORY AND EXPERIMENTAL EVIDENCE

There are various stories stating that BHT may have a life-saving impact on accidental hypothermia. One of the most popular incidents occurred in 1963 in which a young boy drowned in a cold river in Norway.[3] Through careful warming of his body, he was successfully brought from the verge of death due to hypothermia to a complete recovery. Afterward, some of the animal experiments in the 1980s reported that 34°C provides some degree of cerebral cell protection.[2]

In the 1990s, BHT was applied in human trial studies. Since 2000, it has been shown to be effective against cardiac arrest in adults.[4] In 2010, BHT was endorsed in the American Heart Association guideline for adult cardiac arrest,[5] as well as in the guideline for Hypoxic Ischemic Encephalopathy (HIE) in newborns.[6] The following reasons were indicated in the BHT guidelines for adults and newborns. In adults, BHT prevents cerebral edema, inhibits cerebral metabolism to reduce the amount of oxygen consumption, and improves homeostasis of intracerebral Ca^{2+} to reduce cerebral nerve damage. In newborns with HIE, BHT is said to preserve oxygen supply through cerebral ischemia and also prevent ATP deficiency in neuronal cells. In addition, BHT protects against increased free radicals and prevents irreversible nerve cell apoptosis.[5,7] However, there is still very little evidence for the effects of BHT against acute encephalopathy in children.[1,2]

GENERAL PRACTICE FOR BRAIN HYPOTHERMIC THERAPY

Based on the evidence for BHT for adults and newborns, we introduced in children the use of BHT to cytokine storm–related encephalopathy, with a primary symptom status epilepticus. Moreover, we applied it in near-drowning based on the evidence, introduced by its use in hypoxic ischemic encephalopathy in neonates.

In our treatment strategies for acute encephalopathy and status epilepticus, we enforced the management of central nervous system together with the treatment of the whole body organ systems.[1] Central nervous system management may prevent irreversible cerebral nerve cell apoptosis. Therefore, it is for this reason that the BHT team was combined with the ICU and related members of the patient transport systems.

In Japan, the emergency doctor heads off in a helicopter after receiving word of a child with an emergency. They massage the heart and give respiratory care while administering a midazolam nasal spray and intravenous solution as first-line anticonvulsants. BHT is introduced in cases with predicted poor neurologic prognosis, including drowning, cardiac arrest, serious respiratory failure, and status epilepticus lasting 30–45 min. The specialized pediatric ICU always has a prepared bed that is laid with a cooling blanket to introduce BHT promptly.

General management with BHT, anesthetic management, respiratory care, circulation, and body temperature control are all taken care of in the ICU. Intracranial pressure is also controlled as per the requirement with a neurosurgeon. Cooling is done simultaneously for the body's cooling blanket and the head cooling system.

Commonly, the classification of clinical hypothermia is divided into 4 degrees (Table 29.1). We currently use "mild hypothermia" defined between the 35 and 32°C. To maintain body temperature, the temperature of the urinary bladder is brought to 34.5°C. Hypothermia persists for 48 h, and then the body temperature increased at a pace of 0.5° every 12 h. Steroid pulse therapy is administered together with the concomitant use of other drugs including anesthetics and mannitol.[1] Fig. 29.1 is a diagram of the process for BHT. BHT is performed in three stages. The first one is the introduction stage, the next is the cooling stage, and the final stage is the rewarming stage. The target is to keep the body temperature of the urinary bladder at 34.5°C for 48 h. Concomitant monitoring during BHT includes respiration, an ECG, CVP, and oxygen saturation. A portable electroencephalogram (EEG), with a scalp skin oxygen saturation device (INVOS), a Bispectral index (BIS) monitor, and an intracranial pressure monitor are available when necessary.

EEGs undergo dramatically rapid changes during the three stages of BHT (Fig. 29.2).

In the introduction stage, we see irregular high-voltage slow wave activity. During the cooling stage, this changes to "suppression and burst pattern." At that time, the body temperature is retained at 34.5°C. Rewarming stage of the body begins by suspending the use of anesthetics. In recovery examples, there is a gradual appearance of basic background waves in the EEG. For useful EEG managing "suppression and bursts" during the cooling stage, a BIS monitor is placed on the forehead by an anesthesiologist when administering general anesthesia.

There are concerns with the use of hypothermia as adverse events such as cardiac arrhythmia, low blood pressure, coagulation abnormalities, severe infection, and abnormalities in hematopoiesis. The more severe the degree of hypothermia, the greater the chance that adverse effects may occur but may still happen with mild hypothermia.

TABLE 29.1
Classification of Clinically Hypothermia

Normothermia	35.0–37.0°C
Mild hypothermia	35.0–32.0°C
Moderate hypothermia	32.0–28.0°C
Severe hypothermia	Below 28.0

CONCLUSION

We anticipate that in the future there will be additional evidence that will help establish the role of BHT in the treatment of acute encephalopathy in childhood,

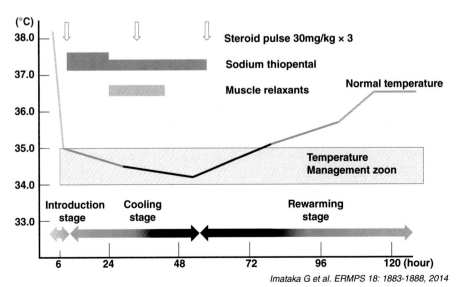

Imataka G et al. ERMPS 18: 1883-1888, 2014

FIG. 29.1 Clinical process for mild brain hypothermia therapy. (From Imataka G, wake H, Yamanouchi H, et al. Brain hypothermia therapy for status epilepticus in childhood. *Eur Rev Med Pharmacol Sci*. 2014;18:1883–1888.)

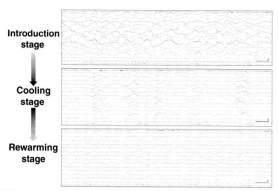

Introduction stage

↓

Cooling stage

↓

Rewarming stage

FIG. 29.2 Electroencephalogram changes during three stages of brain hypothermic therapy.

by developing criteria how to be safely used and an understanding of the possible outcomes separating the potential injury stemming from the cause of the underlying etiology as well as the symptoms i.e., status epilepticus.

REFERENCES

1. Imataka G, wake H, Yamanouchi H, et al. Brain hypothermia therapy for status epilepticus in childhood. *Eur Rev Med Pharmacol Sci.* 2014;18:1883–1888.
2. Imataka G, Arisaka O. Brain hypothermia therapy for childhood acute encephalopathy based on clinical evidence (Review). *Exp Ther Med.* 2015;10:1624–1626.
3. Kvittingen TD, Naesse A. Recovery from drowning in fresh water. *Br Med J.* 1963;18:1315–1317.
4. Bernard SA, Gray TW, Buist MD. Treatment of comatose survivors of out-of-hospital cardiac arrest with induced hypothermia. *N Engl J Med.* 2002;346:557–563.
5. Holzer M. Targeted temperature management for comatose survivors of cardiac arrest. *N Engl J Med.* 2010;363:1256–1264.
6. Perlman JM, Wyllie J, Kattwinkel J, et al. Part 11: Neonatal resuscitation: 2010 international consensus on cardiopulmonary resuscitation and emergency cardiovascular care science with treatment recommendations. *Circulation.* 2010;122:S516–S538.
7. Shankaran S, Pappas A, McDonald SA, et al. Childhood outcomes after hypothermia for neonatal encephalopathy. *N Engl J Med.* 2012;366:2085–2092.

CHAPTER 30

Neurosurgical Interventions for Encephalitis-Related Seizures and Epilepsy

TOMONORI ONO, MD, PHD • RYOKO HONDA, MD • KEISUKE TODA, MD, PHD • HIROSHI BABA, MD, PHD

INTRODUCTION

Encephalitis, an inflammatory process involving the brain, causes a number of neurologic symptoms, including seizures. Etiologically, the majority of pathogens reported to cause encephalitis are viruses.[1] However, noninfectious immune-mediated mechanisms can also contribute to the development of encephalitis.[2] Seizures frequently occur in the acute stage of encephalitis but may recur as a sequela in the late stage following resolution (postencephalitic epilepsy, PEE).[1] Seizures in the acute stage are often resistant to conventional antiepileptic drugs (AEDs), often evolving to status epilepticus (SE). Recurrent seizures in the late stage are also highly drug-registrant.[3] Accordingly, surgical treatment is an alternative for some patients with medically refractory seizures. To date, surgical treatments have been performed for controlling encephalitis-related seizures mainly in PEE and a specific form of progressive immune-mediated epilepsy called Rasmussen encephalitis (RE). On the other hand, although the number is small, some case studies have described neurosurgical attempts to control SE in the early stage of disease. The purpose of this article is to provide a review of neurosurgical interventions for acute and chronic encephalitis-related seizures and to discuss their rationales based on the pathophysiologic mechanisms.

NEUROSURGICAL INTERVENTIONS FOR ACUTE ENCEPHALITIS AND STATUS EPILEPTICUS

The most common form of acute encephalitis is that caused by viral infection, most predominantly due to herpes simplex virus (HSV) type 1 in both children and adults where a viral pathogen is isolated.[1,2] Pathologically, an acute inflammatory process of the brain parenchyma characterized by infection of neural cells with perivascular inflammation, neuronal destruction, and tissue necrosis is centered primarily in the gray matter and localized to the mesial temporal structures.[4] This also determines the clinical manifestations suggesting the diagnosis.[4] Symptoms of HSV encephalitis include fever, headache, focal neurologic deficits, confusion/hallucination, and disturbance of consciousness, among others.[1,5] Seizures are the most common feature, seen in roughly 40%–60% of cases and potentially evolving into the serious complication of SE.[1,6] Predictors for the occurrence of seizures include young age, lower level of consciousness, and the presence of cortical involvement on neuroimaging.[1]

Antiviral drugs (principally acyclovir) and adjunctive corticosteroid in addition to AEDs are the current conventional therapies.[6] In extremely progressive cases, brain edema accompanying intracerebral necrosis and hemorrhage occurs acutely and medical management may fail to control brain herniation. To date, over 50 cases have been described in which the neurosurgical intervention of external decompression was used with or without temporal lobectomy to achieve relief from this life-threatening situation.[7] Several case studies have documented surgical resection of the affected cerebral lesion in the early stage of disease, successfully suppressing refractory SE or seizures in patients with acute viral and noninfectious encephalitis.[8–11]

Conventional emergency treatment of SE involves high-dose suppressive therapy with AEDs and anesthetic agents, regardless of the cause. This therapy often faces difficulty in controlling seizures or in the discontinuation of pharmacotherapy, increasing the rate of complications associated with intensive care, such as drug-induced hypotension and cardiorespiratory depression, pneumonia, deep vein thrombosis, and

TABLE 30.1
Pathophysiology of Postencephalitic Epilepsy (PEE) and Rasmussen Encephalitis (RE)

	PEE	RE	MTLE
Possible cause/ etiology	Viral infection (e.g., HSV-1; VZV) Autoimmune (autoantibodies, e.g., NMDAR; VGKC) Unknown	Viral infection Unknown pathogen Autoimmune (cytotoxic T cell–mediated)	Febrile status epilepticus No specific cause
Neuropathologic feature	Perivascular and meningeal lymphocytic infiltration T cells (CD3+ and CD8+) Abundant activated macrophage-microglial cells Microglial nodules Astrocytosis Viral genome	Perivascular and meningeal lymphocytic infiltration T cells (CD8+, granzyme B+) Microglial nodules Astrocytosis Neuronal cell loss	Hippocampal neuronal cell loss Gliosis Fiber sprouting
Postulated mechanism of epileptogenesis	Neurodegeneration (after tissue necrosis and apoptosis) Neuroinflammation (microglial activation) Cytokines	Neurodegeneration (T cell–induced apoptosis) Neuroinflammation (microglial activation) Cytokines	Neurodegeneration Synaptic remodeling Aberrant circuitry Gene modification Excitatory/inhibitory imbalance Neuroinflammation
References	1–4,6,13,18,19	22–24,26	18,23

HSV-1, herpes simplex virus type 1; *MTLE*, mesial temporal lobe epilepsy; *NMDAR*, N-methyl-D-aspartate receptor; *VGKC*, voltage-gated potassium channel; *VZV*, varicella-zoster virus.

line sepsis.[8] Furthermore, the cooccurrence of acute encephalitis and SE represents the highest risk factor for PEE.[3] Although still controversial, neurosurgical interventions are considered as a last option when multiple life-threatening or highly comorbid conditions are present.

NEUROSURGICAL INTERVENTIONS FOR POSTENCEPHALITIC EPILEPSY

Surgical treatments play an important role in the management of PEE, which is highly medically intractable. According to previous reports of relatively large series, in patients manifesting temporal lobe epilepsy (TLE) who underwent unilateral anterior temporal lobectomy with resection of mesial temporal structures, the postoperative seizure-free rate was calculated as around 40%.[12-15] However, this rate is much lower than that of mesial TLE (more than 70%).[16,17] Intracranial electroencephalography (EEG) recording and additional extratemporal resections may occasionally be required, but this appears associated with worse seizure outcomes.[13-15] This may be because the anatomical distribution of lesions in acute encephalitis is

relevant to putative epileptogenic foci in PEE.[1] Asymmetrical bilateral temporal lobe involvement is usually seen accompanied by insular and cingular invasions on magnetic resonance imaging (MRI), probably because of selective limbic system vulnerability in acute encephalitis.[5,13] The largest study of preoperative evaluations showed that most patients with PEE are categorized as showing bilateral TLE or extratemporal lobe and/or multifocal epilepsy based on EEG.[13] Multifocal and/or bilateral epileptic activity thus probably leads to a higher difficulty of controlling seizures even after focal surgical resection in patients with PEE.

If epileptogenic lesions are unilaterally widespread or hemispheric and severe neurologic comorbidity is present, more extensive surgery including hemispheric surgery (HES) may be considered in PEE, similar to the chronic state of RE and hemiconvulsion-hemiplegia syndrome.

The pathogenesis of PEE remains unclear. However, in addition to the epileptogenic neurodegenerative changes suggested in mesial TLE, a specific process may contribute to the development of epilepsy in PEE (Table 30.1). In the previous studies, significant features suggesting chronic encephalitis and inflammation with the presence of a viral genome were histopathologically identified in resected tissue from patients with HSV-1-related PEE who underwent temporal lobectomy.[18,19] Hence, differing from mesial TLE, chronic encephalitis and persistent inflammation possibly stimulated by residual viral pathogen may influence the development of epilepsy and therapeutic difficulty in PEE. This may also account for the situation in which focal surgical resection is unlikely to suppress unprovoked seizures, similar to RE.

As other surgical interventions, callosotomy or vagus nerve stimulation (VNS) may provide palliative relief in terms of seizure frequency and severity in patients not indicated for resective surgery because of generalized seizures and widespread EEG findings at the presurgical evaluation. However, the number of case studies focusing only on PEE and not including other infections remains small.[20]

RASMUSSEN ENCEPHALITIS
Pathological and Clinical Background Targeted by Current Medical Treatments

RE is a rare inflammatory brain disorder associated with progressive cerebral hemiatrophy, hemiparesis, cognitive decline, and refractory focal epilepsy.[21,22] The autoimmune or inflammatory processes are considered to be fundamental mechanisms in this disease. Neuropathologic features described from the surgical specimens show characteristics of inflammatory changes including perivascular and leptomeningeal lymphocytic infiltration, microglial nodules, astrocytosis, and neuronal degeneration.[21] Cytotoxic T cells, which are mostly CD8-positive and often granzyme B-positive, are thought to play a major pathologic role in RE.[23] These cytotoxic T cells attack neurons and astrocytes after recognizing unknown antigens and induce apoptosis of those cells and thus progressive cerebral tissue atrophy.[23,24] Microglial activation and release of inflammatory mediators, as other neurobiological processes in RE, play complex roles in the breakdown of the blood-brain barrier, impairment of the extracellular environment, glutamate release, neurogenesis, and eventual epileptogenesis.[25]

Clinically, serial MRI studies allow identification of the area of neuroinflammation and progression of the disease. Characteristic MRI findings develop from (1) focal cortical swelling with cortical/subcortical signal changes usually affecting the frontotemporal region; (2) insular or perirolandic cortical atrophy; (3) atrophy of the head of the caudate nucleus; and finally (4) progressive gray and white matter atrophy across the hemisphere.[21] Positron-emission tomography and single photon emission computed tomography also detect inflammatory or epileptogenic lesions.

The therapeutic rationales of immunomodulatory treatments for RE are based on the immune-mediated process of the disease. Current immunomodulatory treatments for RE include corticosteroids, intravenous immunoglobulins, and immunosuppressants (tacrolimus and azathioprine).[21-24] A recent prospective randomized study comparing the effects of long-term immunotherapy with tacrolimus and immunoglobulins reported that patients receiving immunomodulatory therapy were protected against functional or structural damage to the brain compared with untreated historical controls but were not protected against refractory epilepsy.[22] Surgical treatment thus remains important for patients suffering from seizures in RE.

Neurosurgical Interventions for Rasmussen Encephalitis

Currently, the most effective neurosurgical intervention for RE is HES including functional hemispherectomy and hemispherotomy, which were recently developed to minimize surgical complications.[26] According to larger studies, 65%–80% of patients with RE receiving HES became seizure free.[27-30] Surgical indications usually include (1) frequent drug-resistant disabling seizures from the affected hemisphere; (2) the presence of unilaterally widespread/diffuse destructive lesion on MRI; (3) progressive and irreversible neurologic deficits such as hemiparesis and aphasia; (4) a situation in which the expected benefits to activities of daily living from seizure freedom outweigh postoperative neurologic consequences such as hemianopia and deterioration of hemiparesis, especially fine motor function. Most candidates undergoing HES thus seem to be at the advanced stage of RE. In cases with involvement of the language-dominant side, the decision to perform surgery may be complicated. Basically, HES can be indicated for any patients with aphasia, regardless of age. In younger children under 4 years of age, the indication should primarily be based on seizure severity and motor assessment, rather than language considerations.[24] However, in cases of patients without severe language disability and guaranteed language transfer, decisions would be dependent on not only the clinical course of seizures and language disability but also expected functional outcomes after HES. As options not burdened with severe morbidity, but considered as palliative treatments, focal cortical resection, multiple subpial transection, corpus callosotomy, and VNS can be alternatives for patients with RE unsuitable for HES.[21]

CONCLUSIONS AND FUTURE DIRECTIONS

To date, only a limited number of studies have separately investigated the efficacy of neurosurgical treatments for encephalitis-related seizures and epilepsy. Resective surgery, preferably extensive, is feasible for selected patients with PEE, although postoperative seizure outcomes are not as favorable as those in patients with other etiologies. This may be because the epileptogenic lesion is likely widespread or multiple although the temporal lobe and mesial temporal structures are susceptible to acute encephalitic activity. Palliative surgeries including callosotomy and VNS may be available for patients unsuited to resective surgery.

For patients with RE, HES is strongly recommended as an option for controlling refractory disabling seizures and disease progression if postoperative comorbidity is acceptable.

Neurosurgical interventions at the early stage of encephalitis are still less established but can be considered under the limited situation of refractory SE.

Basically, the application of neurosurgical intervention should be determined by taking into account the individual etiology, postulated pathophysiology, and clinical condition, regardless of stage. The influence of surgery timing on prognosis has not yet been fully clarified. For example, whether less-invasive focal resection of an inflammatory lesion can prevent the progression of disease is still unclear. Based on the pathophysiology and therapeutic rationale, multimodal treatment together with immunomodulatory therapy should be considered for immune-mediated encephalitis such as RE. Further experience and studies are required.

ACKNOWLEDGMENTS

We wish to thank all staff in the Department of Neurosurgery at National Nagasaki Medical Center and all members of the Nagasaki Epilepsy Group. Tomonori Ono acknowledges grant support from the Japan Epilepsy Research Foundation (2016–18).

REFERENCES

1. Misra UK, Tan CT, Kalita J. Viral encephalitis and epilepsy. *Epilepsia.* 2008;49:13–18. http://dx.doi.org/10.1111/j.1528-1167.2008.01751.x.
2. Granerod J, Ambrose HE, Davies NWS, et al. Causes of encephalitis and differences in their clinical presentations in England: a multicentre, population-based prospective study. *Lancet Infect Dis.* 2010;10:835–844. http://dx.doi.org/10.1016/S1473-3099(10)70222-X.
3. Singh TD, Fugate JE, Hocker SE, Rabinstein AA. Postencephalitic epilepsy: clinical characteristics and predictors. *Epilepsia.* 2015;56:133–138. http://dx.doi.org/10.1111/epi.12879.
4. Johnson RT. State-of-the-art clinical article acute community-acquired sinusitis. *Clin Infect Dis.* 1996;23:219–226.
5. Eran A, Hodes A, Izbudak I. Bilateral temporal lobe disease: looking beyond herpes encephalitis. *Insights Imaging.* 2016;7:265–274. http://dx.doi.org/10.1007/s13244-016-0481-x.
6. Sellner J, Trinka E. Seizures and epilepsy in herpes simplex virus encephalitis: current concepts and future directions of pathogenesis and management. *J Neurol.* 2012;259:2019–2030. http://dx.doi.org/10.1007/s00415-012-6494-6.
7. Safain MG, Roguski M, Kryzanski JT, Weller SJ. A review of the combined medical and surgical management in patients with herpes simplex encephalitis. *Clin Neurol Neurosurg.* 2015;128:10–16. http://dx.doi.org/10.1016/j.clineuro.2014.10.015.
8. Weimer T, Boling W, Pryputniewicz D, Palade A. Temporal lobectomy for refractory status epilepticus in a case of limbic encephalitis. *J Neurosurg.* 2008;109:742–745. http://dx.doi.org/10.3171/JNS/2008/109/10/0742.
9. Barros P, Brito H, Ferreira PC, et al. Resective surgery in the treatment of super-refractory partial status epilepticus secondary to NMDAR antibody encephalitis. *Eur J Paediatr Neurol.* 2014;18:449–452. http://dx.doi.org/10.1016/j.ejpn.2014.01.013.
10. Halling G, Giannini C, Britton JW, et al. Focal encephalitis following varicella-zoster virus reactivation without rash in a healthy immunized young adult. *J Infect Dis.* 2014;210:713–716. http://dx.doi.org/10.1093/infdis/jiu137.
11. Almeida V, Pimentel J, Campos A, et al. Surgical control of limbic encephalitis associated with LGI1 antibodies. *Epileptic Disord.* 2012;14:345–348. http://dx.doi.org/10.1684/epd.2012.0515.
12. O'Brien TJ, Moses H, Cambier D, Cascino GD. Age of meningitis or encephalitis is independently predictive of outcome from anterior temporal lobectomy. *Neurology.* 2002;58:104–109.
13. Trinka E, Dubeau F, Andermann F, et al. Clinical findings, imaging characteristics and outcome in catastrophic post-encephalitic epilepsy. *Epileptic Disord.* 2000;2:153–161.
14. Lee JH, Lee BI, Park SC, et al. Experiences of epilepsy surgery in intractable seizures with past history of CNS infection. *Yonsei Med J.* 1997;38:73–78.
15. Davies K, Hermann B, Wyler A. Surgery for intractable epilepsy secondary to viral encephalitis. *Br J Neurosurg.* 1995;9:759–762.http://dx.doi.org/10.1080/02688699550040729.
16. Englot DJ, Rolston JD, Wang DD, Sun PP, Chang EF, Auguste KI. Seizure outcomes after temporal lobectomy in pediatric patients. *J Neurosurg Pediatr.* 2013;12:134–141. http://dx.doi.org/10.3171/2013.5.PEDS12526.
17. Josephson CB, Dykeman J, Fiest KM, et al. Systematic review and meta-analysis of standard vs selective temporal lobe epilepsy surgery. *Neurology.* 2013;80:1669–1676. http://dx.doi.org/10.1212/WNL.0b013e3182904f82.
18. Jay V, Hwang P, Hoffman HJ, Becker LE, Zielenska M. Intractable seizure disorder associated with chronic herpes infection: HSV1 detection in tissue by the polymerase chain reaction. *Childs Nerv Syst.* 1998;14:15–20. http://dx.doi.org/10.1007/s003810050167.

19. Lellouch-Tubiana A, Fohlen M, Robain O, Rozenberg F. Immunocytochemical characterization of long-term persistent immune activation in human brain after herpes simplex encephalitis. *Neuropathol Appl Neurobiol.* 2000;26:285–294. http://dx.doi.org/10.1046/j.1365-2990.2000.00243.x.

20. Cendes F, Ragazzo PC, da Costa V, Martins LF. Corpus callosotomy in treatment of medically resistant epilepsy: preliminary results in a pediatric population. *Epilepsia.* 1993;34:910–917.

21. Dubeau F, Andermann F, Wiendl H, Bar-Or A. Rasmussen's encephalitis (chronic focal encephalitis). In: Engel JJ, Pedly TA, eds. *Epilepsy: A Comprehensive Textbook.* Philadelphia: Lippincott Williams & Wilkins, A Wolters Kluwer Business; 2008:2439–2453.

22. Bien CG, Tiemeier H, Sassen R, et al. Rasmussen encephalitis: incidence and course under randomized therapy with tacrolimus or intravenous immunoglobulins. *Epilepsia.* 2013;54:543–550. http://dx.doi.org/10.1111/epi.12042.

23. Varadkar S, Bien CG, Kruse CA, et al. Rasmussen's encephalitis: clinical features, pathobiology, and treatment advances. *Lancet Neurol.* 2014;13:195–205. http://dx.doi.org/10.1016/S1474-4422(13)70260-6.

24. Bien CG, Granata T, Antozzi C, et al. Pathogenesis, diagnosis and treatment of Rasmussen encephalitis: a European consensus statement. *Brain.* 2005;128:454–471. http://dx.doi.org/10.1093/brain/awh415.

25. Vezzani A, French J, Bartfai T, Baram TZ. The role of inflammation in epilepsy. *Nat Rev Neurol.* 2011;7:31–40. http://dx.doi.org/10.1038/nrneurol.2010.178.

26. Bien CG, Schramm J. Treatment of Rasmussen encephalitis half a century after its initial description: promising prospects and a dilemma. *Epilepsy Res.* 2009;86:101–112. http://dx.doi.org/10.1016/j.eplepsyres.2009.06.001.

27. Delalande O, Bulteau C, Dellatolas G, et al. Vertical parasagittal hemispherotomy: surgical procedures and clinical long-term outcomes in a population of 83 children. *Neurosurgery.* 2007;60:19–32. http://dx.doi.org/10.1227/01.NEU.0000249246.48299.12.

28. Moosa ANV, Gupta A, Jehi L, et al. Longitudinal seizure outcome and prognostic predictors after hemispherectomy in 170 children. *Neurology.* 2013;80:253–260. http://dx.doi.org/10.1212/WNL.0b013e31827dead9.

29. Pulsifer MB, Brandt J, Salorio CF, Vining EPG, Carson BS, Freeman JM. The cognitive outcome of hemispherectomy in 71 children. *Epilepsia.* 2004;45:243–254. http://dx.doi.org/10.1111/j.0013-9580.2004.15303.x.

30. Kossoff E, Vining E, Pillas D, et al. Hemispherectomy for intractable unihemispheric epilepsy etiology vs outcome. *Neurology.* 2003:887–890. http://dx.doi.org/10.1212/01.WNL.0000090107.04681.5B.

CHAPTER 31

Rehabilitation After Acute Encephalopathy in Childhood

HIROSHI ARAI, MD • SATORI HIRAI, MD • YUKIHIRO KITAI, MD

OVERVIEW

Acute encephalopathy deprives infants or young children of not only the present function but also future possibility of typical development. During the acute and subacute phase, rehabilitation is provided to reduce temporary symptoms such as spasticity, dystonia, hypotonia, and hyperkinesia. At the same time, the future outcome should be estimated by close assessment of neurologic and physical status to determine the adequate goal and to plan long-term, individualized interventions. Developmental outcomes depend on the type of encephalopathy, severity of brain injury, the time of the onset, complications such as epilepsy and contractures, and environment where the affected children are involved.

In this chapter, outcomes of the survivors of three representative types of encephalopathy are described. In addition, comprehensive interventions for them including rehabilitation, medication, and environmental adjustment are discussed.

ACUTE ENCEPHALOPATHY WITH BIPHASIC SEIZURES AND LATE REDUCED DIFFUSION

Acute encephalopathy with biphasic seizures and late reduced diffusion (AESD) is the most frequently diagnosed encephalopathy in childhood in Japan.[1] The onset is usually under 2 years of age. Long-term sequelae include mild to severe motor and intellectual disability and epilepsy. Actually, 70%–90% of the affected children become able to walk independently, and higher brain dysfunction will be the major issue to treat.[2,3] Prolonged seizure at the onset, loss of consciousness 24 h after the onset, higher creatinine and LDH levels, and lower platelet counts in the acute phase were reported to correlate with poor prognosis.[4,5]

The affected children lose total postural control during the acute phase. Spasticity, dystonia, and dysphasia may coexist and diminish spontaneously except for the severest cases.[6] In the following weeks, various hyperkinetic movements are observed, which are considered as exaggerated voluntary movements modified by severe truncal hypotonia. Such apparently involuntary movements subside within a month or two from the onset, and hypotonia remains. During the following several months, gross motor functions are gradually restored and higher brain dysfunction becomes evident. Especially, frontal lobe symptoms such as perseveration, attention deficit, and disinhibition are observed to various extents. Asymmetry is also one of the major problems when the child has hemispheric involvement. Not only hemiplegia but also hemiasomatognosia and hemispatial neglect are observed.[7] Epileptic seizures usually appear several months after the onset, and impair the children's quality of life and development seriously. Although their duration is short, they are frequent (often daily or hourly) and intractable.[8]

We found two factors that related to the long-term motor outcome. One was the extent of cerebral white matter injury. Severe atrophy of the cerebral white matter related to poor gross motor outcome. The other was the recovery speed of hypotonia. Of 19 children who could walk independently within 2 years from the onset, 18 could hold the heads up at 2 months after the onset and could sit alone within 6 months (Fig. 31.1). That means those who could not control their heads within 2 months nor sit alone within 6 months from the onset have little possibility to be able to walk independently.[9]

If the affected children have extensive white matter lesion and cannot hold the head up at 2 months after the onset, the goal of the intervention will be "to move with a walker under a person's guidance." Generally, crutches or a powered wheelchair cannot be practical for those children because of higher brain dysfunction. If the affected children can hold the head up within 2 months and can sit without support within 6 months, the goal will not be recovery of gross motor function but improvement of higher brain dysfunction and

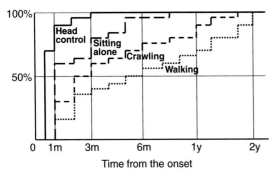

FIG. 31.1 Recovery ratios of gross motor functions in 19 children who became able to walk independently within 2 years from the onset of acute encephalopathy with biphasic seizures and late reduced diffusion. *m*, month(s); *y*, year(s).

environmental adjustment at home and school (or nursery). At the school-going stage, mild motor dysfunction and mild to moderate intellectual impairment must be taken into account. Measurement of the detailed intelligence scale is desirable to disclose specific developmental problems of the children and to help their families accept their condition. Proper understanding of the children's ability is necessary to plan individualized programs at school. Too difficult lecture or too much homework for the children will exhaust them and deprive them of developing self-confidence.

The rehabilitation program during the recovery phase (until around 6 months from the onset) is prescribed based on neurologic impairments. Injury of cerebral white matter generally extends over bilateral frontal and parietal lobes, except perirolandic regions.[10] Bilateral frontal lobe lesions cause hypotonia, impairment of motor planning and anticipatory postural adjustment, and reduced motivation. Bilateral parietal lobe lesions cause impairment of sensory association. As a result, the first target of physical therapy is antigravity postural control. Preparation of concrete base of support and adjustment of body alignment are necessary to transmit somatic sensory information to the sensory area properly. Practice of the way to sustain or change postures makes children learn how to control their bodies. For example, therapists put the child on the firm floor in the sitting position, guide the center of the pressure just above the ischial bone, straighten the back, and tilt the trunk laterally, facilitating the abdominal and back muscles to teach the tightening activity. Such a therapy may be coupled with reaching activity of the hand to enhance motivation and anticipatory postural adjustment. If

the child has unilateral lesion, approach for the asymmetry should be introduced early and intensively, as is the case with adult stroke. Hemiplegia after AESD is considered to be a good indication for constraint-induced movement therapy (CIMT) or hand-arm bimanual intensive training (HABIT).[11] Enrichment of the environment is also necessary to accelerate development.[12] For example, toys to enhance interest, low tables to hold for standing, and chairs to support proper sitting position should be introduced to the family and the nursery.

Medications for involuntary movement or spasticity should be decreased during the subacute phase without delay because most of them aggravate hypotonia and drowsiness. Antiepileptic drugs tend to be increased for controlling frequent seizures, but they should be adjusted weighing the relative merits of seizure control and adverse effects. Especially, high-dose benzodiazepines must be avoided. We experienced some children who became able to walk independently after reduction of benzodiazepines.

HEMORRHAGIC SHOCK AND ENCEPHALOPATHY

Most children with hemorrhagic shock and encephalopathy (HSE) have extensive brain injury[13] and become severely rigospastic. As a result, various complications occur. Scoliosis and hip dislocation appear even in early childhood. Severe and untreatable dysphasia is often accompanied by gastroesophageal reflux (GER) and causes aspiration pneumonia. Generally, secondary epilepsy is intractable.

Multimodal interventions should be administered constantly from the acute phase. Adequate positioning, range of motion exercise, and medication are indispensable to prevent contracture and deformity. As for the positioning, constant supine position aggravates total asymmetrical extensor pattern of the trunk and the extremities that causes scoliosis and hip dislocation. Sitting or semisitting position with flexed hips and knees relieves hypertonus of the whole body and enhances the movement of thorax and diaphragm, which improves respiratory function. To increase the variation of daily posture, a prone-standing flame or a semistanding walker with a saddle may be introduced. A prone-standing position facilitates symmetrical extensor activity of perispinal muscles, which may help to prevent scoliosis. Upright position of the upper body also contributes to the prevention of GER.

Several types of muscle relaxants are prescribed to reduce marked hypertonus. The first-line oral

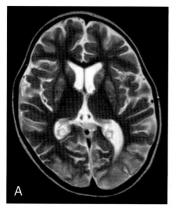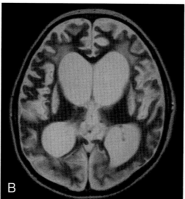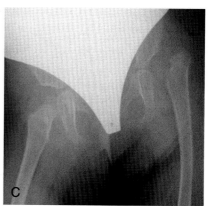

FIG. 31.2 **(A** and **B)** Axial T2-weighted MR images of multifocal injury **(A)** and diffuse injury **(B)** of the brain caused by hypoxic ischemic encephalopathy. **(C)** Early dislocation of the left hip joint found in an infant with diffuse injury of the brain.

medication may be benzodiazepines, and the second-line includes baclofen, tizanidine, and dantrolene. Combination of these drugs with hypnotics or sedatives may be an ordinary regimen, but excessive medications often result in drowsiness, dysphasia, and aspiration pneumonia. Intramuscular botulinum toxin injection and intrathecal baclofen infusion are usually effective and have the advantage of lower adverse effects than oral medications. If the hip is dislocated, reduction surgery is performed to maintain a symmetrical posture. Supine surgery will be indicated when Cobb's curve exceeds 50 degrees.[14] Early gastrostomy and introduction of parenteral semisolid food are desirable to prevent GER and aspiration pneumonia.[15]

HYPOXIC ISCHEMIC ENCEPHALOPATHY

Brain injury from hypoxic ischemic encephalopathy (HIE) can be divided into two types: multifocal and diffuse, while some intermediate cases exist.[16] Multifocal injury includes bilateral putamen and watershed regions of cerebral hemispheres. Diffuse injury includes almost whole cerebral hemispheres and central gray matters. In the severest case, brainstem and cerebellum are also involved (Fig. 31.2A and B).

Children with multifocal injury may have involuntary movements, cortical blindness, and higher brain dysfunction.[17] Injury of bilateral putamen causes fluctuation in postural tone, dystonia, and choreoathetotic movements. Watershed infarction causes impairment of motor planning and postural adjustment, dysarthria, and visual impairment. Spastic paresis may be present if corticospinal tracts are also involved. Overall outcomes

are variable from mild higher brain dysfunction with mild motor impairment to global developmental deficit with severe motor impairment. At first, the affected children have only very narrow central vision, and they are considered as totally blind because young children cannot describe how they can see. Visual impairment improves gradually to some extent, but peripheral vision is likely to remain impaired. Gross motor function recovers rapidly during 6 months from the onset. If the affected children cannot walk 6 months after the onset, they can hardly walk independently in the future.[16]

Physical therapy after HIE with multifocal injury is intended to improve postural control and to stabilize muscle tone. The affected children are induced to learn trunk control and how to support their body with the extremities. Walkers and braces may be induced to practice walking. Occupational and optometric therapies are also important to attain daily life mobility and manipulation. Enrichment of the visual clues in the environment is necessary for the children to move and to manipulate things by themselves. For examples, vividly colored toys and books with large fonts are introduced. It is better to gather foods in one plate to utilize central vision. Adjustment of spoons and forks is also desirable to be held easier by dystonic hands.

Children with diffuse injury become severely rigospastic. Complications tend to appear early, including bone fractures and secondary deformity such as hip dislocation[16] (Fig. 31.2C). Interventions are almost the same as those for HSE, but they should be begun earlier. Dysphasia and respiratory insufficiency are marked when brainstem was involved. Such children cannot live without assisted ventilation, parenteral nutrition, and continuous monitoring of vital signs. In these days, home ventilation system and associated social support have become popular in Japan, and they can go back to home and live with their family. After they come home, rehabilitation is delivered at home. Goals of interventions are to maintain respiratory function and to prevent contracture and deformity. Especially, seating equipment should be made early and arranged as they grow.

SUMMARY

The goal and the strategy of rehabilitation to children after acute encephalopathy should be determined based on appropriate evaluation of neurologic impairment and proper estimation of the outcome. Interventions must be comprehensive and multimodal. Not only rehabilitation but also medication, neuromodulation, psychologic intervention, and surgery should be taken into account. Environmental adjustment is the key to improve participation to school and social life.

REFERENCES

1. Hoshino A, Saitoh M, Oka A, et al. Epidemiology of acute encephalopathy in Japan, with emphasis on the association of viruses and syndromes. *Brain Dev.* 2012;34:337–343.
2. Takanashi J, Oba H, Barkovich AJ, et al. Diffusion MRI abnormalities after prolonged febrile seizures with encephalopathy. *Neurology.* 2006;66:1304–1309.
3. Takanashi J. Two newly proposed infectious encephalitis/encephalopathy syndromes. *Brain Dev.* 2009;31:521–528.
4. Hayashi N, Okumura A, Kubota T, et al. Prognostic factors in acute encephalopathy with reduced subcortical diffusion. *Brain Dev.* 2012;34.
5. Azuma J, Nabatame S, Nakano S, et al. Prognostic factors for acute encephalopathy with bright tree appearance. *Brain Dev.* 2015;37(2):191–199.
6. Lee S, Sanefuji M, Torio M, et al. Involuntary movements and coma as the prognostic marker for acute encephalopathy with biphasic seizures and late reduced diffusion. *J Neurol Sci.* 2016;370:39–43.
7. Okumura A, Suzuki M, Kidokoro H, et al. The spectrum of acute encephalopathy with reduced diffusion in the unilateral hemisphere. *Eur J Paediatr Neurol.* 2009;13:154–159.
8. Ito Y, Natsume J, Kidokoro H, et al. Seizure characteristics of epilepsy in childhood after acute encephalopathy with biphasic seizures and late reduced diffusion. *Epilepsia.* 2015;56:1286–1293.
9. Hirai S, Arai H. Rehabilitation and epilepsy. In: Shiomi M, ed. *Acute Encephalitis and Encephalopathy.* Tokyo: Nakayama Shoten Co., Ltd; 2011:80–83. [in Japanese].
10. Takanashi J. Neuroradiological findings in acute encephalopathy with biphasic seizures and late reduced diffusion (AESD). *No To Hattatsu.* 2008;40:128–132. [in Japanese].
11. Gordon AM, Hung YC, Brandao M, et al. Bimanual training and constraint-induced movement therapy in children with hemiplegic cerebral palsy: a randomized trial. *Neurorehabil Neural Repair.* 2011;25(8):692–702.
12. Morgan C, Darrah J, Gordon AM, et al. Effectiveness of motor interventions in infants with cerebral palsy: a systematic review. *Dev Med Child Neurol.* 2016;58(9):900–909.
13. Levin M, Hjelm M, Kay JD, et al. Haemorrhagic shock and encephalopathy: a new syndrome with a high mortality in young children. *Lancet.* 1983;8341:64–67.
14. White 3rd AA, Panjabi MM. The clinical biomechanics of scoliosis. *Clin Orthop Relat Res.* 1976;118:100–112.
15. Miyazawa R, Tomomasa T, Kaneko H, Arakawa H, Shimizu N, Morikawa A. Effects of pectin liquid on gastroesophageal reflux disease in children with cerebral palsy. *BMC Gastroenterol.* 2008;8:11.
16. Kitai Y, Ohmura K, Hirai S, Arai H. Long-term outcome of childhood hypoxic-ischemic encephalopathy. *No To Hattatsu.* 2015;47:43–48. [in Japanese].
17. Kurihara M, Shishido A, Yoshihashi M, Fujita H, Kohagizawa T, Ida H. Long-term prognosis of children with hypoxic encephalopathy. *No To Hattatsu.* 2014;46:265–269. [in Japanese].

Index

Note: Page numbers followed by "f" indicate figures, "t" indicate tables and "b" indicate boxes.

Printed in the United States
By Bookmasters